DIAGNOSIS AND THERAPY IN CLINICAL DERMATOLOGY

Comprehensive Guide to Morphologic Recognition, Decision Pathways, & Skin Conditions for Primary Care Physicians

Ramon C. Henson, MD

Trademark Disclaimer

All brand names, product names, drug names, certification names, and registered trademarks mentioned in this textbook are the property of their respective owners. Their use in this publication does not imply endorsement, affiliation, or sponsorship by the trademark owner, nor does it imply that the trademark owner has reviewed, approved, or is in any way associated with this work. All trademarked names and registered marks appearing in this textbook are used solely for purposes of identification and educational reference, without any intent of trademark infringement.

Medical Disclaimer

This textbook is intended solely for educational and informational purposes and is designed to support the continuing professional development of licensed healthcare providers. The clinical content presented herein reflects information believed to be accurate and current at the time of publication; however, medicine evolves rapidly, and readers are advised that new research findings, updated clinical practice guidelines, and revised regulatory approvals may alter or supersede information contained in this work after its publication date.

Nothing in this publication constitutes medical advice, clinical guidance specific to any individual patient, or a substitute for the independent professional judgment of a licensed and qualified healthcare provider. No clinician-patient relationship is established, implied, or intended by the use of this textbook or any portion thereof. All clinical decisions, including but not limited to diagnosis, therapeutic selection, drug dosing, and patient monitoring, must be individualized based on thorough and direct assessment of the patient, the totality of current published evidence, applicable clinical practice guidelines, institutional protocols, and the informed professional judgment of the responsible clinician.

Drug information, dosages, treatment protocols, and therapeutic recommendations presented in this publication are offered for educational reference only and must be independently verified against current prescribing information, pharmacopeial references, and applicable regulatory approvals prior to clinical application. The author and publisher have made every reasonable effort to ensure the accuracy and completeness of the information presented; nevertheless, they expressly disclaim all liability for any adverse outcomes, clinical errors, patient harm, loss, or injury alleged to arise, directly or indirectly, from the use, misuse, or application of any information, recommendation, protocol, or clinical guidance contained in this publication.

TABLE OF CONTENT

PREFACE

Dermatology occupies a peculiar position among the clinical disciplines. Its diagnostic method is almost entirely visual, its therapeutic decisions are made at the bedside within minutes of that visual assessment, and yet its teaching literature has long separated the two halves of that process into different books: an atlas for recognition, a formulary for treatment. A clinician holding both open at once, trying to reconcile a photograph on one page with a dosing table on another, experiences the central frustration this book was written to resolve.

This textbook treats diagnosis and therapy as a single continuous act of clinical reasoning rather than two separate skills. Every major condition covered here is presented the way it is actually encountered in practice: a pattern is recognized, that pattern is tested against its most dangerous or most common look-alikes, and a management decision follows directly from that resolution. The book's integrated feature, the Morphology-to-Management System, makes this continuity explicit. At every major disease topic, a structured callout carries the reader from the named morphologic pattern through its variation across skin tones, ages, and body sites, through the look-alike conditions that most often cause diagnostic error, to the definitive first-line-through-escalation treatment decision the pattern triggers, and finally to a single high-yield anchor finding that locks the pattern in memory. A dedicated Morphology-to-Management Master Atlas at the end of the book consolidates every one of these patterns into a single cross-referenced, indexed reference the reader can scan during a clinic day or before a difficult case.

The decision to fuse recognition and management this tightly was driven by where diagnostic error in dermatology actually originates. It is rarely a failure to notice a lesion. It is far more often a failure to discriminate between two or three conditions that share a superficial morphology, compounded by the fact that many of the discriminating features that matter most vary systematically by skin tone and have been inconsistently represented in the dermatologic literature. This book addresses that gap directly: presentation variance across the full range of skin pigmentation is treated as a first-class element of every pattern discussion, not an addendum.

This is a book for the primary care physician who sees dermatologic complaints daily but trained in a different discipline, for the nurse practitioner and physician assistant building independent competency in skin disease, for the resident and medical student constructing a durable clinical framework, and for any clinician who wants a single authoritative reference that does not force a choice between recognizing a condition and knowing what to do about it. Content throughout is grounded in current society guidelines and the primary literature, presented as confident clinical prose in the tradition of a definitive reference rather than an examination-preparation workbook. The chapters are organized to build from foundational skin biology and diagnostic method through the major disease categories in the order a clinician actually encounters them, closing with dedicated treatment of special populations, dermatologic emergencies, and office-based procedures.

It is the author's hope that this book earns a permanent place on the desk rather than the shelf — opened not once before an examination, but repeatedly, in the middle of a clinical day, when a pattern on a patient's skin needs to be turned quickly and reliably into the right next step.

CHAPTER 1: SKIN STRUCTURE, FUNCTION, AND THE LANGUAGE OF DERMATOLOGIC DIAGNOSIS

Learning Objectives

1. Describe the structural organization of the epidermis, dermis, and subcutaneous compartment and relate each layer to a specific category of clinical disease.
2. Explain the barrier, thermoregulatory, sensory, and immunologic functions of the skin and the clinical consequences that follow when each is disrupted.
3. Identify the primary and secondary morphologic lesion types used throughout dermatologic diagnosis and apply standardized descriptive terminology to a clinical finding.
4. Use anatomic distribution and lesion configuration as independent diagnostic variables that narrow a differential diagnosis before any laboratory or histologic data are obtained.
5. Apply the Morphology-to-Management System framework to translate a recognized pattern into a structured, evidence-based management decision.

Structure and Function of the Skin

The skin is the largest organ of the body and the only one whose entire surface is available for direct visual and tactile examination at the bedside, which is precisely what makes dermatology a discipline built on pattern recognition rather than instrumented measurement. Because every diagnostic clue in this specialty arrives through the examiner's own eyes and fingers, an accurate mental model of cutaneous architecture is not academic background information; it is the working vocabulary that converts an undifferentiated red patch into a specific, namable disease process. A clinician who understands that the epidermis is avascular, for example, immediately understands why a purely epidermal process such as psoriasis blanches completely under diascopy, while a clinician who understands that the dermis carries the cutaneous vasculature understands why a vasculitic lesion does not blanch at all. The anatomy is the diagnosis in waiting.

Overview of Cutaneous Architecture and Its Clinical Relevance

The skin is organized into three principal compartments stacked from superficial to deep: the epidermis, a stratified squamous epithelium that provides the physical and chemical barrier to the external environment; the dermis, a connective tissue layer that supplies mechanical strength, vascular and nerve supply, and the bulk of the skin's appendageal structures; and the subcutaneous fat, or hypodermis, which provides thermal insulation, mechanical cushioning, and a metabolically active endocrine depot. Each compartment gives rise to a distinct family of disease. Epidermal disease produces scale, because scale is nothing more than abnormally retained or abnormally produced stratum corneum. Dermal disease produces induration, erythema that may or may not blanch, and a texture that is palpable before it is always visible. Subcutaneous disease produces deep, often ill-defined nodularity and, when inflammatory, the deep tenderness characteristic of panniculitis. Learning to ask, at the bedside, which compartment a finding originates in is the single most efficient triage step available to the examiner, because it immediately restricts the differential diagnosis to a fraction of the more than two thousand named cutaneous conditions.

Barrier Function and the Stratum Corneum

The outermost epidermal layer, the stratum corneum, is composed of terminally differentiated corneocytes embedded in a lipid matrix dominated by ceramides, free fatty acids, and cholesterol arranged in a highly ordered lamellar structure. This lipid organization is what gives the barrier its selective permeability, allowing the skin to restrict water loss outward while excluding most environmental antigens, microorganisms, and irritants from penetrating inward. Because ceramide composition and lamellar organization are frequently abnormal in atopic dermatitis, the resulting barrier defect is not a downstream consequence of the eczema but a primary driver of it, permitting transepidermal water loss to rise and environmental allergens to penetrate deeply enough to engage the cutaneous immune system, which in turn perpetuates the inflammatory cycle. Filaggrin, a structural protein that aggregates keratin filaments during terminal differentiation and is subsequently degraded into natural moisturizing factor, illustrates this link directly: loss-of-function mutations in the gene encoding filaggrin, FLG, produce both the dry, scaling skin of ichthyosis vulgaris and a markedly increased risk of atopic dermatitis, because a single structural defect degrades barrier integrity and immune surveillance simultaneously.

Thermoregulatory, Sensory, and Immunologic Roles

Beyond its barrier function, the skin regulates core body temperature through eccrine sweat production and through vasodilation or vasoconstriction of the dermal vascular plexuses, a function whose failure explains the heat intolerance seen in extensive burns or widespread erythroderma, where the sheer surface area of disrupted skin overwhelms thermoregulatory reserve. Cutaneous sensory nerve endings mediate touch, pressure, temperature, and pain, and their density and distribution explain why pruritus is concentrated in specific anatomic regions in certain diseases, such as the scalp and extensor surfaces in dermatitis herpetiformis. Finally, the skin functions as a peripheral immune organ in its own right, a concept formalized as skin-associated lymphoid tissue, in which epidermal Langerhans cells, dermal dendritic cells, resident memory T cells, and an extensive innate immune apparatus survey the barrier continuously, ready to mount a response to breach long before a systemic immune reaction would otherwise be triggered.

Compartment	Dominant Cell Type	Primary Clinical Signature When Diseased
Epidermis	Keratinocyte	Scale, crust, epidermal fragility (blistering at the dermoepidermal junction or above)
Dermis	Fibroblast, endothelial cell, perivascular immune cell	Induration, erythema (blanching or non-blanching), palpable texture
Subcutis	Adipocyte	Deep nodularity, panniculitis-pattern tenderness, contour change

KEY POINT: Identifying which cutaneous compartment a lesion originates in is the fastest available triage step in dermatologic diagnosis and should precede any attempt at a specific diagnosis.

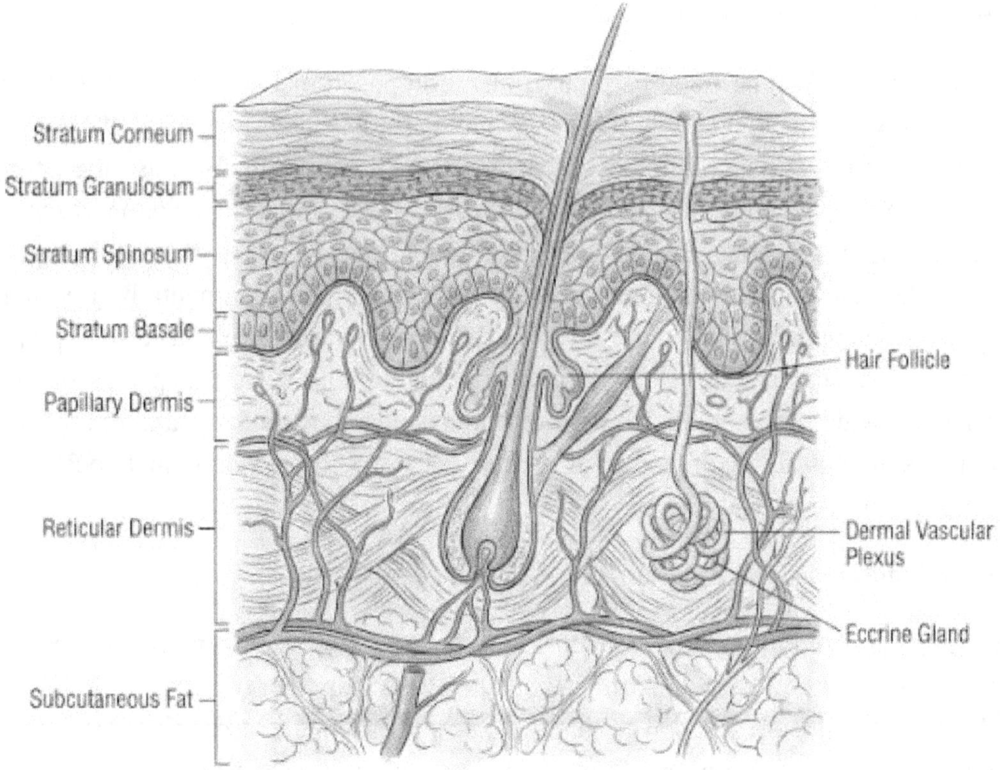

The Epidermis, Dermis, and Subcutaneous Compartments

Epidermal Keratinocyte Differentiation and Turnover

The epidermis renews itself continuously through a program of keratinocyte differentiation that begins with mitotically active basal cells anchored to the basement membrane and ends, roughly four weeks later, with anucleate corneocytes shed from the skin surface. Each stage of this journey is marked by a characteristic protein expression profile, and disease frequently announces itself by disrupting this timeline rather than any single protein in isolation. In psoriasis, keratinocyte transit time collapses from approximately twenty-eight days to three or four days, driven by an interleukin-17 and interleukin-23 dominated inflammatory axis; the epidermis simply does not have time to complete normal terminal differentiation, and the result is the thick, adherent, silvery scale composed of retained nuclei and incompletely processed keratin that defines the disease morphologically. Because this accelerated turnover is a direct histologic correlate of interleukin-17 pathway activity, the same mechanistic link that explains the scale also explains why interleukin-17 and interleukin-23 inhibition produces such rapid clinical clearance in appropriately selected patients.

Dermal Connective Tissue and Vascular Supply

The dermis is divided into a superficial papillary layer, composed of loosely organized type III collagen and rich in the capillary loops that supply the overlying avascular epidermis, and a deeper reticular layer, dominated by thick type I collagen bundles that confer tensile strength. Because the epidermis has no blood supply of its own, every inflammatory or neoplastic process that depends on vascular delivery of immune cells, oxygen, or nutrients must first involve the dermis, which is why erythema, whether from vasodilation in inflammation or from angiogenesis in neoplasia, is fundamentally a dermal event even when the visible lesion appears to sit on the surface. The dermal vascular plexus also explains the clinical utility of diascopy: pressing a glass slide against an erythematous lesion displaces blood from patent dermal vessels and produces blanching, whereas erythema caused by extravasated red blood cells outside the vessel wall, as in vasculitis or a purpuric drug eruption, does not blanch because there is no intravascular blood left to displace.

The Subcutaneous Fat Compartment and Its Clinical Significance

The hypodermis is organized into fat lobules separated by fibrous septa carrying larger vessels and nerves, and this septal-lobular architecture is directly responsible for the two major clinical patterns of panniculitis. Erythema nodosum, a septal panniculitis, produces tender, ill-defined, deep nodules typically confined to the pretibial surface because inflammation concentrated in the fibrous septa produces a diffuse, poorly demarcated clinical lesion, whereas lobular panniculitides such as those associated with pancreatic disease or alpha-1 antitrypsin deficiency produce more discrete nodules with a tendency toward central liquefactive necrosis and drainage, because the inflammatory process is confined within, and eventually destroys, individual fat lobules. Recognizing this septal-versus-lobular distinction at the bedside, based on lesion demarcation and tenderness pattern, allows a clinician to narrow a broad systemic differential diagnosis before any tissue is obtained.

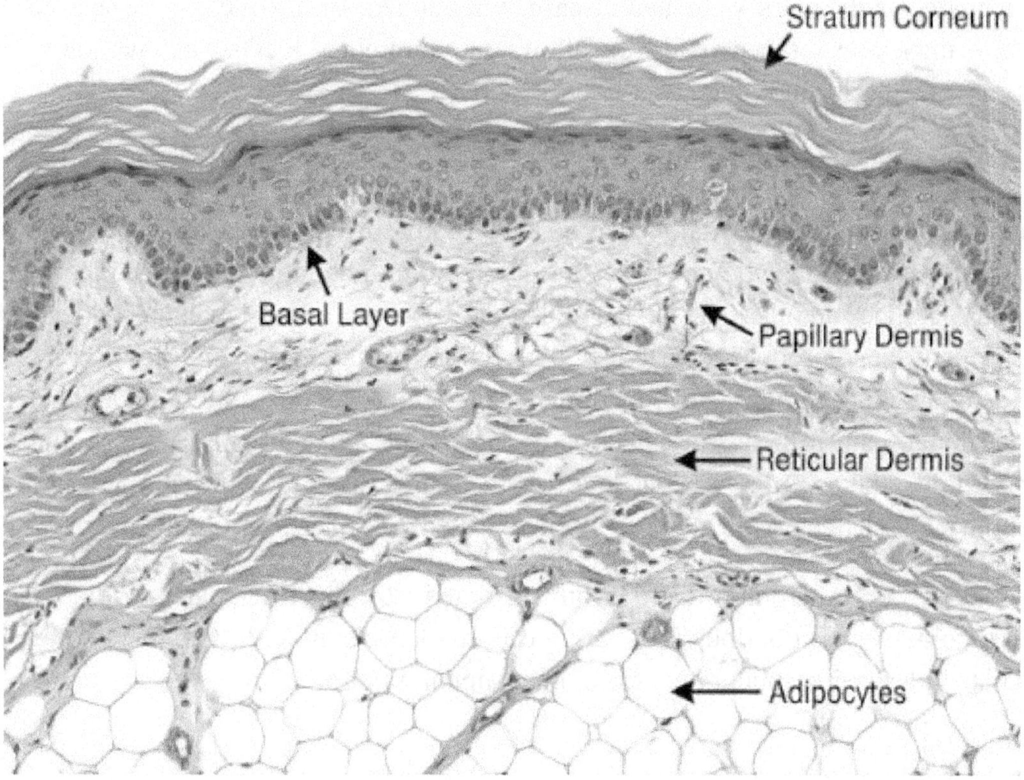

Skin Appendages: Hair, Nail, and Glandular Structures

The Pilosebaceous Unit and Hair Growth Cycle

The pilosebaceous unit couples the hair follicle to its associated sebaceous gland and arrector pili muscle, and this coupling explains why acne, a disease of the pilosebaceous unit rather than of the epidermis generally, is anatomically restricted to sites with high sebaceous gland density such as the face, chest, and back. Hair follicles themselves cycle asynchronously through anagen, a growth phase lasting two to six years on the scalp; catagen, a brief regression phase; and telogen, a resting phase lasting roughly three months before the hair is shed and the cycle restarts. Because only a small fraction of scalp follicles are in telogen at any given time under normal conditions, a process that synchronously shifts a large proportion of follicles into telogen, such as the physiologic stress of childbirth, severe illness, or rapid weight loss, produces a delayed but dramatic shedding two to three months later, a pattern that is best understood by the growth-cycle mechanism rather than memorized as an isolated clinical fact.

Nail Unit Anatomy

The nail unit comprises the matrix, which generates the nail plate and is therefore responsible for its thickness and surface texture; the nail bed, which is closely applied to the plate and gives it its pink color through the underlying vascular supply; and the surrounding proximal and lateral nail folds, which form a seal against the external environment. Damage localized to the matrix produces surface abnormalities of the plate, such as the pitting of psoriasis or the longitudinal ridging of lichen planus, while damage confined to the nail bed produces changes in color and adherence, such as onycholysis or the oil-drop discoloration characteristic of psoriatic nail disease, without necessarily altering the surface texture of the plate itself. This matrix-versus-bed distinction allows the examiner to localize nail pathology anatomically before ever arriving at a specific diagnosis.

Eccrine and Apocrine Glandular Function

Eccrine glands are distributed essentially over the entire body surface, are most dense on the palms, soles, and axillae, and produce a hypotonic sweat used for thermoregulation, whereas apocrine glands are restricted to the axillae, areolae, and anogenital region, become functional only after puberty under androgenic influence, and produce a protein-rich secretion that is odorless until metabolized by resident cutaneous bacteria. This anatomic and functional segregation explains why hidradenitis suppurativa, a disease of terminal hair follicles in apocrine-bearing skin, is confined to the axillae, groin, and inframammary folds and essentially never involves the palms or soles, while primary hyperhidrosis, an eccrine phenomenon, characteristically does involve the palms, soles, and axillae together.

CLINICAL PEARL: Anatomic distribution restricted to apocrine-bearing skin (axillae, groin, inframammary folds) versus distribution favoring eccrine-dense skin (palms, soles) is often sufficient by itself to separate hidradenitis suppurativa from other suppurative folliculitides.

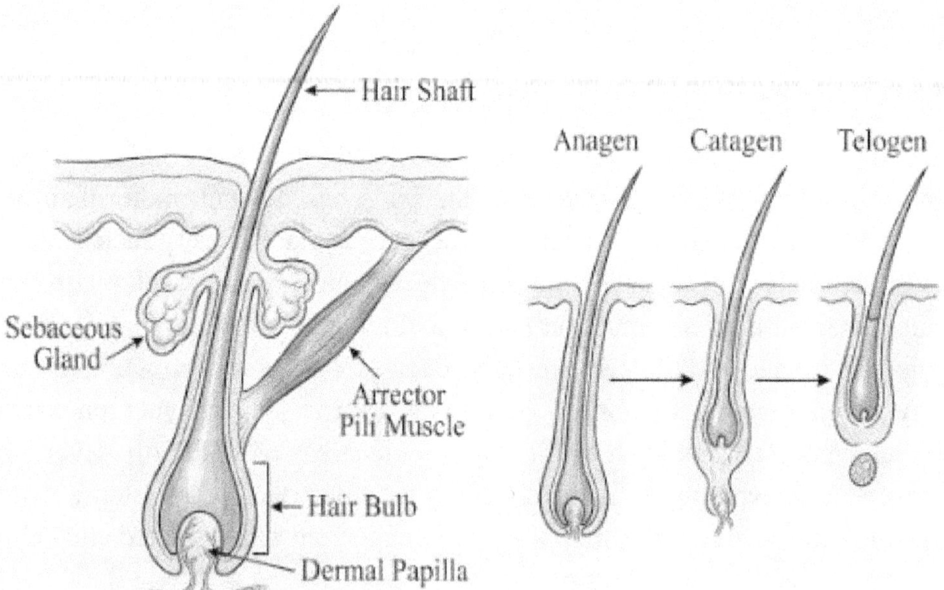

Immunologic and Barrier Function of the Skin

Innate Immune Surveillance in the Epidermis

Keratinocytes are not passive structural cells; they express pattern recognition receptors, including Toll-like receptors, that detect microbial and damage-associated molecular patterns and respond by secreting antimicrobial peptides such as cathelicidin and beta-defensins, along with a cascade of proinflammatory cytokines that recruit neutrophils and dendritic cells. This innate response occurs within the epidermis itself, ahead of any adaptive immune involvement, which is why a superficial bacterial infection can be walled off as impetigo without ever engaging the dermis, while a deeper breach that reaches the dermal vasculature recruits a broader systemic inflammatory response and produces cellulitis.

Adaptive Immune Populations and the Skin-Associated Lymphoid Tissue

Langerhans cells, dendritic antigen-presenting cells resident within the epidermis, continuously sample the barrier environment and migrate to regional lymph nodes to present processed antigen to naive T cells, a process central to the sensitization phase of allergic contact dermatitis. Once sensitized, antigen-specific memory T cells persist within the skin itself as tissue-resident memory cells rather than recirculating exclusively through blood, which explains why a previously sensitized individual develops a dermatitis reaction at the site of allergen re-exposure within hours to a day or two, far faster than a primary sensitization response, which typically requires ten to fourteen days to develop.

Clinical Consequences of Barrier Disruption

Because barrier integrity and immune surveillance are mechanistically coupled rather than independent systems, any process that compromises the stratum corneum, whether an inherited structural defect, chronic mechanical trauma, or an acquired inflammatory disease, increases both transepidermal water loss and antigen penetration simultaneously. This coupling is the mechanistic explanation for the well-documented clinical progression sometimes called the atopic march, in which early barrier-driven eczema increases sensitization to food and environmental allergens through percutaneous exposure, with a subset of affected children subsequently developing allergic rhinitis and asthma; the skin, in this model, functions as the initiating organ for a broader systemic atopic phenotype rather than as an isolated target organ.

THE MORPHOLOGY-TO-MANAGEMENT SYSTEM — Foundational Pattern: The Well-Demarcated Erythematous Plaque With Silvery Scale

The Pattern: A well-demarcated, erythematous plaque surmounted by thick, adherent, silvery-white scale, most often over extensor surfaces, the scalp, and the gluteal cleft.

Presentation Variance: In lighter skin tones the plaque is bright salmon-pink to red beneath the scale; in darker skin tones the erythema is frequently violaceous to gray-brown rather than red, and post-inflammatory dyspigmentation, both hyperpigmentation and hypopigmentation, is far more prominent and often outlasts the active plaque, which can lead an examiner unfamiliar with this variation to underestimate disease activity in patients with richly pigmented skin.

Trap Logic: Nummular eczema produces a similarly round, scaly plaque but favors the extremities of an already xerotic or atopic patient, itches more intensely, and lacks the tightly adherent micaceous scale of psoriasis; tinea corporis produces central clearing with an active, scaling leading edge on potassium hydroxide preparation, whereas psoriatic scale is uniform across the plaque without central clearing.

Management Pivot: Limited disease is managed first-line with a mid- to high-potency topical corticosteroid, often paired with a vitamin D analog to limit steroid-related atrophy on prolonged use; extensive, refractory, or joint-involving disease escalates to phototherapy or a systemic agent, with interleukin-17 and interleukin-23 inhibitors now favored over older systemic agents in patients with moderate to severe disease given their combination of high efficacy and favorable safety profile, a decision that should be confirmed against current society guidelines and payer-specific protocols.

Pattern Anchor: Micaceous, uniformly adherent scale over extensor surfaces, without central clearing, is the single most discriminating anchor separating psoriasis from its closest morphologic mimics.

The Language of Dermatologic Diagnosis: Primary and Secondary Morphology

Primary Lesion Morphology

Dermatologic description begins with the primary lesion, the earliest and most characteristic manifestation of a disease process before secondary change or external manipulation has occurred. A macule is a flat, non-palpable change in color under one centimeter; a patch is the same finding over one centimeter. A papule is a palpable, elevated lesion under one centimeter, and a plaque is a palpable elevation over one centimeter, typically formed by the coalescence of papules or by primary plaque formation, as in psoriasis. A nodule is a palpable lesion with substantial depth, often extending into the dermis or subcutis, distinguishing it from a papule by its three-dimensional character rather than its diameter alone. Vesicles and bullae are fluid-filled elevations distinguished from each other, like macules and patches, by a one-centimeter size threshold, while a pustule is a circumscribed elevation containing purulent material, which may be either infectious or sterile, as in pustular psoriasis.

Secondary Changes and Their Diagnostic Weight

Secondary changes develop after the primary lesion has evolved, either through the natural course of disease or through external manipulation, and they carry substantial diagnostic weight of their own. Scale reflects abnormal keratinization, as already discussed; crust represents dried serum, blood, or purulent exudate on the skin surface and often signals a preceding vesicular or erosive process, as in impetigo, where the characteristic honey-colored crust forms from dried serous exudate. Erosion denotes a partial-thickness epidermal defect that heals without scarring, whereas an ulcer extends into the dermis and heals with scarring, a distinction with direct prognostic implications. Lichenification, a thickened, hyperpigmented, exaggeration of normal skin markings, develops specifically from chronic rubbing and scratching, making its presence itself a marker of a pruritic process of substantial duration, most classically atopic dermatitis or lichen simplex chronicus.

Color, Palpation, and the Tactile Examination

Color description in dermatology must be calibrated to the patient's baseline skin tone rather than described in absolute terms, because erythema that appears bright red in lightly pigmented skin frequently appears violaceous, gray, or simply darker than the surrounding skin in richly pigmented skin, a distinction with direct consequences for disease recognition and severity scoring across the literature. Palpation supplies information unavailable from inspection alone: induration signals a dermal or deeper process, fluctuance signals a fluid collection, and blanching under diascopy separates vascular erythema from extravasated purpura, as introduced earlier in this chapter. A complete morphologic description integrates primary lesion type, secondary change, color calibrated to baseline pigmentation, and palpatory findings into a single reproducible clinical vocabulary that can be communicated precisely between clinicians.

Primary Lesion	Defining Feature	Representative Condition
Macule / Patch	Flat, non-palpable; <1 cm / >1 cm	Vitiligo, café-au-lait macule
Papule / Plaque	Palpable, elevated; <1 cm / >1 cm	Lichen planus papule, psoriatic plaque
Nodule	Palpable with substantial depth	Dermatofibroma, cutaneous lymphoma deposit
Vesicle / Bulla	Fluid-filled; <1 cm / >1 cm	Herpes simplex vesicle, bullous pemphigoid bulla
Pustule	Circumscribed, purulent contents	Folliculitis, pustular psoriasis

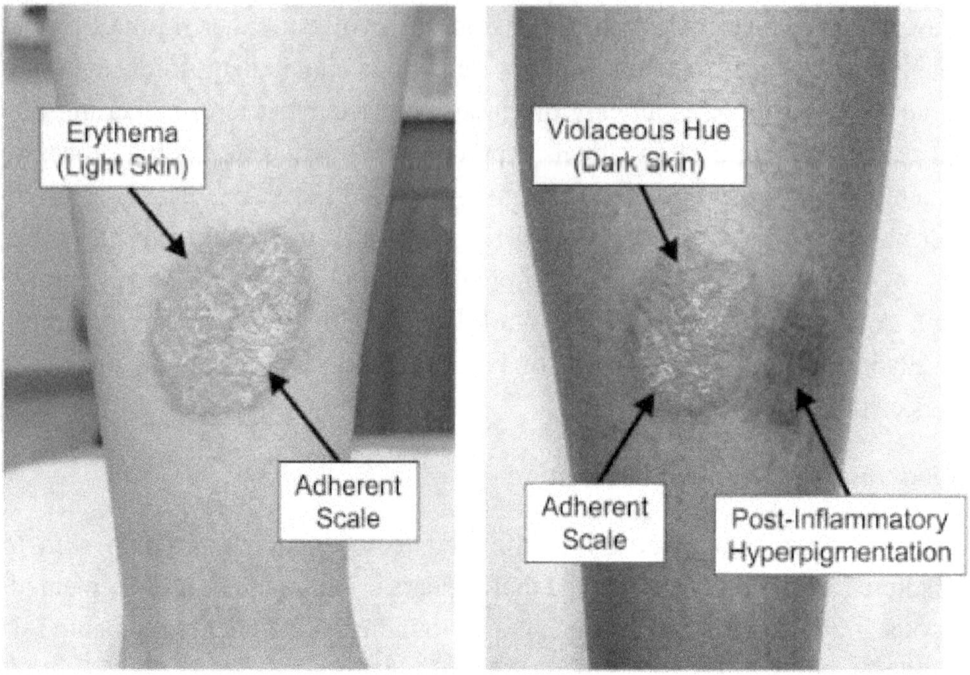

Distribution, Configuration, and Diagnostic Pattern Recognition

Anatomic Distribution as a Diagnostic Clue

The anatomic location of an eruption is rarely incidental. Extensor surface predominance suggests psoriasis; flexural predominance in an infant or child suggests atopic dermatitis; a photodistributed pattern sparing the upper eyelids, the area beneath the chin, and the postauricular skin suggests a photosensitive process such as cutaneous lupus or a drug-induced photoreaction, because these specific sites are shadowed from direct ultraviolet exposure by normal facial anatomy. A dermatomal distribution restricted to a single, sharply demarcated unilateral band is essentially diagnostic of herpes zoster, reflecting reactivation of latent varicella-zoster virus within a single sensory ganglion and its corresponding cutaneous territory, and this anatomic reasoning alone is often sufficient to establish the diagnosis before any laboratory confirmation is obtained.

Configuration: Annular, Linear, Grouped, and Dermatomal Patterns

Configuration describes the arrangement of multiple lesions or the shape of a single lesion's border and functions as an independent diagnostic axis from morphology and distribution. An annular, or ring-shaped, configuration with an active, scaling border and central clearing suggests tinea corporis, while an annular configuration without scale and with a firm, non-scaling border suggests granuloma annulare, and expanding annular erythema following a tick bite suggests erythema migrans; three annular conditions with entirely different pathophysiology, distinguished largely by the presence, absence, and character of surface change within the ring. A linear configuration suggests either an exogenous cause, such as contact dermatitis from a plant allergen dragged across the skin, or a process following an embryologic developmental line, as in linear lichen planus following the lines of Blaschko. Grouped, or herpetiform, vesicles clustered on an erythematous base are characteristic of herpes simplex and varicella-zoster infection, reflecting the pattern of viral spread within a localized region of skin innervated by an infected sensory nerve.

Integrating Morphology, Distribution, and History

No single diagnostic axis, morphology, distribution, or configuration, is reliably sufficient in isolation; diagnostic accuracy rises sharply when all three are integrated with a focused history covering onset, evolution, associated symptoms, and relevant exposures. This integration is the organizing principle behind the Morphology-to-Management System introduced in this book: rather than presenting morphology as an isolated recognition exercise, each disease-specific chapter carries the reader from pattern recognition through the discriminating features that separate genuine look-alikes to the management decision the resolved pattern demands, so that recognition and treatment remain a single continuous clinical act rather than two disconnected skills.

THE MORPHOLOGY-TO-MANAGEMENT SYSTEM — Foundational Pattern: The Expanding Annular Lesion

The Pattern: A slowly expanding, roughly annular erythematous lesion with a distinct border, evolving over days to weeks rather than appearing acutely.

Presentation Variance: Erythema migrans is frequently less apparent or entirely absent in darker skin tones and may present instead as a subtle bruise-like or violaceous patch, a variance strongly implicated in delayed recognition and delayed treatment of early Lyme disease in patients with richly pigmented skin. Granuloma annulare's flesh-colored to violaceous ring is more easily overlooked against darker baseline pigmentation, which can delay recognition of an otherwise benign, self-limited process.

Trap Logic: Tinea corporis is discriminated by an active, scaling leading edge confirmed on potassium hydroxide preparation; granuloma annulare lacks surface scale entirely and is composed of firm, non-scaling papules coalescing into a ring; erythema migrans lacks scale, expands more rapidly than tinea, and occurs in the setting of a known or presumed tick exposure, often but not always with a preceding bite recalled by the patient.

Management Pivot: Tinea corporis is treated with a topical antifungal for limited disease or an oral agent for extensive or recalcitrant disease; granuloma annulare is often observed without treatment given its tendency toward spontaneous resolution, with topical or intralesional corticosteroid reserved for symptomatic or cosmetically concerning lesions; erythema migrans requires prompt oral antimicrobial therapy targeted at Borrelia burgdorferi, with the specific agent and duration confirmed against current guideline recommendations and regional resistance patterns.

Pattern Anchor: Surface change within the ring, scale present in tinea, scale absent in granuloma annulare and erythema migrans, is the fastest single discriminator, after which expansion rate and exposure history separate the latter two.

Introduction to the Morphology-to-Management System

Why Diagnosis and Therapy Are Treated as One Process in This Book

Traditional dermatologic teaching has often separated visual recognition from management decision-making, an artifact of how atlases and formularies have historically been published as distinct products rather than a reflection of how the diagnosis actually unfolds in practice. This book rejects that separation. Every major disease-specific topic in the chapters that follow includes at least one instance of the Morphology-to-Management System, a structured five-part callout that carries the reader from a named morphologic pattern through its clinically important variation across skin tones, ages, and body sites, through the specific look-alike conditions most likely to cause diagnostic confusion, to a definitive management decision, and finally to a single anchor finding that consolidates the entire pattern into one memorable clinical fact.

How to Read the Five-Part Pattern Callout

The Pattern names the morphologic finding in the same standardized vocabulary introduced earlier in this chapter. Presentation Variance addresses how that same pattern can look meaningfully different depending on the patient's skin tone, age, or the anatomic site involved, a component included specifically to counter the documented underrepresentation of darker skin tones in dermatologic teaching materials and the diagnostic delay that underrepresentation produces. Trap Logic identifies the specific conditions most often confused with the pattern in question and states the discriminating feature that separates them, rather than simply listing a differential diagnosis without guidance on how to resolve it. Management Pivot states the definitive treatment decision the resolved pattern triggers, structured from first-line therapy through the threshold for escalation. Pattern Anchor distills the entire callout into the single most clinically decisive finding, intended to be the detail that remains in memory long after the surrounding prose has been forgotten.

Using the Morphology-to-Management Master Atlas

Every pattern introduced across this book's twenty-five chapters is indexed a second time in the Morphology-to-Management Master Atlas at the end of the book, organized by disease category and cross-referenced back to the chapter in which it first appears. The Atlas is designed to function as a rapid-lookup reference during an active clinical day, allowing a clinician who recalls a pattern but not its full discussion to locate the discriminating trap logic and management pivot within seconds, without paging back through the entire chapter in which the pattern was originally introduced.

EVIDENCE: Documented underrepresentation of darker skin tones in dermatologic textbooks and teaching materials has been directly linked to delayed recognition and delayed treatment of common conditions in patients with richly pigmented skin, a finding that has informed the deliberate inclusion of presentation variance as a mandatory element of every pattern discussed in this book.

Skin Structure and Function Across the Lifespan

The anatomic and functional principles introduced in this chapter are not static; they shift predictably across the lifespan, and each shift produces its own characteristic pattern of disease susceptibility. A clinician who understands why neonatal skin behaves differently from adult skin, and why aged skin behaves differently again, is equipped to recognize disease patterns that would otherwise appear anomalous when judged against an adult baseline alone.

Neonatal and Infant Skin

The neonatal stratum corneum is thinner and less well organized than the adult barrier, particularly in infants born preterm, producing a higher ratio of surface area to body mass and a correspondingly greater risk of transcutaneous water loss, temperature instability, and systemic absorption of topically applied agents. This immaturity is directly responsible for the practice of restricting potent topical corticosteroids and certain antiseptic agents in the neonatal period, since a percutaneous absorption rate that would be clinically negligible in an adult can produce measurable systemic drug levels in a premature infant. Neonatal sebaceous glands, by contrast, are transiently enlarged and hyperfunctional under the influence of maternal and placental androgens that cross into fetal circulation, which explains the self-limited neonatal acne and the greasy scale of infantile seborrheic dermatitis that pediatric clinicians encounter almost universally in the first months of life, both of which resolve spontaneously as maternal hormonal influence wanes over the following weeks to months.

Skin Changes of Aging

Chronologic aging and cumulative ultraviolet exposure act on the skin through overlapping but distinguishable mechanisms, and separating the two is diagnostically useful. Intrinsic, chronologic aging produces a gradual flattening of the dermoepidermal junction, a reduction in dermal collagen and elastin turnover, and a decline in Langerhans cell density, changes that collectively thin the skin, reduce its immune surveillance capacity, and increase its fragility to shear forces, producing the easy bruising and skin tears characteristic of elderly skin even at sites shielded from the sun. Photoaging, superimposed on this intrinsic process at sun-exposed sites, produces a histologically distinct pattern of elastotic degeneration, in which normal collagen is replaced by disorganized, basophilic elastotic material, clinically manifesting as coarse wrinkling, mottled pigmentation, and the substantially elevated risk of keratinocyte carcinoma and melanoma that concentrates specifically at chronically sun-exposed sites such as the face, dorsal hands, and forearms rather than distributing uniformly over the body surface.

Patient Education Across the Lifespan

Because both barrier fragility and photoaging-driven malignancy risk are cumulative and substantially modifiable, patient counseling calibrated to life stage is a core component of dermatologic care rather than an adjunct to it. Counseling for a new parent should emphasize fragrance-free emollients and avoidance of unnecessary topical agents on neonatal skin given its heightened percutaneous absorption. Counseling across the adult lifespan should emphasize consistent broad-spectrum photoprotection, since ultraviolet exposure is the single most modifiable risk factor for both photoaging and keratinocyte carcinoma, and counseling for the older adult should additionally address fall risk and mechanical skin protection given the increased fragility of thinned, photoaged, and chronologically aged skin. Each of these counseling points recurs throughout later chapters at the specific disease for which it is most clinically relevant.

PATIENT EDUCATION: Daily broad-spectrum sunscreen use, begun in childhood and sustained across the lifespan, remains the single most effective and most modifiable intervention available for reducing lifetime risk of photoaging and keratinocyte carcinoma.

Dermoscopy of Erythematous Scaling Plaque

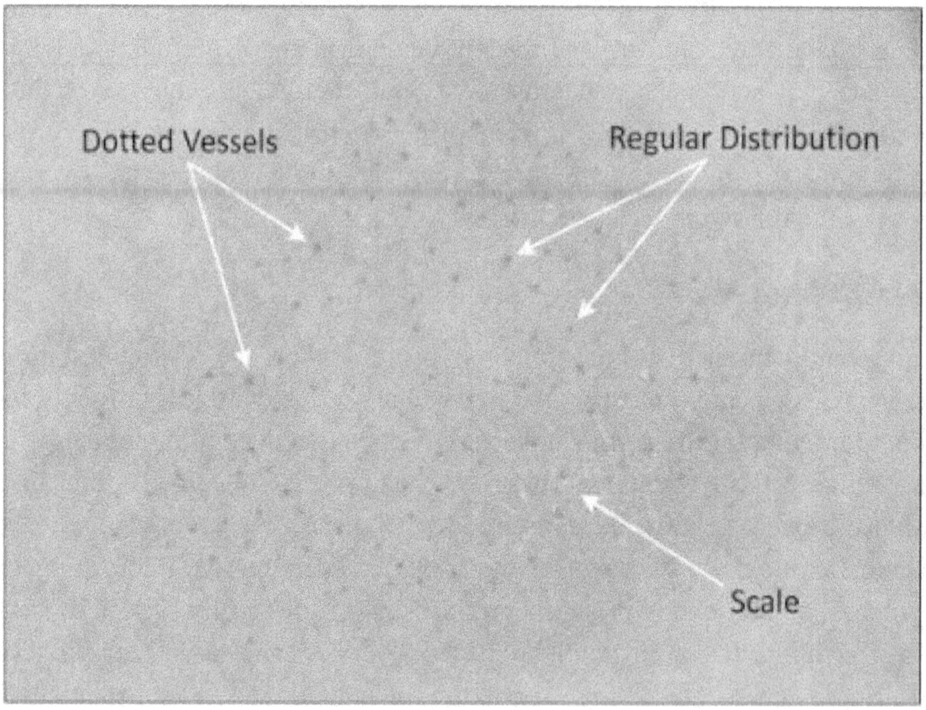

Clinical Case: Building the Diagnostic Language at the Bedside

A 34-year-old woman presents with a three-week history of an itchy rash on both elbows and knees that she initially attributed to dry skin. On examination, well-demarcated, erythematous plaques with thick, adherent, silvery scale are present symmetrically over both extensor elbows and knees, with several smaller similar plaques scattered over the scalp margin. Gentle scraping of a plaque produces multiple small bleeding points once the scale is removed, a finding sometimes referred to by the eponym-free descriptive term pinpoint bleeding on scale removal. She reports mild nail pitting on inspection of her fingernails but no joint pain, swelling, or morning stiffness.

Working through the diagnostic language introduced in this chapter, the examiner first localizes the process to the epidermis and superficial dermis based on the scale and the pinpoint bleeding on removal, which reflects the thinned suprapapillary epidermis and dilated papillary dermal capillaries characteristic of psoriasis. The primary lesion is a plaque; the secondary change is adherent scale; the distribution is extensor and scalp-predominant; the configuration is symmetric rather than linear or annular. Working through the Trap Logic component of the pattern callout introduced earlier in this chapter, nummular eczema is excluded by the absence of prominent xerosis or an atopic history, and tinea corporis is excluded by the symmetric, bilateral, extensor-predominant distribution, which would be unusual for a dermatophyte infection, along with the absence of central clearing. The nail pitting further supports psoriasis rather than an eczematous process, since nail pitting reflects psoriatic involvement of the proximal nail matrix and is not a typical feature of eczema.

Following the Management Pivot for this pattern, limited plaque psoriasis of this distribution and severity is appropriately managed first-line with a mid-potency topical corticosteroid applied to affected areas, combined with a vitamin D analog to allow steroid-sparing maintenance therapy and to limit the risk of cutaneous atrophy from prolonged topical steroid use. The absence of joint symptoms is documented explicitly, since psoriatic arthritis can precede, accompany, or follow cutaneous disease, and periodic reassessment for joint involvement at follow-up is a standard component of longitudinal psoriasis management. The patient is counseled that involvement of more than five to ten percent of body surface area, or inadequate response to topical therapy, would prompt consideration of phototherapy or a systemic agent, and she is scheduled for reassessment in four to six weeks.

CAUTION: Nail pitting and other nail matrix changes should prompt a directed joint examination and history at every visit, since psoriatic arthritis can develop at any point in the disease course independent of cutaneous severity and is frequently underrecognized when attention is confined to the skin alone.

A second, brief case illustrates how the same diagnostic language resolves a different foundational pattern. A 9-year-old boy is brought in for a single expanding pink ring on his forearm, first noticed five days earlier as a small red spot at the site of a recalled insect bite and now measuring nearly six centimeters across with a faint central clearing. There is no surface scale on close inspection, and the border, while distinct, is flat rather than raised or vesicular. His family recalls a recent camping trip in a wooded area but did not observe an embedded tick.

Applying the annular-lesion pattern introduced earlier in this chapter, the absence of surface scale is the first and fastest discriminator, and it excludes tinea corporis before any potassium hydroxide preparation is performed, since a dermatophyte infection of this size and duration would be expected to show at least a subtly scaling leading edge. The expansion rate, roughly five to six centimeters within five days, is faster than the indolent growth typical of granuloma annulare, which more often evolves over weeks rather than days, and the recent wooded exposure raises specific concern for a tick-borne process even without a recalled bite, since the tick vector responsible for early Lyme disease is frequently small enough to go unnoticed and attaches for a period of time before detachment. Following the Management Pivot for this pattern, empiric oral antimicrobial therapy targeted at Borrelia burgdorferi is initiated promptly on clinical grounds in an endemic region, without waiting for serologic confirmation, since early treatment shortens the clinical course and reduces the risk of later disseminated disease, and the family is counseled on monitoring for associated symptoms such as fever, joint pain, or facial weakness that would prompt more urgent reevaluation.

CLINICAL PEARL: When an annular lesion is expanding over days rather than weeks and surface scale is absent, an infectious or tick-associated cause should be presumed and treated empirically in an endemic region rather than deferred pending serologic confirmation.

THE MORPHOLOGY-TO-MANAGEMENT SYSTEM — Foundational Patterns of the Diagnostic Language

Patterns Introduced This Chapter: The well-demarcated erythematous plaque with silvery scale (psoriasis and its mimics) and the expanding annular lesion (tinea corporis, granuloma annulare, and erythema migrans).

Cross-Cutting Anchor: Surface change, scale present versus scale absent, is the fastest single discriminator across both foundational patterns introduced in this chapter, and this same first question, is there surface scale, will recur as the opening discriminator in the disease-specific chapters that follow.

Summary and Key Concepts

The skin is organized into epidermal, dermal, and subcutaneous compartments, each of which gives rise to a distinct and predictable family of clinical disease, making compartment localization the fastest available diagnostic triage step.

Barrier function and cutaneous immune surveillance are mechanistically coupled; disruption of one reliably potentiates the other, a relationship that underlies conditions ranging from atopic dermatitis to the broader atopic march.

Standardized morphologic vocabulary, primary lesion type, secondary change, distribution, and configuration, converts a visual impression into reproducible clinical data and forms the diagnostic language used throughout this book.

Color description must be calibrated to the patient's baseline skin tone, since erythema and other primary findings present differently across the pigmentation spectrum, with direct consequences for diagnostic accuracy and timeliness of treatment.

The Morphology-to-Management System, introduced in this chapter and applied throughout the book, treats pattern recognition and management decision-making as a single continuous clinical process rather than two separate skills.

CHAPTER 2: THE DERMATOLOGIC HISTORY, EXAMINATION, AND DIAGNOSTIC APPROACH

Learning Objectives

1. Elicit a dermatologic history that captures onset, evolution, symptom character, and exposures relevant to the differential diagnosis.
2. Perform a complete, systematic skin examination that reliably identifies incidental findings outside the presenting complaint.
3. Apply bedside diagnostic aids, including diascopy, the Wood lamp, and potassium hydroxide preparation, to narrow a differential diagnosis before biopsy.
4. Construct a working differential diagnosis by integrating morphology, distribution, configuration, and history into a ranked list of probable diagnoses.
5. Document dermatologic findings using standardized descriptive language that communicates precisely between clinicians.

The Dermatologic History

A dermatologic history differs from a general medical history primarily in the weight it assigns to temporal evolution and external exposure, because most skin disease is either driven by an identifiable external trigger or defined by a characteristic pattern of change over time that the patient can describe even when the current examination captures only a single moment in that evolution. A rash that appeared abruptly over hours and is spreading rapidly suggests a different process, and a different urgency, than one that has been present unchanged for months, and a history that fails to establish this timeline forces the examiner to interpret a static snapshot without the dynamic context that often supplies the diagnosis.

Onset, Evolution, and Symptom Character

Onset should be characterized as acute, over hours to days, or insidious, over weeks to months, because this distinction alone reorganizes the differential diagnosis before a single lesion is examined. Evolution should capture whether the eruption is spreading, static, or resolving, and whether individual lesions are changing character over time, since a fixed drug eruption recurs in the same anatomic location with each re-exposure while a viral exanthem evolves through a predictable sequence of morphologic stages over days. Symptom character, particularly the presence, timing, and severity of pruritus, carries substantial diagnostic weight: intensely pruritic eruptions concentrate in a relatively short list of conditions dominated by eczematous and urticarial processes, while relatively asymptomatic eruptions redirect attention toward infectious, neoplastic, or drug-related causes that do not typically activate cutaneous pruritic pathways to the same degree.

Exposure History and Systemic Review

A directed exposure history, covering new medications, topical products, occupational and recreational contacts, travel, and household or intimate contacts with similar findings, is disproportionately productive in dermatology relative to general internal medicine, because a substantial fraction of dermatologic disease is either directly caused by or substantially modified by an identifiable external exposure. Medication history requires particular precision, since drug eruptions can appear days to weeks after a medication is started and may persist for a period after the medication is discontinued, a delay that frequently causes patients to overlook a causal medication started well before symptom onset. A brief systemic review, covering fever, joint symptoms, mucosal involvement, and weight change, screens for the systemic disease processes that dermatologic findings not infrequently herald before other organ involvement becomes clinically apparent.

Past Dermatologic and Family History

A history of prior similar episodes, prior diagnosed skin conditions, and a family history of atopic disease, psoriasis, or autoimmune skin disease meaningfully shifts pretest probability toward conditions with a recognized hereditary or recurrent pattern. Atopic dermatitis, psoriasis, and several of the porphyrias each carry substantial heritability, and a family history positive for any of these conditions should be actively sought rather than passively noted, since patients frequently do not volunteer family history unless specifically asked in the context of a skin complaint.

KEY POINT: A precise timeline of onset and evolution is frequently more diagnostically productive in dermatology than the physical examination performed in isolation, because morphology at a single moment cannot substitute for the trajectory of change over time.

The Structured Skin Examination

Lighting, Positioning, and Complete Surface Examination

An adequate dermatologic examination requires even, bright lighting, ideally natural or full-spectrum artificial light rather than the yellow-tinted lighting common in many examination rooms, because color assessment, particularly the distinction between erythema and dyspigmentation, is unreliable under poor lighting conditions. A complete examination includes the scalp, palms, soles, nails, and mucosal surfaces, sites that are frequently omitted when the examination is restricted to the presenting complaint alone but that not infrequently carry the finding that clarifies the diagnosis, as when scalp involvement confirms psoriasis in a patient presenting with an isolated extremity plaque or when oral mucosal lesions confirm lichen planus in a patient presenting with cutaneous papules alone.

Systematic Sequence and Incidental Findings

A systematic head-to-toe sequence, rather than an examination confined to the area the patient points to, reliably identifies incidental findings, some benign and some clinically significant, that the patient has not mentioned, either because they are asymptomatic or because the patient did not recognize their significance. A pigmented lesion with irregular borders discovered incidentally on the back during an examination for an unrelated complaint is a common and important example of this principle in practice, and the systematic full-skin examination is the mechanism by which such findings are reliably captured rather than missed.

Palpation and Special Maneuvers

Palpation should assess induration, warmth, tenderness, and fluctuance, each of which supplies information unavailable from visual inspection alone, as introduced in the discussion of dermal and subcutaneous disease in the previous chapter. Special maneuvers extend the examination further: the Darier sign, in which stroking a lesion produces localized urtication, supports a diagnosis of mastocytosis; the Nikolsky sign, in which lateral pressure on perilesional skin produces separation of the epidermis, supports a diagnosis of a superficial blistering disease such as pemphigus vulgaris or staphylococcal scalded skin syndrome; and the Auspitz sign, pinpoint bleeding on removal of adherent scale, supports psoriasis, as demonstrated in the case presented in the previous chapter.

Examination Maneuver	Technique	Diagnostic Significance
Diascopy	Compress lesion with a glass slide	Distinguishes vascular erythema (blanches) from extravasated purpura (does not blanch)
Nikolsky Sign	Apply lateral shear pressure to perilesional skin	Positive in superficial blistering diseases (pemphigus, staphylococcal scalded skin syndrome)
Darier Sign	Stroke a lesion firmly	Positive (urtication) supports cutaneous mastocytosis
Auspitz Sign	Gently remove adherent scale	Pinpoint bleeding supports psoriasis

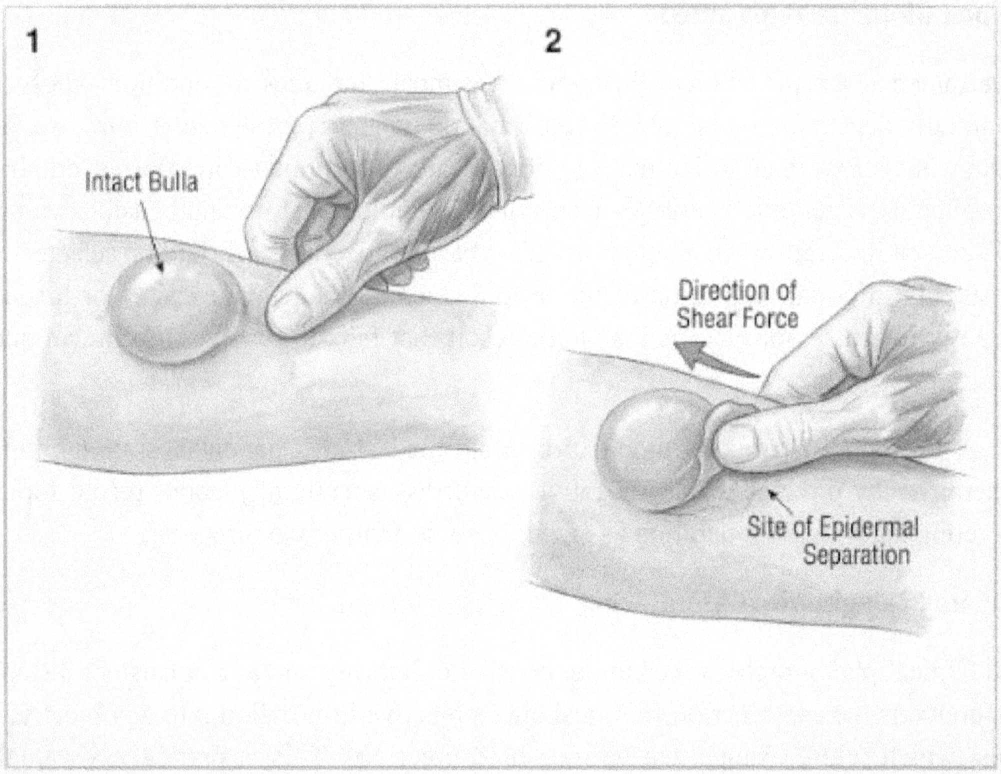

Diagnostic Aids at the Bedside

Dermoscopy as a Bedside Extension of the Naked Eye

Dermoscopy magnifies the skin surface while eliminating surface reflection, either through polarized light or through direct contact with a fluid interface, and in doing so reveals subsurface vascular and pigment structures invisible to unaided inspection. This additional layer of structural information is why dermoscopy has become a standard extension of the physical examination for pigmented lesion assessment, discussed in detail in the chapter devoted to melanoma, and why it is increasingly applied to inflammatory and infectious conditions as well, where characteristic vascular patterns can support or refute a clinical impression before biopsy is undertaken.

Potassium Hydroxide Preparation and Wood Lamp Examination

A potassium hydroxide preparation dissolves keratinocyte cell walls while leaving fungal elements intact, allowing direct microscopic visualization of hyphae or spores from a scale scraping within minutes, and this rapid, inexpensive test should precede empiric antifungal therapy whenever the clinical picture leaves genuine diagnostic uncertainty. Wood lamp examination exploits characteristic fluorescence patterns produced by specific organisms and pigment changes under long-wave ultraviolet light: certain dermatophyte infections of the hair shaft fluoresce green, erythrasma fluoresces coral red due to porphyrin production by the causative organism, and vitiligo demonstrates an enhanced, sharply demarcated white fluorescence that can reveal the true extent of depigmentation beyond what is visible under ambient light, information that directly affects both diagnosis and treatment planning.

Deciding When Biopsy Is Warranted

Biopsy is warranted when the clinical differential diagnosis includes a condition whose management differs substantially depending on histologic confirmation, when a pigmented lesion raises any suspicion for melanoma, when a presumed inflammatory process fails to respond to appropriate empiric therapy, or when the morphology is genuinely ambiguous despite a complete history and bedside evaluation. Biopsy technique, discussed in detail in the chapter on office-based procedures, should be selected to sample the most diagnostically informative portion of the lesion, since an inadequately sited or inadequately deep biopsy frequently returns a nonspecific histologic result that fails to resolve the clinical question it was intended to answer.

CAUTION: A potassium hydroxide preparation performed after a patient has already applied topical antifungal therapy may produce a false-negative result; ask specifically about recent topical treatment before interpreting a negative preparation as excluding a dermatophyte infection.

Photography and Longitudinal Monitoring

Standardized clinical photography, taken under consistent lighting and at a consistent distance and angle at each visit, converts the examination from a single subjective impression into an objective longitudinal record against which future change can be measured precisely. This is particularly valuable for three categories of finding: a pigmented lesion being monitored for morphologic change rather than immediately biopsied, an inflammatory dermatosis being tracked for treatment response over a course of therapy, and a slowly progressive process, such as morphea or early cutaneous lymphoma, whose diagnosis often depends on demonstrating change over months rather than on any single examination finding. Digital dermoscopic photography adds a further layer of precision for pigmented lesion monitoring, since it captures the subsurface structures described earlier in this chapter in addition to the surface appearance, allowing subtle structural change to be detected before it becomes apparent to the unaided eye.

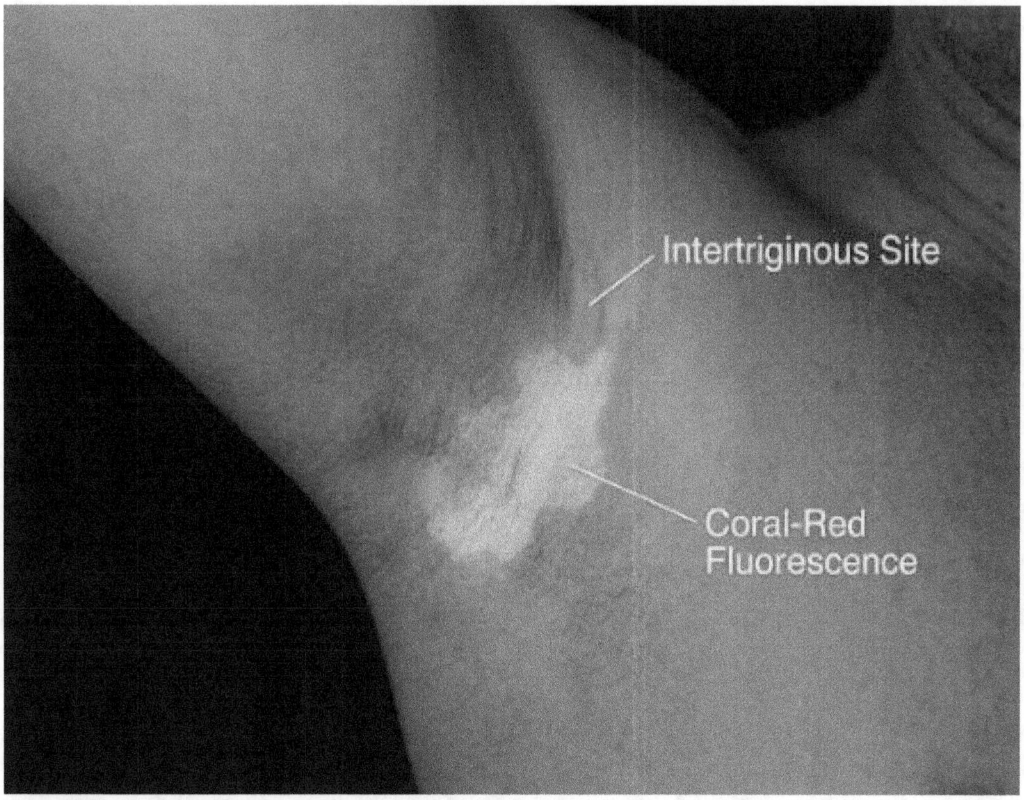

Special Populations in History-Taking and Examination

The Pediatric History and Examination

History-taking in the pediatric patient depends substantially on parental or caregiver observation rather than patient self-report, and specific questions about feeding, growth, sleep disruption from pruritus, and daycare or school exposures often yield more diagnostically useful information than direct questioning of a young child. Examination technique must also adapt to the child's tolerance: a systematic sequence performed calmly and, where possible, with the caregiver holding the child, reduces movement and distress and improves both the completeness and the accuracy of the examination, and deferring an uncomfortable maneuver such as a mucosal examination to the end of the visit, after rapport has been established, frequently improves cooperation without sacrificing examination completeness.

The Geriatric History and Examination

Older adults frequently carry multiple concurrent dermatologic findings, some clinically significant and some incidental, and a complaint-focused history risks anchoring on the presenting concern while overlooking a coexisting finding of greater clinical importance, such as a keratinocyte carcinoma discovered incidentally during examination for an unrelated eczematous complaint. Medication review is disproportionately important in this population given the higher prevalence of polypharmacy and the correspondingly higher likelihood that a cutaneous eruption represents a drug reaction, and skin fragility related to the aging changes discussed in the previous chapter requires gentler examination technique, particularly during palpation and any bedside maneuver involving shear force, to avoid iatrogenic skin tears.

Adapting History and Examination Across Skin Tones

Because color-based descriptive language calibrated to lighter skin does not transfer reliably to richly pigmented skin, as introduced in the previous chapter, history-taking should include specific questions about symptom character, pruritus, warmth, and tenderness that do not depend on color description, since these symptom-based findings remain diagnostically reliable regardless of baseline pigmentation. Examination technique should likewise prioritize palpation for induration and warmth, and should use natural light or full-spectrum lighting specifically calibrated to reveal subtle erythema and dyspigmentation in darker skin tones, since standard examination-room lighting has been shown to obscure clinically important color change in this population more often than in lighter skin.

PATIENT EDUCATION: Caregivers of pediatric patients and family members of older adults with cognitive impairment should be specifically asked about changes they have observed over time, since they frequently notice evolution the patient cannot report directly.

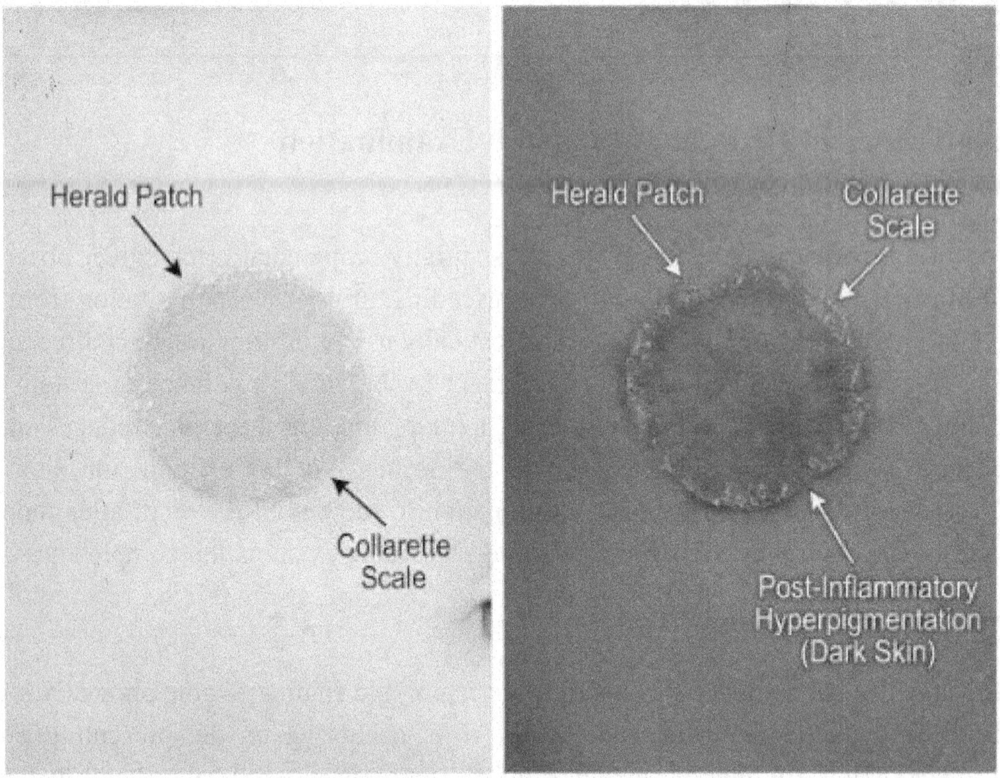

THE MORPHOLOGY-TO-MANAGEMENT SYSTEM — Foundational Pattern: The Acute, Widespread, Fine Papulosquamous Eruption

The Pattern: A sudden onset, generalized eruption of small, oval, fine-scaling papules and thin plaques distributed along skin cleavage lines on the trunk, often preceded by a single larger lesion appearing days to weeks earlier.

Presentation Variance: In darker skin tones the individual lesions are frequently inverse in color relative to the classic description, appearing hyperpigmented or violaceous-brown rather than salmon-pink, and can be more papular and less obviously scaling than the same eruption in lighter skin, a variation that has led to underdiagnosis in richly pigmented patients when clinicians rely on descriptions calibrated to lighter skin alone.

Trap Logic: Guttate psoriasis produces a similar generalized fine-scaling papular eruption but favors more uniformly distributed, thicker, more adherent scale without the herald patch or Christmas-tree distribution along cleavage lines; secondary syphilis produces a similar generalized papulosquamous eruption but characteristically involves the palms and soles, a site this pattern otherwise spares, and warrants serologic testing whenever that palmoplantar involvement is present.

Management Pivot: This is typically a self-limited eruption resolving over six to eight weeks without specific antiviral or antifungal therapy; management is supportive, directed at associated pruritus with emollients, oral antihistamines, or a short course of topical corticosteroid, with reassurance regarding the expected time course; palmoplantar involvement, mucosal involvement, or a positive relevant exposure history should prompt serologic testing to exclude secondary syphilis before this benign course is assumed.

Pattern Anchor: A preceding herald patch and distribution along truncal cleavage lines, together with palmoplantar sparing, is the anchor combination that separates this self-limited eruption from its two most consequential mimics.

Constructing and Refining the Differential Diagnosis

Ranking Probability Before Ordering Tests

A differential diagnosis in dermatology should be constructed as a ranked list reflecting the integrated weight of morphology, distribution, configuration, and history introduced across this chapter and the previous one, rather than an unranked list of every condition that could theoretically produce a similar appearance. Ranking probability before ordering any test focuses subsequent evaluation efficiently: a bedside potassium hydroxide preparation is appropriately the next step when a scaling annular lesion is the leading diagnosis, whereas a punch biopsy is appropriately the next step when an ambiguous inflammatory or neoplastic process is the leading concern, and conflating these two evaluation pathways wastes both time and diagnostic yield.

Using Trap Logic to Resolve Close Calls

When two or three conditions remain closely ranked after history and examination, the Trap Logic component of the Morphology-to-Management System, introduced in the previous chapter and applied throughout this book, supplies the specific discriminating feature that resolves the close call without requiring additional testing in many cases. This same discriminating-feature logic underlies the bedside maneuvers introduced earlier in this chapter: diascopy resolves the question of blanching, potassium hydroxide preparation resolves the question of fungal elements, and a directed reexamination of palms, soles, and mucosa resolves the question of syphilitic involvement in the pattern just discussed.

When to Escalate Beyond the Bedside

Escalation beyond bedside evaluation, to biopsy, laboratory testing, or specialist referral, is warranted when the differential diagnosis includes a condition with materially different management depending on the answer, when the presentation is atypical for the leading diagnosis, when empiric first-line therapy fails to produce the expected response, or when red flag features are present, including rapid progression, mucosal involvement, systemic symptoms, or any suspicion of a blistering or necrotizing process, each of which is addressed in the chapter on dermatologic emergencies.

Diagnostic Algorithm: The Generalized Papulosquamous Eruption

1. Confirm generalized distribution and fine papulosquamous morphology, and specifically examine palms, soles, and oral mucosa.
2. If palms, soles, or mucosa are involved, obtain serologic testing for syphilis before proceeding further.
3. If palms, soles, and mucosa are spared, ask specifically about a preceding solitary herald lesion and assess scale character and distribution along cleavage lines.
4. If the herald-patch history and cleavage-line distribution are present, manage supportively with reassurance regarding an expected six-to-eight-week course.
5. If the eruption instead shows thicker, more uniform, more adherent scale without a herald patch, reconsider guttate psoriasis and evaluate for a preceding streptococcal pharyngitis.

Cognitive Pitfalls in Dermatologic Diagnosis

Because dermatologic diagnosis depends so heavily on rapid visual pattern matching, it is particularly susceptible to a specific set of cognitive biases that can produce confident but incorrect conclusions well before the structured history and examination sequence described in this chapter has been completed. Recognizing these pitfalls explicitly is as important a diagnostic skill as recognizing the morphologic patterns themselves.

Anchoring on the Presenting Complaint

Anchoring occurs when an initial impression, often formed within the first few seconds of visual inspection, is allowed to dominate subsequent information gathering, so that history and examination findings that would otherwise argue against the initial impression are unconsciously discounted rather than weighted appropriately. This bias is compounded when a patient arrives with a self-diagnosis, such as the patient in the case presented later in this chapter who assumed his own eruption was ringworm, since a clinician can unconsciously adopt the patient's framing rather than independently reconstructing the differential diagnosis from the history and examination as described earlier in this chapter.

Premature Closure and the Value of the Second Look

Premature closure occurs when a clinician accepts the first diagnosis that adequately explains the presenting findings without actively testing that diagnosis against its closest mimics, the Trap Logic step that has been emphasized throughout this chapter and the previous one. A deliberate second look, specifically directed at the discriminating features that would distinguish the leading diagnosis from its next most probable alternative, is a simple and effective countermeasure to premature closure and should be treated as a routine step in every dermatologic evaluation rather than reserved for cases that already feel diagnostically uncertain.

Base Rate Neglect and Atypical Presentations

Base rate neglect occurs when a rare but memorable condition is assigned disproportionate weight in the differential diagnosis relative to its actual prevalence, often because it was recently encountered, discussed, or read about, while a common condition presenting atypically is correspondingly underweighted. Because common conditions presenting atypically are, in absolute terms, encountered far more often than rare conditions presenting classically, an atypical presentation of a common disease should generally remain higher on a ranked differential diagnosis than a classic presentation of a rare one, particularly in a primary care or general dermatology setting rather than a tertiary referral practice enriched for unusual disease.

Confirmation Bias During Bedside Testing

Confirmation bias can subtly distort the interpretation of bedside diagnostic aids themselves: a potassium hydroxide preparation examined with strong prior expectation of a positive result can lead an examiner to interpret ambiguous keratin debris or cotton fibers as hyphae, and a Wood lamp examination performed with strong prior expectation of a specific fluorescence pattern can similarly bias color interpretation under an inherently subjective viewing condition. Deliberately considering, before performing a bedside test, what a negative result would mean for the differential diagnosis, rather than only what a positive result would confirm, is a practical safeguard against this bias and reinforces the ranked, multi-hypothesis approach to the differential diagnosis emphasized throughout this chapter.

KEY POINT: A deliberate second look for Trap Logic discriminating features, performed as a routine step rather than only when uncertainty is already felt, is one of the most effective available countermeasures to premature diagnostic closure.

Teledermatology and Remote Diagnostic Assessment

Store-and-forward and live-video teledermatology have become a routine part of dermatologic practice, and the structured history, examination, and documentation principles developed throughout this chapter apply directly to the remote encounter, with several modifications specific to the limitations of a camera-mediated examination.

Image Quality and Its Effect on Diagnostic Accuracy

Diagnostic accuracy in store-and-forward teledermatology depends heavily on image resolution, focus, and lighting, and a poorly lit or poorly focused image can obscure precisely the morphologic detail, fine scale, subtle color change, or border characteristics, that the structured examination approach in this chapter identifies as diagnostically decisive. Patients submitting images for remote evaluation should be given specific, simple instructions: use natural, indirect light rather than direct flash, which tends to wash out fine surface texture and can distort color rendering, capture the lesion at both a close range that shows morphologic detail and a wider range that shows anatomic distribution, and include a size reference, such as a coin, when lesion dimension is clinically relevant.

Recognizing the Limits of the Remote Examination

A remote examination cannot replicate palpation, cannot reliably assess subtle color change without calibrated lighting, and cannot perform bedside diagnostic aids such as diascopy, potassium hydroxide preparation, or the Nikolsky and Darier maneuvers described earlier in this chapter. A teledermatology encounter should therefore explicitly identify which components of the standard structured examination cannot be performed remotely and should set a correspondingly lower threshold for requesting in-person follow-up when the differential diagnosis includes a condition whose distinction depends on one of those unavailable maneuvers, tenderness, induration, or fluctuance, blanching under diascopy, or a positive Nikolsky sign, rather than proceeding to a remote diagnosis and management plan built on incomplete information.

Calibrating Diagnostic Confidence Across Skin Tones Remotely

The color-calibration challenge introduced earlier in this chapter is magnified in the remote setting, where variable camera white balance, ambient lighting, and image compression can each independently distort color rendering in ways that disproportionately affect the assessment of subtle erythema and dyspigmentation in richly pigmented skin. A remote evaluator should weight symptom-based history, tenderness, warmth, pruritus intensity, and rate of change more heavily relative to color description when assessing a patient with darker skin tone through a remote platform, and should maintain a lower threshold for requesting an in-person visit specifically to resolve color-dependent diagnostic questions in this population.

Cognitive Pitfall	Example in This Chapter	Countermeasure
Anchoring	Assuming tinea corporis based on patient self-diagnosis	Independently reconstruct the differential from history and examination
Premature Closure	Accepting the first adequate diagnosis without testing mimics	Deliberate second look for Trap Logic discriminating features
Base Rate Neglect	Overweighting a rare condition recently encountered elsewhere	Rank by prevalence-adjusted probability, not recency or memorability

CAUTION: A remote encounter that cannot perform palpation, diascopy, or a Nikolsky maneuver should explicitly flag that limitation in the documentation and set a low threshold for in-person follow-up whenever the differential diagnosis depends on one of these unavailable findings.

Documentation and Communication of Dermatologic Findings

Structured Documentation Format

Dermatologic documentation should follow a consistent structure: primary lesion type, secondary change, color calibrated to the patient's baseline skin tone, distribution, configuration, and any positive or negative special maneuvers, in that order, so that a subsequent reader, whether the same clinician at a later visit or a consulting specialist, can reconstruct the examination without ambiguity. Photographic documentation, when available and consented to by the patient, substantially improves the reliability of longitudinal comparison, particularly for slowly evolving pigmented lesions where subtle change over months is the diagnostically decisive finding.

Communicating Findings to Other Clinicians

Referral and consultation communication should specify the same structured elements rather than a general descriptive term such as rash, which conveys almost no diagnostic information to the receiving clinician, and should explicitly state the differential diagnosis under consideration and the specific question the referral is intended to answer, since a referral framed around a specific question is substantially more likely to receive a focused and clinically useful response than one framed as an open-ended request for evaluation.

CLINICAL PEARL: Replacing the word rash with a structured morphologic description in every note and referral is one of the highest-yield habits a clinician managing dermatologic disease can adopt, since it converts an ambiguous visual impression into reproducible clinical data.

Continuity of Care Across Multiple Visits

Chronic dermatologic conditions are frequently followed across many visits, sometimes by different clinicians within the same practice, and documentation that consistently records body surface area involved, distribution, and response to the specific therapy most recently prescribed allows a subsequent clinician to assess trajectory accurately rather than reconstructing the treatment history from memory or from an incomplete medication list. This is particularly important for conditions managed with sequential escalation through a defined treatment ladder, such as psoriasis or atopic dermatitis, where the specific agents already tried, and the specific reason each was discontinued, whether for inadequate efficacy, intolerance, or cost, materially changes the appropriate next step and should never require the patient to reconstruct that history unaided at each new visit.

Standardized clinical photography integrated into the medical record, rather than stored separately or omitted entirely, closes the loop on this continuity requirement by allowing a subsequent clinician to compare the current examination directly against a documented prior state rather than relying solely on the prior clinician's descriptive text, which, however carefully structured, cannot capture every detail a photograph preserves. A consistent practice of structured description paired with photographic documentation, applied at every dermatologic encounter regardless of perceived acuity, is the single habit most likely to improve diagnostic accuracy and continuity of care across the remainder of this book's disease-specific chapters.

Clinical Case: Integrating History, Examination, and Bedside Testing

A 22-year-old man presents with a two-week history of an oval, mildly scaling patch on his chest that he initially thought was ringworm and treated with an over-the-counter antifungal cream without improvement. Over the past four days, he has noticed multiple smaller, similar oval lesions appearing on his trunk, arranged in a pattern he describes as following the lines of his ribs. He denies fever, joint pain, or oral lesions, and reports no new sexual partners or medications. On examination, a two-centimeter oval, fine-scaling patch with a collarette of scale at its inner border is present on the right chest, with numerous smaller similar lesions distributed symmetrically over the trunk along horizontal skin lines, sparing the palms, soles, and oral mucosa entirely.

Applying the structured history-taking approach introduced in this chapter, the two-week timeline with a larger initial lesion followed by a secondary eruption of smaller lesions corresponds directly to the herald-patch pattern described in the Rhythm Layer callout earlier in this chapter, and the failure to improve with an empiric antifungal argues against tinea corporis despite the patient's own initial impression, since an inadequate response to appropriate topical antifungal therapy should prompt reconsideration of the working diagnosis rather than escalation to a more potent antifungal agent. The structured examination, performed systematically rather than confined to the area of greatest concern, confirms palm, sole, and mucosal sparing, which argues against secondary syphilis, and the cleavage-line distribution and collarette scale support the herald-patch pattern over guttate psoriasis.

Following the Management Pivot for this pattern, the patient is reassured that this represents a self-limited eruption expected to resolve over the coming weeks, and he is offered a low-potency topical corticosteroid and an oral antihistamine for symptomatic pruritus. Given the absence of any risk factors or examination findings suggesting syphilis, serologic testing is not pursued, though the patient is counseled explicitly that any subsequent development of palmoplantar lesions, oral lesions, or systemic symptoms should prompt immediate reevaluation, an explicit safety-netting instruction that closes the loop on the one differential diagnosis in this case that would materially change management if it were in fact present.

EVIDENCE: Failure of a presumed dermatophyte infection to respond to an adequately applied topical antifungal after two to four weeks should prompt reconsideration of the working diagnosis rather than automatic escalation to a more potent antifungal agent, since inadequate response is more often a marker of an incorrect diagnosis than of undertreatment.

This case also illustrates the value of explicit safety-netting language in documentation and patient communication: rather than closing the encounter with an unqualified diagnosis, the clinician records the specific findings that would change the working diagnosis and communicates them directly to the patient, so that the patient becomes an active participant in monitoring for the features, palmoplantar or mucosal involvement in this instance, that would prompt earlier reevaluation than a routine follow-up interval would otherwise allow.

Clinical Case: Avoiding Premature Closure in an Atypical Presentation

A 61-year-old woman with well-controlled type 2 diabetes presents with a three-month history of a slowly enlarging, mildly itchy patch on her lower leg that her primary care clinician has treated twice with a topical antifungal cream for presumed tinea corporis, without improvement. She reports the area is now larger and slightly more indurated than when it was first noticed, though it remains only mildly symptomatic. On examination, a five-centimeter, annular, yellow-brown plaque with a slightly atrophic, telangiectatic center and a faintly raised border is present on the anterior shin. There is no scale at the border on close inspection, and a potassium hydroxide preparation performed at this visit is negative.

Applying the cognitive-pitfall framework introduced in this chapter, the initial working diagnosis of tinea corporis appears to have anchored the two prior treatment courses, and the persistence of the lesion despite adequate topical antifungal therapy should itself have prompted the second look and reconsideration of the working diagnosis emphasized earlier in this chapter, rather than a second empiric treatment course of the same class. Applying the structured examination approach instead, the absence of an active scaling border argues against a dermatophyte infection, and the atrophic, telangiectatic, yellow-brown quality of the plaque, together with the patient's diabetes, is far more consistent with necrobiosis lipoidica, a granulomatous process associated with diabetes mellitus that characteristically favors the anterior shin and is frequently misdiagnosed as tinea corporis or a resolving bruise before the diagnosis is considered.

Following the Management Pivot for this pattern, biopsy is obtained to confirm the diagnosis given both its atypical appearance for tinea and the diagnostic and prognostic implications of confirming an underlying granulomatous process, and the biopsy confirms necrobiosis lipoidica. Management centers on optimizing glycemic control, protecting the atrophic, fragile plaque from trauma given its propensity to ulcerate, and a trial of potent topical or intralesional corticosteroid for the active, expanding border, with the patient counseled that the disease often has a chronic, slowly evolving course only partially responsive to treatment. This case illustrates directly how anchoring on an initial diagnosis, reinforced by two rounds of ineffective treatment rather than diagnostic reconsideration, delayed recognition of a condition whose management differs substantially from that of the originally presumed tinea corporis.

CLINICAL PEARL: A dermatologic diagnosis that fails to respond to two sequential courses of appropriately selected first-line therapy should be actively reconsidered rather than treated a third time with the same therapeutic class.

Both cases presented in this chapter share a common structure that recurs throughout the remainder of this book: a plausible initial impression, a specific piece of history or examination that argues against premature acceptance of that impression, and a resolution reached by systematically applying the discriminating logic built into the Morphology-to-Management System rather than by additional testing performed reflexively. Readers are encouraged to approach each disease-specific chapter that follows with this same discipline, treating the Trap Logic component of every pattern callout not as supplementary detail but as the step that most directly determines diagnostic accuracy at the bedside.

THE MORPHOLOGY-TO-MANAGEMENT SYSTEM — Bedside Diagnostic Method

---

Pattern Introduced This Chapter: The acute, widespread, fine papulosquamous eruption with cleavage-line distribution, and its two most consequential mimics, guttate psoriasis and secondary syphilis.

Cross-Cutting Anchor: Palmoplantar and mucosal involvement is the single fastest bedside discriminator that must be actively sought, not passively awaited, whenever a generalized papulosquamous eruption is being evaluated.

Summary and Key Concepts

A precise timeline of onset, evolution, and symptom character frequently carries as much diagnostic weight as the physical examination itself and should never be abbreviated in favor of examination alone.

A complete, systematic skin examination, including scalp, palms, soles, nails, and mucosa, reliably captures incidental findings that a complaint-focused examination misses.

Bedside diagnostic aids, diascopy, potassium hydroxide preparation, Wood lamp examination, and dermoscopy, resolve many diagnostic questions without requiring biopsy.

A differential diagnosis should be constructed as a ranked probability list integrating morphology, distribution, configuration, and history, with Trap Logic supplying the discriminating feature that resolves close calls.

Structured documentation using standardized descriptive language, rather than the generic term rash, communicates dermatologic findings precisely and improves the value of specialist referral.

CHAPTER 3: PRINCIPLES OF DERMATOLOGIC THERAPEUTICS

Learning Objectives

1. Select an appropriate topical vehicle based on lesion morphology, anatomic site, and chronicity.
2. Apply topical corticosteroid potency classification to match agent strength to disease severity and anatomic site while minimizing cutaneous atrophy risk.
3. Compare the major classes of systemic dermatologic therapy, including their mechanisms, monitoring requirements, and principal toxicities.
4. Describe the mechanism, indications, and safety considerations of phototherapy in inflammatory skin disease.
5. Apply a structured treatment-escalation framework that matches disease severity to therapeutic intensity while minimizing cumulative treatment burden.

Topical Therapy: Vehicles, Potency, and Absorption

Topical therapy remains the foundation of dermatologic treatment because it delivers an active agent directly to the diseased tissue while minimizing systemic exposure, but its efficacy depends as much on the vehicle carrying the active ingredient as on the active ingredient itself, a principle frequently underappreciated outside dermatology.

Matching Vehicle to Lesion and Site

Ointments, being occlusive and largely free of preservatives and emulsifiers, maximize drug penetration and hydration and are preferred for thick, lichenified, or chronically dry lesions and for use on non-hair-bearing, non-intertriginous skin, but their greasy texture limits patient acceptance on the face or in warm climates. Creams, an emulsion of oil and water, are better tolerated cosmetically and are appropriate for acute or subacute inflammatory lesions and for intertriginous sites where occlusion would promote maceration. Lotions, gels, foams, and solutions carry progressively less oil content and greater alcohol or propylene glycol content, making them preferred for hair-bearing areas such as the scalp, where an ointment or cream would mat the hair and reduce adherence to treatment; gels and solutions can, however, produce a stinging or burning sensation on eroded or fissured skin due to their alcohol content, an important counseling point that affects adherence.

Site-Dependent Absorption and Systemic Risk

Percutaneous absorption varies by more than an order of magnitude across anatomic sites because it is governed directly by stratum corneum thickness: the eyelids, genitalia, and intertriginous folds absorb topical agents far more efficiently than the palms and soles, where the stratum corneum is markedly thicker. This anatomic variation is the mechanistic basis for restricting higher-potency topical corticosteroids on the face, genitalia, and intertriginous folds, where the same concentration and potency that would be appropriate and safe on the trunk or extremities can produce atrophy, striae, or systemic absorption sufficient to suppress the hypothalamic-pituitary-adrenal axis, particularly in infants and young children whose surface-area-to-body-mass ratio further amplifies this risk, as introduced in the discussion of neonatal skin in the first chapter of this book.

Occlusion and Enhanced Delivery

Occlusive dressing over a topical agent, whether through plastic wrap, a hydrocolloid dressing, or simply thick application under cotton gloves or socks, increases hydration of the stratum corneum and can increase percutaneous absorption of the underlying agent severalfold, a technique used deliberately to enhance efficacy in thick, recalcitrant plaques such as chronic lichenified eczema or thick psoriatic plaques on the palms and soles, but one that correspondingly increases the risk of local and systemic corticosteroid adverse effects and should be used for a limited, defined duration with explicit follow-up rather than as an indefinite maintenance strategy.

Vehicle	Key Characteristic	Preferred Use
Ointment	Occlusive, minimal preservatives, maximal penetration	Thick, lichenified, or dry lesions on non-intertriginous skin
Cream	Oil-in-water emulsion, cosmetically acceptable	Acute/subacute inflammation, intertriginous sites
Gel/Solution	Alcohol-based, minimal residue	Scalp and other hair-bearing areas
Foam	Rapid spreading, cosmetically elegant	Scalp and large surface area application

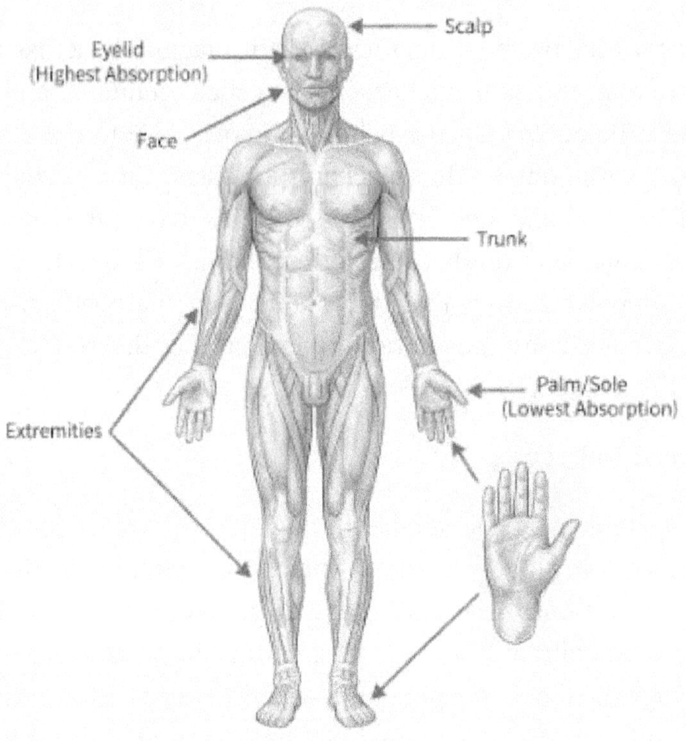

Topical Corticosteroids and Steroid-Sparing Agents

Potency Classification and Site-Matched Selection

Topical corticosteroids are classified into seven potency classes, from superhigh potency to lowest potency, based on standardized vasoconstrictor assay data, and matching potency class to anatomic site and disease severity is the single most important determinant of both efficacy and adverse effect risk. As a general framework, low-potency agents are reserved for the face, eyelids, genitalia, and intertriginous folds, where thin stratum corneum and often occluded anatomy predispose to atrophy; mid-potency agents are appropriate for the trunk and extremities in most inflammatory dermatoses; and high- to superhigh-potency agents are reserved for thick, lichenified plaques, palmoplantar disease, or short, closely monitored courses for severe or recalcitrant disease elsewhere on the body.

Local and Systemic Adverse Effects

Cutaneous atrophy, telangiectasia, striae, and perioral or periocular steroid dermatitis develop with prolonged use of inappropriately potent agents at vulnerable sites, and these changes, particularly striae, are frequently irreversible once established, which is why potency and duration limits should be set explicitly at the time a topical corticosteroid is prescribed rather than left open-ended. Systemic absorption sufficient to produce hypothalamic-pituitary-adrenal axis suppression is uncommon with appropriate use but becomes a genuine concern with high-potency agents used over large body surface areas, under occlusion, or in infants, and any of these circumstances should prompt either a lower-potency substitute or explicit time-limited, closely monitored use of the higher-potency agent.

Steroid-Sparing Topical Agents

Topical calcineurin inhibitors, tacrolimus and pimecrolimus, inhibit T-cell activation without producing cutaneous atrophy, making them particularly valuable for chronic maintenance therapy at atrophy-prone sites such as the face and intertriginous folds, though they carry a boxed warning regarding a theoretical malignancy risk that has not been borne out in long-term post-marketing surveillance and should be discussed transparently with patients rather than allowed to prevent appropriate use. Topical vitamin D analogs, such as calcipotriene, reduce keratinocyte proliferation and are frequently combined with a topical corticosteroid in psoriasis both to enhance efficacy and to allow reduced cumulative steroid exposure through alternating or combination regimens. Topical phosphodiesterase-4 inhibitors and topical Janus kinase inhibitors represent newer steroid-sparing options for atopic dermatitis and, in the case of topical Janus kinase inhibition, for vitiligo, discussed further in the chapters devoted to those conditions.

CAUTION: Potency and duration limits for any topical corticosteroid should be specified explicitly at the time of prescribing, particularly for the face, eyelids, genitalia, and intertriginous folds, since striae and atrophy are frequently irreversible once established.

THE MORPHOLOGY-TO-MANAGEMENT SYSTEM — Therapeutic Principle: Matching Topical Potency to Site and Severity

---

The Pattern: A patient requiring topical corticosteroid therapy for an inflammatory dermatosis involving both a thick, chronic, extremity plaque and a thinner, more acute facial or intertriginous component.

Presentation Variance: Steroid-induced hypopigmentation is far more visually apparent and more distressing to patients with richly pigmented skin, and post-inflammatory dyspigmentation from the underlying disease itself can be difficult to distinguish from treatment-induced hypopigmentation without a clear baseline, making pretreatment counseling and, where feasible, photographic documentation especially important in this population before initiating a potent topical agent.

Trap Logic: Prescribing a single potency for the entire body, rather than site-matched potencies, is the most common prescribing error in topical corticosteroid therapy; a potency appropriate for a thick extremity plaque is frequently excessive for the face or groin, while a potency appropriately conservative for the face is frequently inadequate for a thick, lichenified plaque elsewhere.

Management Pivot: Prescribe two potencies simultaneously with explicit site instructions, for example a mid- to high-potency agent for the trunk and extremities and a low-potency agent or a steroid-sparing calcineurin inhibitor for the face and intertriginous folds, with an explicit maximum duration for the higher-potency agent and a scheduled reassessment before renewal.

Pattern Anchor: One potency does not fit the whole body; site-matched dual prescribing is the anchor practice that prevents both undertreatment and atrophy.

Systemic Therapeutics in Dermatology

Conventional Systemic Immunomodulators

Methotrexate, an antimetabolite that inhibits dihydrofolate reductase and reduces lymphocyte proliferation at the low weekly doses used in dermatology, remains a mainstay for moderate to severe psoriasis and select other inflammatory dermatoses, with hepatotoxicity and myelosuppression as its principal monitored risks and folic acid supplementation, current complete blood count, and liver function monitoring as standard safeguards, dosed and monitored according to current guideline recommendations. Cyclosporine, a calcineurin inhibitor administered systemically, produces rapid disease control but is generally reserved for short-term use given cumulative nephrotoxicity and hypertension risk with prolonged administration. Systemic retinoids, oral derivatives of vitamin A, normalize keratinocyte differentiation and are used in severe acne, several disorders of keratinization, and select lymphoproliferative skin conditions, with teratogenicity as an absolute contraindication in pregnancy requiring strict pregnancy prevention protocols in patients of childbearing potential, mucocutaneous dryness, and lipid and hepatic monitoring as standard components of therapy.

Monitoring Frameworks for Systemic Agents

Every systemic dermatologic agent carries a defined baseline and interval monitoring protocol, and adherence to that protocol, rather than the choice of agent itself, is frequently what determines whether a serious adverse effect is caught early or allowed to progress. Baseline assessment typically includes relevant infectious disease screening, a complete blood count, and hepatic and renal function testing, with the specific panel and interval determined by the mechanism of the chosen agent and confirmed against current guideline and product labeling recommendations rather than assumed from general principle. Patient-specific risk factors, including alcohol use, preexisting liver or kidney disease, and concurrent hepatotoxic or nephrotoxic medications, should be actively screened for before initiating conventional systemic immunomodulators, since these factors materially change both agent selection and monitoring frequency.

Antimicrobial and Antifungal Systemic Therapy

Systemic antimicrobial and antifungal therapy in dermatology follows the same evidence-based principles as in general infectious disease practice, with the specific agent, dose, and duration guided by the causative organism, site of infection, and current resistance patterns, each addressed in detail within the infectious disease chapters of this book. A recurring dermatology-specific principle is that many cutaneous infections require longer treatment courses than analogous infections at other sites, reflecting the slower turnover of the structures involved, for example the markedly longer courses required to clear a dermatophyte infection of the nail plate compared with a superficial skin infection, given the relatively avascular, slow-growing nature of the nail matrix and plate.

EDUCATIONAL FIGURE: AXIAL BRAIN MRI AND MAJOR NEUROANATOMICAL STRUCTURES

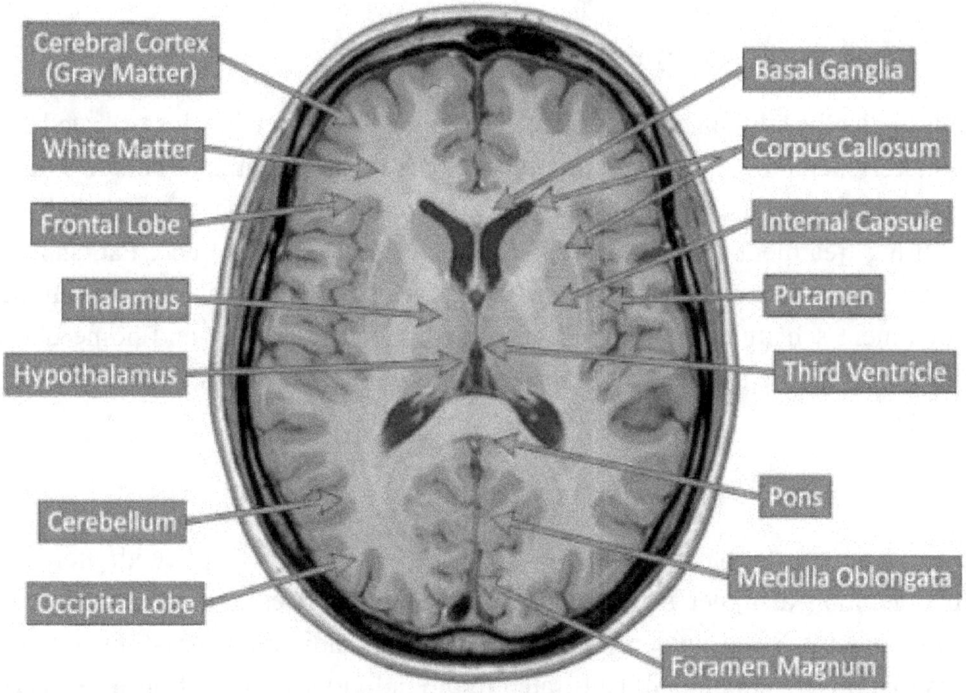

Agent Class	Principal Monitored Risk	Core Monitoring Elements
Methotrexate	Hepatotoxicity, myelosuppression	Complete blood count, liver function testing, folic acid supplementation
Cyclosporine	Nephrotoxicity, hypertension	Blood pressure, renal function, drug level where applicable
Systemic Retinoids	Teratogenicity, dyslipidemia, hepatotoxicity	Pregnancy prevention protocol, lipid panel, liver function testing

Phototherapy

Mechanism and Modalities

Phototherapy delivers a controlled dose of ultraviolet radiation to induce local immunosuppression, reduce pathogenic T-cell activity within the skin, and, for narrowband ultraviolet B specifically, slow keratinocyte proliferation, producing clinical benefit in psoriasis, atopic dermatitis, vitiligo, and several other chronic inflammatory and pigmentary conditions discussed in later chapters. Narrowband ultraviolet B, emitting a tightly restricted wavelength band around 311 nanometers, has become the most widely used modality given its favorable efficacy and safety profile relative to older broadband ultraviolet B and psoralen plus ultraviolet A regimens, the latter reserved for select indications given its association with an increased long-term risk of cutaneous malignancy with cumulative treatment exposure.

Patient Selection and Treatment Protocol

Phototherapy is typically administered two to three times weekly with dose titrated to the individual patient's minimal erythema dose or skin phototype, and a typical treatment course extends over several months before clinical benefit is fully assessed, a time commitment that should be discussed explicitly with patients during treatment selection given its direct effect on adherence. Patients with a history of photosensitive disease, a personal history of skin cancer at high cumulative dose, or an inability to attend the frequent treatment schedule required are generally poor candidates, and home phototherapy units, where available, can improve adherence for appropriately selected, motivated patients unable to attend an in-office schedule.

Safety Considerations Across Skin Types

Starting dose and dose escalation schedule are calibrated to skin phototype, with more richly pigmented skin generally tolerating a higher starting dose and more rapid escalation given greater endogenous photoprotection from increased epidermal melanin, though individual variation within any phototype category means that dosing should still be titrated to the individual patient's observed erythema response rather than assigned by phototype alone. Long-term cumulative ultraviolet exposure across repeated treatment courses should be tracked explicitly in the medical record, since cumulative dose, rather than any single course, is what determines long-term skin cancer risk.

EVIDENCE: Narrowband ultraviolet B has demonstrated a substantially more favorable long-term safety profile than psoralen plus ultraviolet A therapy and has become first-line phototherapy for most inflammatory indications where phototherapy is appropriate.

Home Phototherapy and Adherence Barriers

In-office phototherapy's requirement of two to three visits weekly for several months represents one of the most significant adherence barriers in dermatologic therapy, particularly for patients with inflexible work schedules, limited transportation, or long travel distances to a treatment facility, and this barrier disproportionately affects patients with lower socioeconomic resources, contributing to disparities in access to a therapy that is otherwise highly effective and comparatively inexpensive. Home narrowband ultraviolet B units, prescribed for appropriately selected and adequately trained patients, substantially reduce this adherence barrier while maintaining comparable efficacy to in-office treatment for many patients, and expanding access to this option should be considered explicitly whenever an in-office schedule is likely to be a limiting factor for an otherwise appropriate phototherapy candidate.

PATIENT EDUCATION: Patients beginning phototherapy should be counseled explicitly that a full course typically extends over several months before maximal benefit is assessed, since unrealistic expectations about time to response are a common and preventable cause of early discontinuation.

Biologic and Targeted Systemic Therapy

Cytokine-Targeted Biologic Agents

Biologic agents targeting tumor necrosis factor-alpha, interleukin-17, interleukin-23, and interleukin-12/23 have transformed the management of moderate to severe psoriasis and psoriatic arthritis by achieving rates of near-complete clearance unattainable with conventional systemic agents, while avoiding the hepatotoxicity and nephrotoxicity associated with methotrexate and cyclosporine. Each cytokine target carries its own efficacy, speed of onset, and safety profile, for example interleukin-17 inhibition producing among the most rapid and complete clearance rates but carrying a class-specific caution regarding inflammatory bowel disease exacerbation, information that should directly inform agent selection in a patient with relevant comorbid disease, confirmed against current prescribing information and specialty guideline recommendations.

Targeted Small-Molecule Therapy

Oral Janus kinase inhibitors provide a targeted small-molecule alternative to injectable biologic therapy for select indications, including moderate to severe atopic dermatitis and alopecia areata, working by blocking intracellular cytokine signaling downstream of multiple relevant receptors rather than neutralizing a single extracellular cytokine, and carry their own boxed warning framework regarding thrombosis, malignancy, and major cardiovascular events that requires explicit discussion and risk stratification before initiation, particularly in older patients or those with relevant cardiovascular risk factors.

Pretreatment Screening and Shared Decision-Making

Before initiating any biologic or targeted systemic agent, screening for latent tuberculosis and viral hepatitis is standard given the risk of reactivation under immunosuppression, and this screening should be completed and, where positive, appropriately treated or specialist-comanaged before the biologic agent is started rather than concurrently. Shared decision-making around agent selection should explicitly weigh speed of onset, route and frequency of administration, comorbidity-specific safety considerations, and cost and access, since the most efficacious agent in a controlled trial population is not necessarily the most appropriate agent for a given patient's individual risk profile and life circumstances.

CAUTION: Latent tuberculosis and viral hepatitis screening should be completed, and any positive result appropriately addressed, before initiating biologic or targeted systemic dermatologic therapy, given the risk of reactivation under immunosuppression.

Antibiotic Stewardship in Dermatologic Practice

Dermatology has historically been a substantial contributor to prolonged systemic antibiotic courses, most notably in acne management, where oral tetracycline-class agents have often been prescribed for many months at a time, a practice increasingly recognized as contributing to antimicrobial resistance without proportionate clinical benefit beyond a defined induction period. Current stewardship-oriented practice favors limiting systemic antibiotic courses in acne to the shortest duration consistent with clinical response, typically no more than three to four months, with early introduction of a non-antibiotic maintenance strategy, most often a topical retinoid with or without benzoyl peroxide, to sustain improvement without continued systemic antibiotic exposure. Similar stewardship principles apply to antibiotic selection for cutaneous infections generally, favoring narrow-spectrum agents targeted to the most likely causative organism over broad-spectrum empiric therapy whenever the clinical picture and local resistance patterns permit that narrower selection.

Combination and Sequential Therapy Strategies

Combining agents with complementary, non-overlapping mechanisms and toxicity profiles frequently achieves better disease control at a lower cumulative dose of any single agent than dose-escalating one agent alone, as illustrated by the standard combination of a topical retinoid with benzoyl peroxide in acne, which addresses both abnormal follicular keratinization and Cutibacterium acnes proliferation simultaneously while benzoyl peroxide's antimicrobial mechanism carries no associated resistance risk of its own. Sequential therapy, using an induction-phase agent selected for rapid disease control followed by transition to a different agent selected for long-term maintenance safety, is a related strategy applied throughout dermatology, for example using a short course of a more potent topical corticosteroid to achieve initial control of an inflammatory dermatosis before transitioning to a steroid-sparing agent for sustained maintenance therapy.

EVIDENCE: Limiting systemic antibiotic courses in acne to three to four months, with early transition to a non-antibiotic maintenance regimen, is now widely endorsed as both an antimicrobial stewardship measure and a clinically appropriate treatment strategy, since sustained benefit beyond the induction period is not reliably demonstrated with continued antibiotic use.

Principles of Treatment Selection and Escalation

Matching Therapeutic Intensity to Disease Severity

Treatment selection should match therapeutic intensity to an objective or semi-objective measure of disease severity and body surface area involvement rather than to the mere presence or absence of disease, since limited disease is appropriately managed with topical therapy while extensive, refractory, or quality-of-life-impairing disease warrants earlier escalation to phototherapy or systemic therapy rather than prolonged, incremental topical dose escalation that delays effective treatment.

Escalation Thresholds and Reassessment Intervals

A defined reassessment interval, typically four to twelve weeks depending on the condition and agent, should accompany every new therapy initiated, with an explicit prospective plan for escalation if the expected response is not achieved, rather than open-ended continuation of a therapy that is failing. This structured escalation framework, moving from topical to phototherapy or conventional systemic therapy to biologic or targeted systemic therapy as severity and treatment resistance dictate, recurs throughout the disease-specific Management Pivot components of the Morphology-to-Management System applied in every subsequent chapter of this book.

Deintensification and Long-Term Maintenance

Once disease control is achieved, a deliberate plan for deintensification, whether through reduced application frequency, transition to a steroid-sparing maintenance agent, or extended dosing intervals for a systemic agent, should be considered explicitly rather than continuing peak induction-phase therapy indefinitely, both to reduce cumulative treatment burden and adverse effect risk and to preserve future treatment options should disease activity later increase.

This deintensification planning should be discussed with the patient at the same visit that induction therapy is initiated, framing the treatment course explicitly as induction followed by maintenance rather than presenting maintenance planning only after disease control has already been achieved, since patients who understand from the outset that the initial regimen is not necessarily the long-term regimen are more likely to tolerate a subsequent dose reduction without perceiving it as a loss of effective treatment or a sign that their disease is worsening.

Special Populations in Dermatologic Therapeutics

Pregnancy and Lactation

Several dermatologic therapies carry well-established teratogenic risk and are absolutely contraindicated in pregnancy, most notably systemic retinoids, which require strict, guideline-defined pregnancy prevention protocols in any patient of childbearing potential, including confirmed contraception, regular pregnancy testing, and structured patient counseling documented at each prescription. Methotrexate is similarly contraindicated in pregnancy and requires a washout period before conception is attempted, in men as well as women, given evidence of effects on spermatogenesis and fetal exposure risk. By contrast, many topical therapies, low- to mid-potency topical corticosteroids in particular, have a substantial safety record in pregnancy when used in standard quantities, and denying appropriate topical treatment to a pregnant patient with significant dermatologic disease out of undifferentiated caution can itself cause harm through undertreated disease; each systemic and topical agent should be assessed individually against current pregnancy-specific safety data rather than avoided reflexively as a category.

Pediatric Dosing and Formulation Considerations

Pediatric topical corticosteroid selection must account for the increased percutaneous absorption and higher surface-area-to-body-mass ratio introduced in the first chapter of this book, favoring lower potency classes and shorter treatment durations than would be used for an equivalent adult presentation, with particular caution in the diaper area, where occlusion from the diaper itself compounds absorption risk. Systemic agents used in pediatric dermatology, including selected biologic agents now approved for pediatric atopic dermatitis and psoriasis, require weight-based dosing calculated explicitly rather than extrapolated from an adult dose, and monitoring intervals in children are generally at least as frequent as in adults given more limited long-term pediatric safety data for several newer agents.

Polypharmacy and Drug Interactions in Older Adults

Older adults presenting for systemic dermatologic therapy frequently carry a substantial existing medication burden, and a structured medication reconciliation specifically screening for interactions with the hepatic metabolic pathways used by many systemic dermatologic agents, along with cumulative nephrotoxic or hepatotoxic exposure from other prescribed medications, should precede initiation of any new systemic agent in this population. Reduced hepatic and renal reserve with advancing age can also necessitate dose adjustment or more frequent monitoring even for agents without an absolute age-based contraindication, and baseline functional status and life expectancy should inform the overall intensity of the treatment plan in shared decision-making with the patient.

CAUTION: Systemic retinoids and methotrexate are contraindicated in pregnancy and require structured pregnancy prevention protocols in patients of childbearing potential; do not extend this same reflexive avoidance to low- to mid-potency topical corticosteroids, which have a substantial pregnancy safety record when used appropriately.

Preconception counseling should be initiated well before a planned pregnancy whenever a patient of childbearing potential is being considered for a teratogenic systemic agent, allowing time for the required washout period and for an alternative, pregnancy-compatible regimen to be established and its efficacy confirmed before conception is attempted.

Adherence, Cost, and Access in Treatment Selection

Why Adherence Failure Is Often Mistaken for Treatment Failure

A substantial proportion of apparent topical treatment failure in dermatology reflects inadequate adherence rather than true pharmacologic non-response, driven by factors including inconvenient vehicle choice for the affected site, insufficient quantity prescribed relative to the body surface area being treated, and inadequate counseling on expected time to response. Before escalating therapy for an apparently inadequate response, a structured adherence assessment, including direct, non-judgmental questions about how often and how the medication has actually been applied, should be completed, since escalating to a systemic agent for what is in fact an adherence problem exposes the patient to unnecessary treatment risk and cost without addressing the underlying barrier.

Quantity Prescribing and the Fingertip Unit

Underprescribing of topical agents relative to the body surface area requiring treatment is a common and correctable driver of adherence failure; the fingertip unit, defined as the amount of topical product expressed from a standard tube opening from the distal skin crease to the fingertip, provides a practical, reproducible dosing guide that can be taught directly to patients, with an adult fingertip unit generally sufficient to cover an area equivalent to twice the flat surface of the patient's own hand. Prescribing a quantity calculated explicitly from estimated body surface area and expected treatment duration, rather than a default small quantity, meaningfully improves both adherence and treatment outcomes.

Cost and Insurance Access as Determinants of Real-World Efficacy

A therapy with superior trial efficacy is only as effective as the patient's actual ability to obtain and afford it, and cost, insurance formulary restriction, and prior authorization burden should be discussed explicitly during treatment selection rather than discovered only after a prescription fails to be filled. Generic topical agents and, where clinically appropriate, older, less expensive systemic agents remain valuable options specifically because their lower cost and administrative burden translate into a higher likelihood of sustained real-world adherence, even when a newer agent demonstrates superior efficacy in the controlled conditions of a clinical trial population.

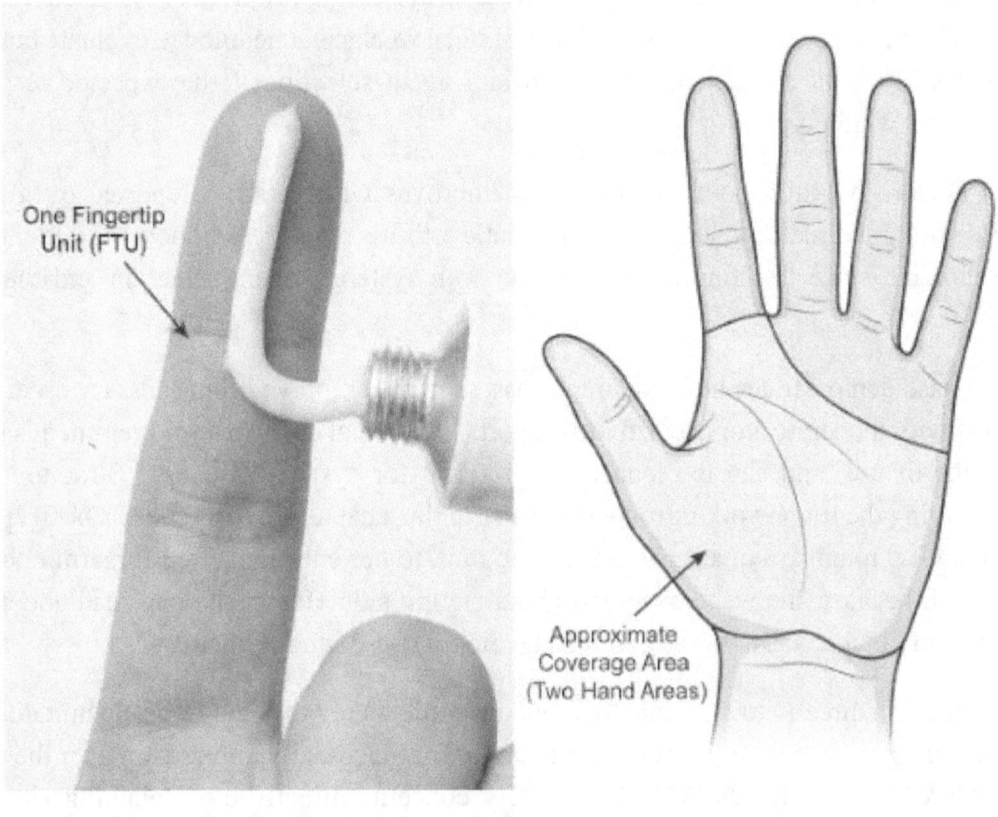

Clinical Case: Structured Treatment Selection and Escalation

A 45-year-old man with plaque psoriasis involving approximately eight percent of his body surface area, including thick plaques on both elbows, knees, and the lower back, has been using a mid-potency topical corticosteroid intermittently for two years with only partial and inconsistent control. He reports the disease affects his ability to wear short sleeves at work and has begun to notice mild lower back stiffness in the mornings that improves with activity.

Applying the treatment-selection framework introduced in this chapter, eight percent body surface area involvement together with an inadequate response to two years of topical therapy meets commonly used thresholds for considering escalation beyond topical therapy alone, rather than continuing further topical dose adjustment. The morning stiffness that improves with activity raises specific concern for inflammatory joint involvement rather than mechanical low back pain, and this finding, per the caution introduced earlier in this chapter regarding periodic joint reassessment in psoriasis, warrants a directed history and examination for psoriatic arthritis and, where appropriate, rheumatologic referral, since confirmed joint involvement would itself favor a systemic agent with demonstrated joint efficacy over a therapy directed at skin disease alone.

Following the structured escalation approach, and pending baseline screening for latent tuberculosis and viral hepatitis as described earlier in this chapter, an interleukin-17 or interleukin-23 inhibitor is a reasonable first systemic agent given the combination of moderate body surface area involvement, inadequate topical response, and possible joint involvement, offering the prospect of near-complete skin clearance together with efficacy against psoriatic arthritis for appropriately selected interleukin-17 pathway agents. A defined reassessment at twelve to sixteen weeks is scheduled to evaluate both cutaneous and joint response, with an explicit plan to reconsider agent selection if the expected response is not achieved within that window.

CLINICAL PEARL: Morning joint stiffness that improves with activity, reported by a patient with psoriasis, should prompt directed evaluation for psoriatic arthritis regardless of how the patient themselves frames the complaint, since this finding can change both systemic agent selection and the urgency of specialist referral.

A second, brief case demonstrates how adherence assessment can prevent unnecessary escalation. A 28-year-old woman with moderate atopic dermatitis reports her topical corticosteroid regimen is not working after three weeks of use, and she is requesting a referral for systemic therapy. Structured adherence questioning, applying the framework introduced earlier in this chapter, reveals she has been applying only a very small quantity, roughly a quarter of a fingertip unit, to her entire affected forearm once every two to three days, both because she was concerned about steroid side effects she had read about online and because a single small tube was not going to last the month if used more liberally.

Rather than proceeding directly to systemic therapy, the clinician reviews the fingertip unit dosing method described in this chapter, prescribes an adequate quantity for twice-daily application over the full affected area for two weeks, and addresses her steroid-safety concerns directly by explaining site-appropriate potency selection and the specific atrophy risks that are relevant to her prescribed regimen and site, as distinct from the more severe risks she had encountered in unfiltered online sources. At a two-week follow-up with correct application confirmed, her dermatitis has substantially improved, illustrating directly that an apparent treatment failure was in fact an adherence and dosing-quantity problem rather than a true pharmacologic non-response, and that systemic escalation would have exposed her to unnecessary risk without addressing the actual barrier to improvement.

KEY POINT: Before escalating from topical to systemic therapy for apparent treatment failure, confirm actual applied quantity and frequency using a concrete reference such as the fingertip unit, since underdosing is a far more common cause of apparent failure than true pharmacologic non-response.

Together, the two cases in this chapter frame the two most common reasons an apparently reasonable dermatologic treatment plan fails in practice: true disease severity outpacing the intensity of therapy selected, addressed through the structured escalation framework, and adequate therapy undermined by inadequate dosing or adherence, addressed through the quantity-and-application assessment described earlier. Distinguishing between these two failure modes before altering a treatment plan is one of the most consequential judgments in dermatologic therapeutics, since the corrective action for each is essentially opposite.

THE MORPHOLOGY-TO-MANAGEMENT SYSTEM — Therapeutic Escalation Framework

Principle Introduced This Chapter: Therapeutic intensity should be matched explicitly to disease severity and body surface area, with a defined reassessment interval and prospective escalation plan built into every new therapy from the outset.

Cross-Cutting Anchor: An inadequate response to an appropriately selected first-line therapy, sustained beyond its expected window of efficacy, is itself an indication for escalation, not a reason to repeat the same therapeutic class.

Summary and Key Concepts

Topical vehicle selection, ointment, cream, gel, foam, or solution, is matched to lesion morphology, chronicity, and anatomic site, and is as important to efficacy as the active ingredient itself.

Topical corticosteroid potency must be matched to anatomic site and disease severity, with explicit potency and duration limits set at the time of prescribing to prevent irreversible atrophy and striae.

Systemic dermatologic agents, conventional immunomodulators, phototherapy, and biologic or targeted small-molecule therapy, each carry defined mechanisms, efficacy profiles, and monitoring requirements that should govern selection.

Biologic and targeted systemic agents require pretreatment screening for latent tuberculosis and viral hepatitis and explicit, comorbidity-informed shared decision-making before initiation.

Treatment selection should match therapeutic intensity to objective disease severity, with a defined reassessment interval and prospective escalation plan built into every new therapy from the outset.

CHAPTER 4: PSORIASIS AND THE PSORIATIC SPECTRUM

Learning Objectives

1. Classify the major clinical subtypes of psoriasis and relate each to its characteristic morphology and distribution.
2. Explain the immunologic mechanism underlying psoriasis and connect it directly to both the histopathologic and clinical features of the disease.
3. Distinguish psoriasis from its principal morphologic mimics using Trap Logic discriminating features.
4. Screen for psoriatic arthritis and the major metabolic and cardiovascular comorbidities associated with moderate to severe disease.
5. Apply a severity- and site-adapted treatment escalation framework, from topical therapy through biologic agents, to a patient with psoriasis.

Definition, Classification, and Epidemiology

Definition and Disease Spectrum

Psoriasis is a chronic, immune-mediated, papulosquamous disease characterized by accelerated, dysregulated keratinocyte proliferation driven by a defined cytokine axis, producing well-demarcated, erythematous, scaling plaques and, in a substantial minority of affected patients, an associated inflammatory arthritis. It is best understood not as a single uniform disease but as a spectrum of related clinical phenotypes, plaque, guttate, inverse, pustular, and erythrodermic, that share a common immunologic mechanism while differing substantially in morphology, distribution, and management implications.

Classification of Clinical Subtypes

Plaque psoriasis, also termed psoriasis vulgaris, accounts for the large majority of cases and is discussed in the Morphology-to-Management System callout introduced in the opening chapter of this book. Guttate psoriasis presents as an eruptive shower of small, drop-shaped papules, often following streptococcal pharyngitis, and is discussed further later in this chapter. Inverse, or flexural, psoriasis involves the axillae, groin, and inframammary folds with smooth, minimally scaling, well-demarcated erythema, since friction and moisture in these sites limit scale accumulation despite the same underlying accelerated keratinocyte turnover. Pustular psoriasis, both generalized and localized palmoplantar forms, reflects a distinct neutrophil-predominant inflammatory pattern superimposed on the same core disease mechanism, and erythrodermic psoriasis represents diffuse involvement of nearly the entire body surface, a dermatologic emergency addressed in detail in the chapter devoted to that topic.

Epidemiology and Global Variation

Psoriasis affects approximately two to three percent of the population in most studied regions, with substantial variation by ancestry and geography, lower prevalence reported in some East Asian and West African populations and higher prevalence in populations of Northern European descent, variation that appears to reflect underlying genetic susceptibility rather than solely environmental or ascertainment differences. Onset shows a bimodal age distribution, with an early peak in the second and third decades of life, often associated with a stronger family history and specific class I human leukocyte antigen associations, and a later peak in the fifth and sixth decades, more often without a strong family history.

Subtype	Characteristic Distribution	Distinguishing Feature
Plaque (Vulgaris)	Extensor surfaces, scalp, gluteal cleft	Well-demarcated plaques with adherent silvery scale
Guttate	Trunk and proximal extremities	Eruptive small drop-shaped papules, often post-streptococcal
Inverse (Flexural)	Axillae, groin, inframammary folds	Smooth, minimally scaling erythema
Pustular	Palms/soles (localized) or generalized	Sterile pustules on erythematous base
Erythrodermic	Diffuse, near-total body surface	Generalized erythema with exfoliation; dermatologic emergency

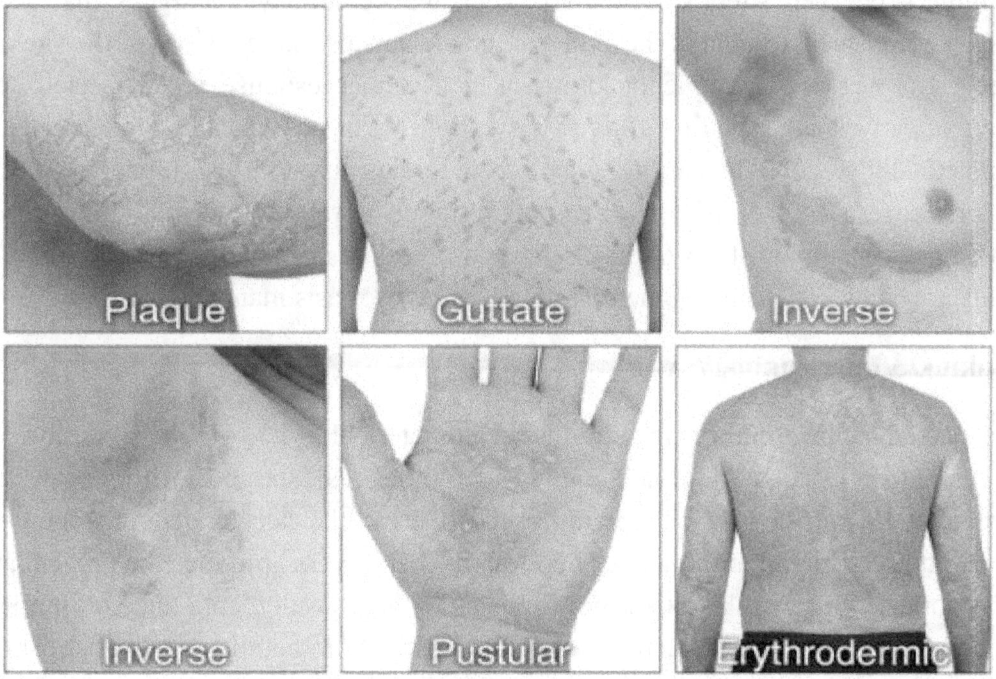

Etiology, Risk Factors, and Pathophysiology

Genetic Susceptibility

Psoriasis demonstrates substantial heritability, with the PSORS1 locus on chromosome 6, encompassing the HLA-Cw6 allele, representing the single strongest and most consistently replicated genetic association, particularly for early onset disease. Additional risk variants implicate genes within the interleukin-23 receptor and interleukin-12/23 signaling pathway, providing direct genetic support for the cytokine-targeted therapies now central to systemic management, discussed in the previous chapter and applied specifically to psoriasis later in this one.

Obesity and Metabolic Contribution to Disease Severity

Obesity contributes to psoriasis through a bidirectional relationship distinct from the simple triggering effect of the environmental factors discussed next in this chapter: adipose tissue is itself an active endocrine and inflammatory organ, secreting proinflammatory adipokines that amplify the same interleukin-23/interleukin-17 axis described later in this chapter, while psoriatic inflammation and its associated sedentary behavior from joint or skin discomfort can in turn promote further weight gain, creating a self-reinforcing cycle. This mechanistic link is the basis for the comorbidity screening and weight-management counseling discussed later in this chapter and explains the clinical observation that meaningful weight loss can measurably improve psoriasis severity independent of any change in topical or systemic anti-psoriatic therapy.

Environmental Triggers

Streptococcal pharyngitis is a well-established trigger for guttate psoriasis, believed to act through molecular mimicry between streptococcal M protein and keratinocyte antigens that activates cross-reactive T cells. Mechanical trauma to the skin can induce new psoriatic lesions at the site of injury after a delay of one to two weeks, a phenomenon known as the Koebner response, which is itself a direct clinical demonstration of how a nonspecific inflammatory trigger can activate the disease-specific cytokine cascade in genetically susceptible skin. Medications including lithium, beta-blockers, and antimalarials can trigger or exacerbate psoriasis, and abrupt systemic corticosteroid withdrawal is specifically associated with precipitating pustular or erythrodermic flares, an important consideration when systemic corticosteroids are being considered, generally avoided, for psoriasis management.

The Interleukin-23/Interleukin-17 Axis

Dendritic cells activated by an initiating stimulus secrete interleukin-23, which drives differentiation and expansion of T helper 17 cells; these cells, along with other resident and infiltrating cell populations, secrete interleukin-17, which acts on keratinocytes to drive the accelerated proliferation, abnormal differentiation, and secondary recruitment of neutrophils that together produce the clinical and histologic phenotype of psoriasis. Because this axis is now understood in molecular detail, the most effective current systemic therapies act directly on interleukin-23 or interleukin-17 rather than on downstream, less specific inflammatory mediators, explaining why these agents achieve substantially higher rates of complete or near-complete skin clearance than earlier, less targeted systemic therapies.

KEY POINT: The interleukin-23/interleukin-17 axis is not merely a laboratory finding; it directly explains the accelerated keratinocyte turnover seen histologically, the Koebner response seen clinically, and the mechanism of the most effective current biologic therapies.

Histopathology

Characteristic Epidermal Changes

Psoriatic plaques demonstrate marked epidermal hyperplasia with regular elongation of the rete ridges, a pattern termed psoriasiform hyperplasia, along with parakeratosis, retained nuclei within the stratum corneum reflecting the accelerated keratinocyte transit time introduced earlier in this chapter, and a diminished or absent granular layer. Munro microabscesses, small collections of neutrophils within the parakeratotic stratum corneum, and spongiform pustules of Kogoj, neutrophil collections within the upper spinous layer, are characteristic and specific findings when present, though their absence does not exclude the diagnosis in an otherwise typical clinical and histologic picture.

Dermal Findings

The papillary dermis shows dilated, tortuous capillary loops extending close to the thinned suprapapillary epidermal plate, the direct histologic correlate of the pinpoint bleeding on scale removal, the Auspitz sign, described in the case presented in the first chapter of this book, along with a superficial perivascular lymphocytic infiltrate. This combination of thinned suprapapillary epidermis and dilated papillary dermal vasculature is what mechanistically explains why gentle removal of adherent scale produces bleeding in psoriasis but not in most of its morphologic mimics, which lack this specific suprapapillary thinning.

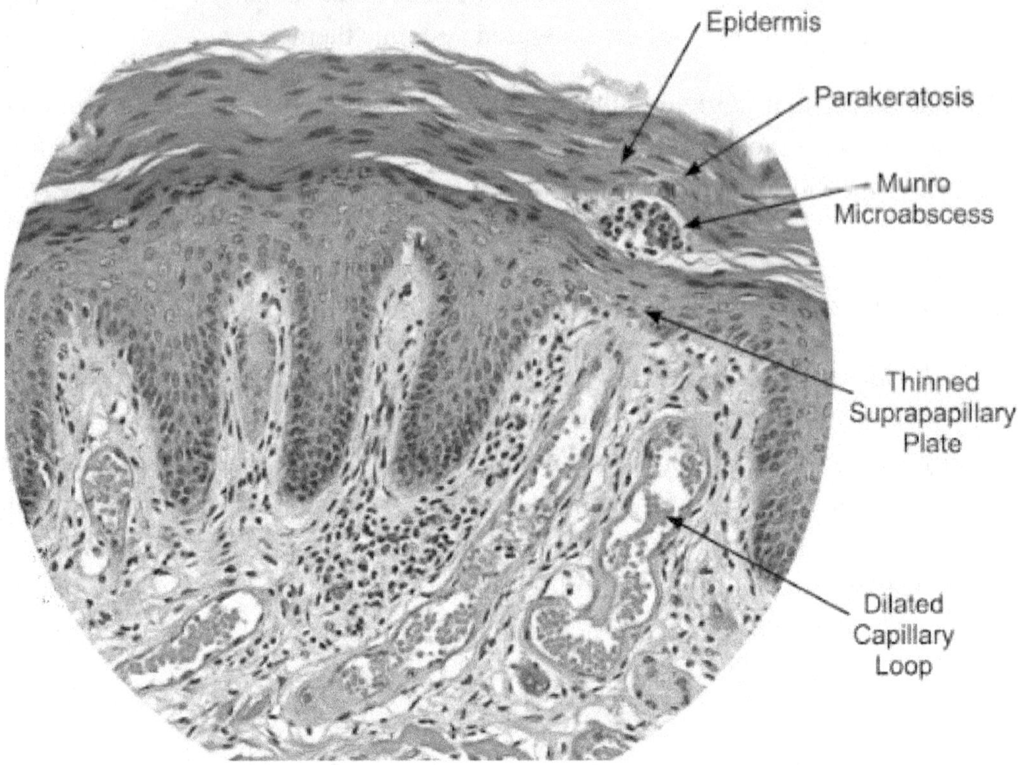

Clinical Presentation and Psoriatic Subtypes

Nail and Scalp Involvement

Nail involvement occurs in a large proportion of patients with psoriasis over the disease course and, as introduced in the first chapter, localizes anatomically to matrix disease, producing pitting, and to nail bed disease, producing onycholysis and the characteristic oil-drop discoloration. Nail involvement carries independent clinical significance beyond cosmetic concern, since it is associated with a substantially increased likelihood of concurrent or future psoriatic arthritis and should therefore prompt specific joint-directed history and examination regardless of overall cutaneous disease severity. Scalp involvement, often among the earliest and most persistent sites of disease, can extend beyond the hairline in a distinctive pattern that helps distinguish psoriasis from seborrheic dermatitis, discussed further in the differential diagnosis section of this chapter.

Guttate Psoriasis

Guttate psoriasis typically presents in children and young adults as an eruptive shower of small, drop-shaped, fine-scaling papules over the trunk and proximal extremities, appearing one to three weeks after streptococcal pharyngitis, a temporal relationship that should be specifically elicited in the history. A substantial proportion of guttate episodes resolve spontaneously, though a meaningful subset of patients subsequently develop chronic plaque psoriasis, and current evidence does not clearly support that treating the antecedent streptococcal infection prevents this progression, though symptomatic pharyngitis should still be treated according to standard infectious disease guidelines on its own merits.

Pustular and Erythrodermic Presentations

Generalized pustular psoriasis presents with widespread sterile pustules on a background of diffuse erythema, frequently accompanied by fever and systemic inflammatory markers, and represents a potentially life-threatening presentation requiring urgent management, addressed in detail in the chapter on dermatologic emergencies. Palmoplantar pustulosis, a more localized and generally less acutely dangerous variant, produces recurrent crops of sterile pustules on the palms and soles that can be substantially disabling functionally even without the systemic risk of the generalized form.

CAUTION: Generalized pustular psoriasis with fever and systemic inflammatory markers is a dermatologic emergency requiring urgent evaluation and treatment; it should never be managed as an outpatient exacerbation of routine plaque psoriasis.

Distinguishing generalized pustular psoriasis from an acute generalized exanthematous pustulosis, a drug-induced pustular eruption discussed further in later chapters, depends heavily on medication history and time course, since the latter typically develops within days of a culprit medication and resolves promptly upon its withdrawal, whereas generalized pustular psoriasis often occurs in a patient with an established psoriasis history or a recognized trigger such as abrupt corticosteroid withdrawal.

Differential Diagnosis and Diagnostic Workup

Distinguishing Psoriasis From Its Principal Mimics

The Trap Logic discrimination between plaque psoriasis, nummular eczema, and tinea corporis was introduced in detail in the Morphology-to-Management System callout in the first chapter of this book and remains the foundational discrimination for this disease. Scalp psoriasis must additionally be distinguished from seborrheic dermatitis, which produces greasier, less adherent, yellowish scale typically confined within the hairline, in contrast to the thicker, drier, silvery scale of psoriasis that frequently extends beyond the hairline onto the forehead and posterior neck. Inverse psoriasis must be distinguished from intertriginous candidiasis, which typically shows satellite pustules beyond the main body of the eruption and responds to potassium hydroxide preparation revealing pseudohyphae, a finding absent in inverse psoriasis.

Confirming the Diagnosis

The diagnosis of psoriasis is usually established clinically based on the morphology, distribution, and history described throughout this chapter, without requiring biopsy in typical presentations. Biopsy is reserved for atypical presentations, for distinguishing psoriasis from cutaneous T-cell lymphoma when clinical uncertainty persists, or for confirming pustular psoriasis when the clinical picture is ambiguous, and the histologic features described earlier in this chapter, when combined with the clinical presentation, are usually sufficient to resolve genuine diagnostic uncertainty.

Presentation Variance Across Skin Tones

Beyond the color variation already introduced in the Morphology-to-Management System callout in the first chapter of this book, psoriasis in richly pigmented skin more often shows thicker plaques with more pronounced scale and a greater tendency toward post-inflammatory dyspigmentation that can persist for months after the active plaque has resolved, occasionally becoming the dominant patient concern even after inflammatory disease activity has been adequately controlled. Severity scoring instruments such as the Psoriasis Area and Severity Index, discussed later in this chapter, were developed and validated predominantly in lighter-skinned populations, and erythema-based components of these scores can underestimate true disease activity in darker skin tones, a limitation clinicians should account for by weighting induration, scale thickness, and patient-reported symptom burden more heavily when assessing severity in this population.

Laboratory Correlates and Baseline Testing

Routine laboratory testing is not required to establish the diagnosis of typical psoriasis, but specific baseline testing becomes relevant once systemic therapy is being considered, following the monitoring framework introduced in the previous chapter: a complete blood count and hepatic function panel before methotrexate, a lipid panel and pregnancy status confirmation before systemic retinoids, and latent tuberculosis and viral hepatitis screening before biologic or targeted systemic therapy. An elevated erythrocyte sedimentation rate or C-reactive protein is nonspecific in psoriasis itself but can support a concurrent diagnosis of psoriatic arthritis when joint symptoms are present, and should prompt rheumatologic correlation rather than being interpreted as a marker of cutaneous disease activity alone.

Severity Assessment and Quality-of-Life Measurement

Body Surface Area and the Palm Method

Body surface area involvement is most practically estimated using the palm method, in which the patient's own palm, including the fingers, is taken to represent approximately one percent of total body surface area, allowing rapid bedside estimation without specialized equipment. This method underlies the commonly used severity thresholds separating limited disease, generally under three percent body surface area, appropriately managed with topical therapy alone, from moderate disease, and extensive disease, generally over ten percent body surface area, which typically warrants consideration of phototherapy or systemic therapy regardless of the specific thresholds used in a given practice setting or guideline.

The Psoriasis Area and Severity Index

The Psoriasis Area and Severity Index combines an assessment of erythema, induration, and scale severity within four body regions with the proportion of each region involved into a single composite score, and is the standard severity measure used in clinical trials and increasingly in specialty practice to document baseline severity and track treatment response objectively over time. While a full Psoriasis Area and Severity Index calculation is more detailed than routine clinical practice typically requires, understanding its components, that severity is assessed as a product of both intensity and extent rather than either alone, usefully informs bedside severity assessment even when the full index is not formally calculated.

Disability and Quality-of-Life Considerations That Override Body Surface Area Thresholds

Body surface area and Psoriasis Area and Severity Index thresholds should not be applied mechanically without considering site-specific and functional impact, since a small area of involvement in a highly visible, sensitive, or functionally important site, the face, genitalia, palms, soles, or scalp, can justify escalation to systemic therapy despite falling below a body-surface-area threshold that would otherwise suggest topical therapy is sufficient. The Dermatology Life Quality Index and similar validated instruments capture this functional and psychosocial dimension directly and should be incorporated into severity assessment and treatment decision-making alongside, rather than instead of, physical severity measures, particularly given the substantial psychosocial burden of psoriasis introduced later in this chapter.

KEY POINT: A patient with limited body surface area involvement at a highly visible or functionally sensitive site can appropriately qualify for systemic therapy despite falling below a body-surface-area threshold that would otherwise suggest topical therapy alone is sufficient.

Reassessing severity using the same instrument at each follow-up visit, rather than switching between different measures or relying on unstructured overall impression, allows treatment response to be tracked objectively over time and provides a clear, documented basis for escalation or deintensification decisions consistent with the structured escalation framework introduced in the previous chapter.

Psoriatic Arthritis and Comorbidity Screening

Recognizing Psoriatic Arthritis

Psoriatic arthritis develops in a substantial minority of patients with cutaneous psoriasis, most often after the onset of skin disease though it can precede or occur concurrently with it, and presents with a range of patterns including asymmetric oligoarthritis, symmetric polyarthritis resembling rheumatoid arthritis, distal interphalangeal joint predominant disease often associated with adjacent nail changes, axial disease resembling ankylosing spondylitis, and dactylitis, diffuse swelling of an entire digit reflecting combined joint and tendon sheath inflammation. Because delayed diagnosis and treatment of psoriatic arthritis is associated with worse long-term joint outcomes, every patient with psoriasis should be screened at intervals for joint symptoms using a brief, validated screening instrument or a structured directed history, regardless of cutaneous disease severity, since joint disease severity does not reliably parallel skin disease severity.

Metabolic and Cardiovascular Comorbidity

Moderate to severe psoriasis is independently associated with an increased risk of obesity, type 2 diabetes, metabolic syndrome, and cardiovascular disease, a relationship believed to reflect shared underlying inflammatory pathways rather than psoriasis simply causing these conditions through a single direct mechanism. This association has direct clinical implications; patients with moderate to severe psoriasis warrant proactive cardiovascular risk factor screening and management at intervals appropriate to their overall risk profile, and successful systemic treatment of psoriatic inflammation may modestly reduce, though does not eliminate, this elevated cardiovascular risk.

Cardiovascular Risk Communication

Communicating cardiovascular and metabolic risk to a patient whose primary concern is their skin requires explicit framing that connects the two, since patients frequently do not intuitively associate a skin condition with cardiovascular risk and may otherwise perceive a cardiovascular risk factor referral as unrelated or unwarranted. Framing this counseling around the shared inflammatory mechanism introduced earlier in this chapter, rather than presenting the referral as an incidental finding unrelated to the visit's purpose, improves patient understanding and, in practice, improves follow-through on the recommended screening and referral.

Psychosocial Impact and Screening for Depression

Psoriasis carries a substantial and often underrecognized psychosocial burden, with elevated rates of depression, anxiety, and impaired quality of life reported across disease severity levels, including in patients with relatively limited body surface area involvement in cosmetically or functionally sensitive locations. Routine screening for depression and quality-of-life impact should be incorporated into psoriasis care rather than reserved for patients who volunteer psychological symptoms, since patients frequently do not spontaneously report this burden despite it substantially affecting their overall wellbeing and treatment adherence.

EVIDENCE: Psoriatic arthritis screening using a brief validated instrument at routine dermatology visits improves detection of joint disease that would otherwise go unrecognized until structural joint damage has already begun, underscoring the value of proactive rather than symptom-triggered screening.

Coordinated care between dermatology and rheumatology, established proactively rather than only after joint damage has already occurred, improves the likelihood that a patient screening positive for psoriatic arthritis is evaluated and, where appropriate, started on joint-directed therapy promptly, and a standing referral pathway between the two specialties within a given practice setting meaningfully shortens this evaluation interval compared with an ad hoc referral process initiated only after screening identifies a concern.

Management and Treatment

Topical and Phototherapy for Limited to Moderate Disease

Limited plaque psoriasis is managed first-line with topical therapy as detailed in the Morphology-to-Management System callout in the first chapter, most often a potent topical corticosteroid combined with a vitamin D analog, applying the site- and potency-matching principles introduced in the previous chapter. Narrowband ultraviolet B phototherapy, discussed in the previous chapter, is an effective option for patients with more extensive disease insufficiently controlled by topical therapy alone but not yet warranting systemic immunomodulation, and remains particularly valuable for patients wishing to avoid systemic medication or for whom systemic therapy carries relative contraindication.

Systemic Therapy for Moderate to Severe Disease

Conventional systemic agents, methotrexate foremost among them, remain appropriate options for moderate to severe disease, particularly where cost or access limits biologic therapy, though biologic agents targeting interleukin-17, interleukin-23, or tumor necrosis factor-alpha now generally achieve substantially higher rates of complete or near-complete skin clearance and, for several interleukin-17 pathway agents specifically, meaningful efficacy against joint disease as well. Agent selection among the biologic classes should weigh joint involvement, relevant comorbidities such as inflammatory bowel disease, which favors avoiding interleukin-17 inhibition, prior treatment history, and patient preference regarding route and frequency of administration, confirmed against current specialty society guidelines.

Special Considerations for Difficult-to-Treat Sites

Scalp, palmoplantar, nail, and genital psoriasis each present specific treatment challenges disproportionate to their body surface area, since these sites are frequently more functionally or psychosocially impactful and often less responsive to standard topical therapy than trunk or extremity disease of equivalent severity. Scalp disease often benefits from a solution or foam vehicle for adherence, as introduced in the previous chapter; nail disease responds slowly and incompletely to any topical therapy given the avascular, slow-growing nature of the nail plate and often requires systemic therapy for meaningful improvement; and genital psoriasis requires lower-potency topical agents given the site-specific absorption considerations discussed previously, often necessitating earlier consideration of systemic therapy when topical options are constrained by site sensitivity.

THE MORPHOLOGY-TO-MANAGEMENT SYSTEM — Scalp Psoriasis Versus Seborrheic Dermatitis Arc

The Pattern: Erythematous, scaling plaques or diffuse scale confined to or extending beyond the scalp and hairline.

Presentation Variance: In patients with tightly coiled hair textures, scale can be more difficult to visualize directly and is more often detected by palpation and by scale accumulation on a comb or brush; post-inflammatory alopecia from chronic scratching is more commonly reported in this population and should not be mistaken for a primary scarring alopecia.

Trap Logic: Seborrheic dermatitis produces greasier, yellowish, less adherent scale typically confined within the hairline with associated facial involvement of the nasolabial folds and eyebrows; psoriasis produces thicker, drier, silvery, more adherent scale that frequently extends beyond the hairline onto the forehead, posterior neck, and periauricular skin.

Management Pivot: Both conditions respond to a corticosteroid solution, foam, or oil formulated for scalp use; seborrheic dermatitis additionally responds to antifungal shampoos targeting Malassezia, while psoriatic scalp disease unresponsive to topical therapy may require the addition of a vitamin D analog scalp solution or escalation to systemic therapy if extensive or resistant.

Pattern Anchor: Extension of scale beyond the hairline onto the forehead and posterior neck favors psoriasis; confinement within the hairline with greasy, yellow scale favors seborrheic dermatitis.

Complications, Prognosis, and Special Populations

Disease Course and Prognosis

Psoriasis follows a chronic, relapsing course for most affected patients, with disease severity fluctuating over time in response to triggers, treatment, and, in some patients, spontaneous variation without a clearly identifiable cause. Early, adequately intensive treatment, particularly in patients with risk factors for psoriatic arthritis such as nail involvement, may reduce the risk or severity of subsequent joint disease, reinforcing the rationale for proactive rather than reactive management discussed throughout this chapter.

Special Populations: Pregnancy and Pediatric Disease

Psoriasis often improves during pregnancy, likely reflecting pregnancy-associated immunologic shifts, though a subset of patients experience worsening, and treatment planning during pregnancy must balance disease control against the pregnancy-specific safety considerations for systemic agents discussed in the previous chapter, with several biologic agents now carrying reassuring, though still evolving, pregnancy safety data that should be reviewed against current guidance at the time of treatment planning. Pediatric psoriasis frequently presents with a higher proportion of guttate and inverse morphology relative to adult-onset disease and requires the pediatric-specific dosing and monitoring considerations for both topical and systemic therapy introduced in the previous chapter.

Impetiginized or superinfected pediatric psoriatic plaques can closely mimic, and be mimicked by, primary impetigo, and distinguishing the two depends on identifying the underlying well-demarcated, adherent-scale plaque characteristic of psoriasis beneath any secondary honey-colored crusting, since treating only the secondary infection without recognizing the underlying psoriatic process leads to recurrence once the antibiotic course ends. Postpartum flares are also well recognized, believed to reflect the reversal of the immunologic shift that produced pregnancy-associated improvement, and patients with a psoriasis history should be counseled about this possibility before delivery so that a flare in the postpartum period is not mistaken for a new or unrelated diagnosis during an already demanding period of newborn care.

Prevention and Long-Term Screening

While the underlying genetic susceptibility to psoriasis cannot be prevented, modifiable trigger avoidance, prompt treatment of streptococcal pharyngitis on its own clinical merits, weight management given the bidirectional relationship between obesity and psoriasis severity, and avoidance of abrupt systemic corticosteroid discontinuation given its association with precipitating severe flares, meaningfully reduces flare frequency and severity for many patients. Long-term screening should include periodic psoriatic arthritis assessment, cardiovascular risk factor screening, and depression screening, as detailed earlier in this chapter, incorporated as standing components of routine follow-up rather than addressed only when a patient raises a specific concern.

A structured annual review, distinct from acute visits addressing active flares, provides a reliable framework for ensuring these longitudinal screening elements are not overlooked amid the more immediate concerns that typically dominate a visit prompted by active disease. This annual review should explicitly document body surface area or Psoriasis Area and Severity Index trend, joint screening results, current cardiovascular and metabolic risk factor status, and quality-of-life impact, creating a longitudinal record that makes gradual change, whether improvement or gradual comorbidity accumulation, apparent in a way that a series of isolated acute visits often fails to capture.

Cutaneous and Infectious Complications of Longstanding Disease

Chronically involved, fissured skin, particularly at palmoplantar and flexural sites, carries an increased risk of secondary bacterial infection, and patients with extensive disease should be counseled on recognizing signs of secondary infection, increasing pain, warmth, purulent drainage, or fever, that would warrant prompt reevaluation rather than continued application of topical anti-inflammatory therapy alone. Erythrodermic progression, discussed in detail in the chapter on dermatologic emergencies, represents the most severe cutaneous complication of longstanding or inadequately controlled disease and carries risks of fluid and electrolyte disturbance, impaired thermoregulation, and secondary infection analogous in some respects to a large surface area burn, underscoring why extensive or rapidly progressing disease warrants urgent rather than routine follow-up.

Clinical Case: Longitudinal Management Across the Psoriatic Spectrum

A 16-year-old girl presents with a two-week eruption of small, scaly, drop-shaped papules over her trunk and upper arms, beginning approximately ten days after a sore throat that resolved without antibiotic treatment. She has no personal or family history of psoriasis and no joint symptoms. Examination confirms numerous 0.5 to 1 centimeter, fine-scaling, salmon-pink papules distributed over the trunk and proximal extremities, sparing the palms, soles, and scalp, with no nail changes.

Applying the diagnostic framework from this chapter, the temporal relationship to antecedent pharyngitis, the drop-shaped morphology, and the trunk-predominant distribution support a diagnosis of guttate psoriasis rather than pityriasis rosea, discussed in the previous chapter, which would be expected to show a herald patch and cleavage-line distribution rather than this more uniform, widespread eruption without a clear preceding solitary lesion. Given her age and the absence of prior psoriasis history, she and her family are counseled that a substantial proportion of guttate episodes resolve spontaneously but that a meaningful minority progress to chronic plaque disease, and she is started on narrowband ultraviolet B phototherapy, an effective option for this widespread but still relatively limited presentation, given her preference to avoid daily topical application to such a large body surface area.

At six-month follow-up, her guttate lesions have resolved, but she has since developed several new well-demarcated plaques with adherent scale on both elbows, confirming the transition to chronic plaque psoriasis anticipated at the initial visit. She is transitioned to topical corticosteroid and vitamin D analog combination therapy for these limited plaques, with an explicit plan, per the escalation framework introduced in the previous chapter, to reconsider phototherapy or systemic therapy if her plaque disease becomes more extensive. She is also asked directly and will continue to be asked at each future visit about joint symptoms and about scalp and nail involvement, given the elevated long-term risk of psoriatic arthritis that accompanies chronic plaque disease even in a patient whose disease began in this comparatively limited guttate form.

CLINICAL PEARL: Guttate psoriasis in a young patient without prior psoriasis history should still prompt counseling about the possibility of progression to chronic plaque disease and should establish a baseline for the joint, scalp, and nail screening that will remain relevant across the remainder of that patient's disease course.

A second, brief case illustrates comorbidity screening in an adult with longstanding disease. A 52-year-old man with a fifteen-year history of plaque psoriasis, previously managed adequately with topical therapy alone, returns for routine follow-up. His plaques remain limited to under five percent body surface area and are well controlled, but a review of his history reveals a body mass index in the obese range, no primary care physician seen in over three years, and no prior lipid or glucose screening. He denies joint symptoms on direct questioning.

Applying the comorbidity screening framework from this chapter, his stable, limited cutaneous disease does not itself require treatment escalation, but his psoriasis diagnosis, combined with elevated body mass index and the absence of recent primary care engagement, identifies him as a patient at meaningfully elevated risk for the metabolic and cardiovascular comorbidities associated with psoriasis independent of cutaneous severity. He is referred for primary care establishment with specific attention to lipid panel, fasting glucose or hemoglobin A1c, and blood pressure screening, and is counseled explicitly that this referral reflects his psoriasis-associated risk profile rather than any change in his skin disease itself, a distinction that helps patients understand why comorbidity screening remains relevant even when their primary complaint, the skin disease, is well controlled.

KEY POINT: Stable, well-controlled cutaneous psoriasis does not eliminate the elevated metabolic and cardiovascular risk associated with the diagnosis; comorbidity screening should continue at routine intervals regardless of current skin disease activity.

THE MORPHOLOGY-TO-MANAGEMENT SYSTEM — The Psoriatic Spectrum

Patterns Introduced This Chapter: The well-demarcated erythematous plaque with silvery scale (introduced in Chapter 1 and expanded here across the full psoriatic spectrum) and scalp psoriasis versus seborrheic dermatitis.

Cross-Cutting Anchor: Extension of adherent, silvery scale beyond a site's natural boundary, beyond the hairline at the scalp, beyond the flexural fold at inverse sites, is the recurring anchor that favors psoriasis over its site-specific mimics throughout this chapter.

Summary and Key Concepts

Psoriasis is a spectrum of related clinical phenotypes, plaque, guttate, inverse, pustular, and erythrodermic, unified by a shared interleukin-23/interleukin-17 immunologic mechanism.

Histopathologic findings, psoriasiform hyperplasia, parakeratosis, and dilated papillary dermal capillaries, directly explain the clinical Auspitz sign and the accelerated keratinocyte turnover characteristic of the disease.

Trap Logic discrimination from nummular eczema, tinea corporis, seborrheic dermatitis, and intertriginous candidiasis depends on specific, site-relevant surface and distribution features rather than gestalt impression alone.

Psoriatic arthritis and metabolic, cardiovascular, and psychosocial comorbidity should be proactively screened at routine visits regardless of cutaneous disease severity, since joint and systemic risk do not reliably parallel skin severity.

Treatment follows a severity- and site-adapted escalation framework, from topical and phototherapy through conventional systemic and biologic agents, with agent selection informed by joint involvement, comorbidity, and patient preference.

CHAPTER 5: ATOPIC DERMATITIS AND THE ECZEMATOUS DERMATOSES

Learning Objectives

1. Describe the barrier-dysfunction and immune-dysregulation mechanisms that together produce atopic dermatitis and connect each to a specific clinical feature.
2. Recognize the age-dependent morphologic presentations of atopic dermatitis, from infancy through adulthood.
3. Distinguish atopic dermatitis from its principal eczematous mimics using Trap Logic discriminating features.
4. Apply a stepwise, severity-adapted treatment escalation framework spanning skin care, topical anti-inflammatory therapy, and systemic and biologic agents.
5. Recognize and manage the infectious and ophthalmologic complications associated with atopic dermatitis.

Definition, Classification, and Epidemiology

Definition and the Eczematous Disease Family

Atopic dermatitis is a chronic, relapsing, intensely pruritic inflammatory skin disease arising from the combination of an impaired epidermal barrier and a dysregulated type 2-skewed immune response, and it is the prototype and most prevalent member of a broader family of eczematous dermatoses that share this same fundamental barrier-plus-inflammation architecture even when their specific triggers differ. Contact dermatitis, discussed in the next chapter, and nummular eczema, discussed later in this chapter, are best understood as variations on this same underlying eczematous mechanism rather than as etiologically unrelated diseases, which is why a clinician who understands the pathophysiology of atopic dermatitis in depth is well equipped to reason through the entire eczematous disease family.

The Atopic Triad and Comorbid Allergic Disease

Atopic dermatitis frequently coexists with allergic rhinitis and asthma, a clustering historically termed the atopic triad, and current evidence increasingly supports the atopic march model introduced in the first chapter of this book, in which early barrier-driven cutaneous sensitization to environmental and food allergens through a disrupted skin barrier promotes subsequent development of allergic airway disease in a meaningful subset of affected children. This model has direct clinical implications: aggressive early barrier repair and inflammation control in infants with atopic dermatitis is an area of active investigation as a possible strategy to reduce the downstream burden of allergic airway disease, reframing dermatitis treatment as having potential systemic preventive value beyond the skin itself.

Epidemiology and Disease Burden

Atopic dermatitis affects a substantial proportion of children in industrialized countries, with prevalence estimates commonly reported in the range of fifteen to twenty percent, and a meaningful minority of affected children continue to have active disease into adulthood, with a further subset experiencing adult-onset disease without a childhood history. Prevalence has risen over recent decades in industrialized nations, a trend commonly attributed to the hygiene hypothesis and related shifts in early-life microbial exposure, though the full explanation for this rise remains an active area of investigation rather than a settled question, and the disease carries a substantial cumulative burden on sleep, mental health, and family quality of life that is frequently underestimated relative to its visible cutaneous severity alone.

Age Group	Characteristic Distribution	Typical Morphology
Infantile (0-2 years)	Face, scalp, extensor extremities	Weeping, crusted, poorly demarcated erythematous patches
Childhood (2-12 years)	Flexural folds (antecubital, popliteal)	Lichenified plaques, less exudative than infantile phase
Adolescent/Adult	Flexural folds, hands, face, neck	Lichenification, dry, thickened, hyperpigmented plaques

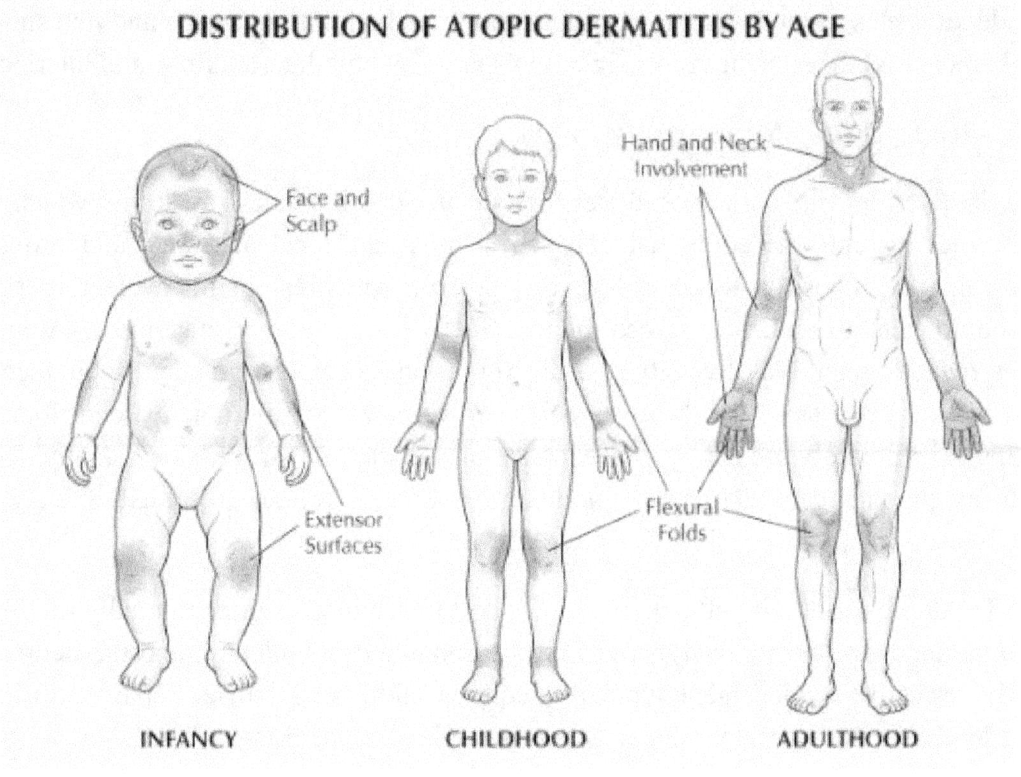

Etiology, Risk Factors, and Pathophysiology

Barrier Dysfunction and the Filaggrin Connection

As introduced in the first chapter of this book, loss-of-function mutations in the gene encoding filaggrin substantially increase the risk of atopic dermatitis by degrading the structural integrity of the stratum corneum and reducing natural moisturizing factor production, elevating transepidermal water loss and permitting deeper penetration of environmental allergens and irritants than an intact barrier would allow. Filaggrin mutations are neither necessary nor sufficient to cause atopic dermatitis on their own, present in only a minority of affected patients and also found in some unaffected individuals, indicating that barrier dysfunction and immune dysregulation act as mutually reinforcing rather than strictly sequential mechanisms, each capable of amplifying the other regardless of which initiates the disease process in a given patient.

Type 2 Immune Dysregulation

Once the barrier is breached, epidermal keratinocytes and resident immune cells release alarmins that activate a type 2-skewed immune response dominated by interleukin-4, interleukin-13, and interleukin-31, each with a distinct and clinically relevant downstream effect: interleukin-4 and interleukin-13 further suppress filaggrin and other barrier proteins, perpetuating the barrier defect in a self-reinforcing cycle, promote immunoglobulin E class switching, which underlies the elevated total and allergen-specific immunoglobulin E levels commonly observed, and interleukin-31 acts directly on cutaneous sensory neurons to drive the intense pruritus that is the disease's most functionally disabling feature. This mechanistic detail directly explains why interleukin-4 receptor alpha blockade, discussed later in this chapter, produces such substantial and rapid improvement in both inflammation and itch simultaneously, since a single receptor blockade interrupts signaling shared by both interleukin-4 and interleukin-13.

The Itch-Scratch Cycle and Microbial Dysbiosis

Interleukin-31-driven pruritus initiates a self-perpetuating itch-scratch cycle in which mechanical scratching further disrupts the epidermal barrier, releases additional alarmins, and provokes further inflammation and itch, a positive feedback loop that explains why breaking the cycle, rather than treating any single component in isolation, is central to effective long-term management. Atopic skin also demonstrates reduced microbial diversity and disproportionate colonization by Staphylococcus aureus compared with unaffected skin, and this dysbiosis is now understood as an active contributor to disease severity rather than a purely secondary consequence of a disrupted barrier, since staphylococcal toxins can function as superantigens that further activate the type 2 immune response already driving the underlying disease.

KEY POINT: Atopic dermatitis pathophysiology is best understood as three mutually reinforcing cycles operating simultaneously, barrier dysfunction, type 2 immune dysregulation, and the itch-scratch cycle, which is why effective management typically requires addressing barrier repair, anti-inflammatory therapy, and pruritus control together rather than any single element alone.

Environmental and lifestyle risk factors, including urban residence, higher socioeconomic status in early epidemiologic studies, smaller family size, and reduced early-life microbial exposure, have each been associated with atopic dermatitis risk in observational research, findings that collectively underpin the hygiene hypothesis referenced earlier in this chapter, though no single environmental factor has been shown to explain the full observed variation in disease prevalence across populations and settings.

Histopathology

Acute and Subacute Histologic Features

Acute atopic dermatitis demonstrates spongiosis, intercellular epidermal edema that can progress to intraepidermal vesiculation when severe, along with a superficial perivascular lymphocytic infiltrate with variable eosinophils, findings that correspond to the weeping, exudative clinical morphology characteristic of acute flares, particularly in the infantile phase described earlier in this chapter. Subacute lesions show a combination of spongiosis and early epidermal thickening, reflecting the transition toward the more chronic histologic pattern described next.

Chronic Histologic Features

Chronic, lichenified atopic dermatitis demonstrates compact hyperkeratosis, irregular epidermal hyperplasia, and coarsening of the papillary dermal collagen with vertically oriented fibrosis, a pattern that directly reflects the chronic mechanical trauma from repetitive scratching described in the itch-scratch cycle discussed earlier in this chapter, distinguishing this histologic pattern from the regular, non-scratch-related epidermal hyperplasia of psoriasis discussed in the previous chapter.

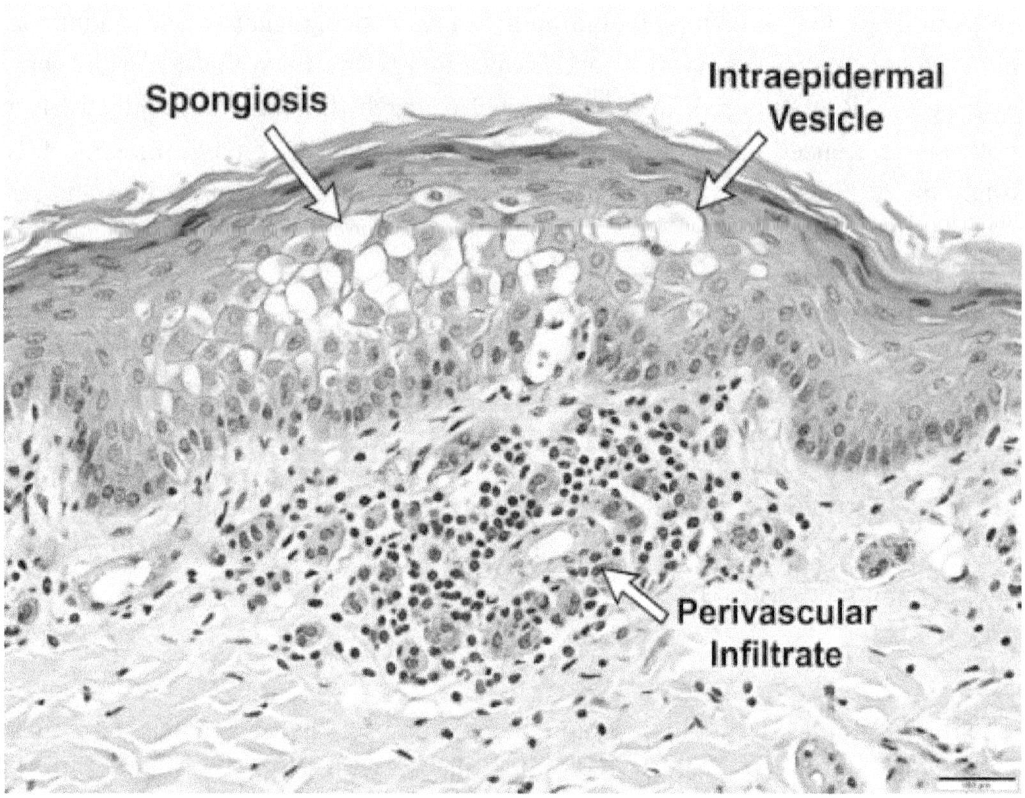

Clinical Presentation Across the Age Spectrum

Infantile Presentation

Infantile atopic dermatitis typically begins between two and six months of age with poorly demarcated, erythematous, often weeping and crusted patches concentrated on the cheeks, scalp, and extensor extremities, a distribution that reflects both the areas most exposed to environmental contact and drool-related irritation and the relative sparing of the diaper area, which benefits from the occlusive, moisture-retentive environment of a diaper that paradoxically protects barrier integrity at that specific site. The intense pruritus characteristic of the disease is present even in this earliest phase and frequently manifests indirectly, as irritability, disrupted sleep, and visible rubbing against bedding or caregivers rather than overt scratching in an infant not yet capable of coordinated scratching movements.

Childhood Presentation

The disease shifts distribution with age, concentrating by early childhood in the flexural folds, the antecubital and popliteal fossae most characteristically, along with the wrists, ankles, and neck, and lesions become progressively more lichenified and less exudative than the infantile phase as chronic scratching produces the thickened, hyperpigmented, exaggerated skin markings described in the first chapter of this book. Periorbital involvement, including an accentuated infraorbital fold sometimes called a Dennie-Morgan fold, and generalized xerosis affecting even clinically uninvolved skin are common associated findings in this age group.

Adolescent and Adult Presentation

Adolescent and adult disease often continues the flexural pattern established in childhood but can also present with a hand-and-neck predominant pattern, particularly in patients with occupational or environmental irritant exposure that compounds the underlying barrier defect, or with a more generalized, chronically lichenified pattern in patients with long-standing, poorly controlled disease. Adult-onset disease without a childhood history, while less common than persistent childhood-onset disease, is increasingly recognized and should not be dismissed diagnostically simply because a patient lacks the classic pediatric history, particularly when the morphology, distribution, and pruritus intensity otherwise fit the pattern described throughout this chapter.

THE MORPHOLOGY-TO-MANAGEMENT SYSTEM — The Flexural Lichenified Plaque Arc

The Pattern: Poorly demarcated, dry, thickened, hyperpigmented or violaceous plaques with exaggerated skin markings, concentrated in the antecubital and popliteal fossae, wrists, and neck, accompanied by intense, often disproportionate pruritus.

Presentation Variance: In darker skin tones, atopic dermatitis frequently presents with more pronounced lichenification and a follicular, papular accentuation rather than the confluent erythema emphasized in classic descriptions, and post-inflammatory hyperpigmentation and hypopigmentation are both common and can persist long after inflammatory activity has resolved, occasionally becoming the dominant concern that brings a patient back for follow-up even after itch and thickening have substantially improved.

Trap Logic: Allergic contact dermatitis, discussed in the next chapter, can mimic flexural atopic dermatitis but typically shows a more sharply demarcated distribution corresponding to a specific contactant exposure pattern rather than the classic flexural symmetry of atopic disease; nummular eczema produces discrete, coin-shaped plaques rather than flexural, poorly demarcated patches; and scabies, discussed in a later chapter, produces intense pruritus with a similar flexural and web-space predominance but is distinguished by burrows, more prominent nocturnal itch intensity, and often a history of similarly affected household contacts.

Management Pivot: First-line management combines liberal emollient use and trigger avoidance with a topical corticosteroid matched to site and severity per the framework introduced in the therapeutics chapter, with a topical calcineurin inhibitor favored for maintenance therapy at atrophy-prone flexural and facial sites; moderate to severe disease refractory to optimized topical therapy escalates to phototherapy or a systemic agent, with interleukin-4 receptor alpha blockade or an oral Janus kinase inhibitor now favored for many patients given their combination of rapid itch relief and high efficacy, confirmed against current guideline recommendations and individual comorbidity profile.

Pattern Anchor: Flexural distribution combined with pruritus intensity disproportionate to visible erythema, and a personal or family history of atopic disease, is the anchor combination that most reliably separates atopic dermatitis from its closest morphologic mimics.

Differential Diagnosis and Diagnostic Workup

Distinguishing Atopic Dermatitis From Related Eczematous Conditions

Nummular eczema presents as sharply demarcated, coin-shaped, intensely pruritic plaques, most often on the extensor extremities of an adult with a background of xerosis, and while it shares the same fundamental barrier-plus-inflammation mechanism as atopic dermatitis, its discrete, round configuration and extensor rather than flexural predominance are the discriminating features emphasized throughout this chapter's diagnostic approach. Seborrheic dermatitis in infancy produces greasy, yellowish scale concentrated on the scalp and face without the intense pruritus of atopic dermatitis, and the two conditions not infrequently coexist in the same infant, requiring the examiner to identify which component is driving a given area of involvement in order to select appropriate therapy for each.

Diagnostic Criteria and the Role of Laboratory Testing

Atopic dermatitis remains a clinical diagnosis based on characteristic morphology, distribution, chronicity, and personal or family atopic history, without a confirmatory laboratory test, though elevated total and allergen-specific immunoglobulin E levels are common supportive findings when obtained. Allergy testing, whether serum-specific immunoglobulin E or skin prick testing, is not routinely required to establish the diagnosis and should be reserved for patients with a specific, clinically suspected trigger or food allergy history, since indiscriminate testing in unselected patients frequently yields clinically insignificant positive results that can lead to unnecessary dietary restriction without proportionate clinical benefit.

When to Consider Biopsy or Referral

Biopsy is rarely required for typical atopic dermatitis and is reserved for atypical presentations or when the differential diagnosis includes a condition requiring histologic distinction, such as cutaneous T-cell lymphoma in an adult with a treatment-refractory eczematous eruption, discussed further in the chapter on cutaneous lymphoma. Referral to allergy and immunology is appropriate when a specific food or environmental trigger is strongly suspected based on history, when disease is severe and refractory to optimized dermatologic management, or when comorbid asthma or allergic rhinitis requires coordinated management alongside the cutaneous disease.

CAUTION: Indiscriminate allergy testing without a specific clinically suspected trigger frequently yields clinically insignificant positive results and can lead to unnecessary, burdensome dietary restriction without proportionate benefit to the underlying skin disease.

Patch testing, discussed in detail in the next chapter, plays a distinct and complementary diagnostic role from the immunoglobulin E-based allergy testing discussed here, since it identifies delayed-type contact allergens rather than the immediate-type food and environmental allergens relevant to atopic dermatitis, and should be considered specifically when a coexisting or superimposed allergic contact dermatitis is suspected, for example in a patient whose distribution pattern includes an area corresponding to a specific product or material contact rather than the classic flexural pattern alone.

Management and Treatment

Foundational Skin Care and Barrier Repair

Liberal, frequent application of a fragrance-free emollient, ideally an ointment or thick cream given the barrier-repair principles introduced in the therapeutics chapter, forms the foundation of management at every severity level and should continue even during periods of good disease control, since maintaining barrier integrity reduces flare frequency independent of any anti-inflammatory therapy in use. Bathing practices should favor lukewarm rather than hot water and prompt post-bath emollient application, sometimes summarized as the soak-and-seal technique, to trap residual moisture within the stratum corneum, and harsh soaps and fragranced products should be avoided given their capacity to further compromise an already impaired barrier.

Topical Anti-Inflammatory Therapy

Topical corticosteroids remain first-line anti-inflammatory therapy for active flares, applied according to the site- and potency-matching principles introduced in the therapeutics chapter, with particular attention to using lower-potency agents at the face and flexural folds given both the atrophy risk and the frequency with which these sites require treatment. Topical calcineurin inhibitors and topical phosphodiesterase-4 inhibitors provide steroid-sparing options particularly valuable for maintenance therapy at atrophy-prone sites and for proactive intermittent application to previously affected areas between flares, a strategy termed proactive therapy that has been shown to reduce flare frequency compared with reactive treatment initiated only after a flare has already become clinically apparent.

Systemic and Biologic Therapy for Moderate to Severe Disease

Moderate to severe disease refractory to optimized topical therapy and phototherapy warrants systemic treatment, and interleukin-4 receptor alpha blockade, which interrupts both interleukin-4 and interleukin-13 signaling as discussed earlier in this chapter, has become a preferred systemic option given its combination of substantial efficacy, rapid pruritus relief, and a favorable safety profile relative to older systemic immunosuppressants such as cyclosporine. Oral Janus kinase inhibitors provide an alternative targeted systemic option with a distinct onset and safety profile, discussed in the general therapeutics chapter, and agent selection between these options should weigh speed of itch relief, route of administration, comorbidity-specific safety considerations, and patient preference in a shared decision-making discussion.

Treatment Tier	Representative Approach	Typical Indication
Foundational	Liberal emollient, gentle skin care, trigger avoidance	All severity levels, continued even during remission
Topical Anti-Inflammatory	Site-matched topical corticosteroid; calcineurin inhibitor for maintenance	Active flares; proactive intermittent use between flares
Phototherapy	Narrowband ultraviolet B	Moderate disease inadequately controlled by topical therapy
Systemic/Biologic	Interleukin-4 receptor alpha blockade; oral Janus kinase inhibitor	Moderate to severe disease refractory to topical therapy and phototherapy

EVIDENCE: Proactive, scheduled intermittent application of a topical anti-inflammatory agent to previously affected sites between flares reduces flare frequency compared with purely reactive treatment initiated only after a new flare becomes apparent.

Complications and Special Populations

Secondary Bacterial and Viral Infection

The combination of a disrupted barrier and Staphylococcus aureus colonization described earlier in this chapter predisposes patients with atopic dermatitis to secondary bacterial infection, presenting as increased weeping, honey-colored crusting, or frank pustules superimposed on existing dermatitis, and appropriate management addresses both the secondary infection and the underlying inflammatory disease rather than antibiotics alone, since treating infection without addressing the underlying barrier and inflammatory drivers frequently leads to prompt recurrence. Eczema herpeticum, a disseminated herpes simplex virus infection superimposed on atopic dermatitis, presents with monomorphic, punched-out vesicles or erosions that can spread rapidly and, particularly in young children, cause systemic illness, representing a dermatologic emergency addressed in detail in the chapter on dermatologic emergencies and warranting prompt antiviral therapy and, in severe cases, hospitalization.

Ophthalmologic and Allergic Complications

Chronic periorbital dermatitis and persistent eye rubbing driven by pruritus are associated with an increased risk of atopic keratoconjunctivitis and, less commonly, keratoconus, a progressive corneal thinning condition, and patients with significant periorbital disease or visual symptoms warrant ophthalmologic referral rather than assuming all periocular complaints reflect dermatitis alone. As discussed earlier in this chapter, comorbid allergic rhinitis, asthma, and food allergy should be screened for as part of comprehensive atopic dermatitis management, with coordinated allergy and immunology or pulmonology involvement when these comorbidities are present or suspected.

Special Populations: Pregnancy and Skin of Color

Atopic dermatitis can worsen during pregnancy for some patients, and treatment planning must balance disease control against the pregnancy-specific safety considerations for systemic agents introduced in the therapeutics chapter, with topical corticosteroids and emollients remaining foundational, generally well-tolerated options throughout pregnancy. As discussed in the Rhythm Layer callout earlier in this chapter, presentation in richly pigmented skin frequently emphasizes follicular accentuation and post-inflammatory dyspigmentation over the confluent erythema described in classic teaching materials, and clinicians should calibrate their diagnostic pattern recognition accordingly rather than under-recognizing disease activity in this population.

CLINICAL PEARL: Monomorphic, punched-out vesicles or erosions spreading rapidly on a background of atopic dermatitis should raise immediate concern for eczema herpeticum and prompt urgent evaluation rather than escalation of routine anti-inflammatory therapy.

Molluscum contagiosum, a poxvirus infection producing discrete, umbilicated papules, occurs with greater frequency and extent in children with atopic dermatitis, likely reflecting both the disrupted barrier and the local immune dysregulation described earlier in this chapter, and surrounding dermatitis at sites of molluscum lesions, sometimes termed molluscum dermatitis, should be managed with continued appropriate anti-inflammatory therapy for the dermatitis component alongside standard observation or treatment of the molluscum lesions themselves according to their own natural history and treatment principles, discussed further in the chapter on viral cutaneous infections.

Prevention, Screening, and Patient Education

Barrier-Focused Prevention Strategies

Early, consistent emollient use in infants at elevated hereditary risk for atopic dermatitis has been studied as a potential preventive strategy given the barrier-centric pathophysiology described throughout this chapter, and while results across trials have been mixed regarding the degree of preventive benefit, consistent emollient use remains a reasonable, low-risk practice in infants with a strong family history of atopic disease. For patients with established disease, identifying and counseling on avoidance of specific individual triggers, harsh soaps, certain fabrics, extremes of temperature and humidity, and, in a subset of patients, specific food or environmental allergens, meaningfully reduces flare frequency when applied consistently.

Patient Education on the Chronic Disease Course

Patients and caregivers benefit from explicit education that atopic dermatitis is typically a chronic, relapsing condition managed rather than cured, with the goal of treatment being sustained control and quality-of-life improvement rather than permanent resolution, framing that helps set realistic expectations and supports sustained adherence to the foundational skin care practices described earlier in this chapter even during periods when the skin appears clear. Education on proper topical medication quantity, using the fingertip unit concept introduced in the therapeutics chapter, and on the specific atrophy and safety profile of the prescribed agents directly addresses the steroid-related anxiety that is a well-documented and correctable barrier to adherence in this patient population.

Psychosocial Support and Sleep

The disproportionate impact of atopic dermatitis on sleep, both the patient's own sleep and that of caregivers in pediatric cases, warrants explicit attention during management planning, since sleep disruption independently affects mood, cognitive function, and family functioning beyond the direct discomfort of the skin disease itself, and improvement in sleep quality following effective treatment is itself a meaningful outcome to track and discuss with patients and families over the course of therapy.

School and workplace accommodation should also be discussed explicitly for patients with visible or functionally limiting disease, since visible facial or hand involvement can carry substantial social and occupational impact that patients may not volunteer without direct inquiry, and connecting patients and families with atopic dermatitis-specific patient advocacy and support resources can provide practical coping strategies and peer support that extend meaningfully beyond what a clinical visit alone can offer.

Nummular Eczema and Related Eczematous Variants

Nummular Eczema

Nummular eczema, briefly introduced earlier in this chapter's differential diagnosis discussion, presents with sharply demarcated, coin-shaped, intensely pruritic plaques studded with fine vesicles or crust in the acute phase, most commonly on the extensor lower extremities of adults with a background of xerosis, and its discrete round configuration distinguishes it clinically from the poorly demarcated, flexural pattern of classic atopic dermatitis even though both conditions share the same underlying spongiotic histopathology and respond to similar anti-inflammatory strategies. Nummular eczema is frequently exacerbated by low ambient humidity, harsh soaps, and hot showers, and management emphasizes the same foundational skin care principles described earlier in this chapter, often with a somewhat higher potency topical corticosteroid given the plaques' tendency toward greater thickness and more intense pruritus than typical flexural atopic dermatitis.

Dyshidrotic Eczema

Dyshidrotic eczema, also termed pompholyx, presents with intensely pruritic, deep-seated vesicles on the lateral aspects of the fingers, palms, and soles, reflecting a distinct clinical pattern within the eczematous disease family that favors these specific acral sites, possibly related to the thicker stratum corneum and higher eccrine gland density at these locations discussed in the first chapter of this book, though the historical implication of sweat gland dysfunction suggested by the term pompholyx is not well supported by current pathophysiologic understanding. Management follows the same anti-inflammatory principles as other eczematous variants, with potent topical corticosteroids often required given the palmoplantar site's relatively reduced percutaneous absorption discussed in the therapeutics chapter, and identification of contributing factors such as nickel exposure or a concurrent dermatophyte infection elsewhere on the body, which can trigger a related vesicular reaction on the hands, should be considered in recurrent or refractory cases.

Asteatotic Eczema in the Older Adult

Asteatotic eczema, sometimes termed eczema craquelé for its characteristic cracked, crazed-pavement surface pattern, develops predominantly in older adults on the lower extremities, reflecting the age-related reduction in sebaceous gland output and barrier lipid production discussed in the first chapter's coverage of skin changes across the lifespan, compounded by low ambient humidity, frequent hot bathing, and diuretic use, each of which further reduces skin surface hydration. Management centers on aggressive emollient use, reduced bathing frequency and water temperature, and humidification of the home environment during dry winter months, with topical corticosteroid reserved for more inflamed areas, illustrating how an eczematous presentation in an older adult often reflects a distinct, largely preventable, environmentally driven mechanism rather than a primary atopic process.

CLINICAL PEARL: A coin-shaped, sharply demarcated eczematous plaque on the extensor lower extremity of an adult with xerosis is more consistent with nummular eczema than with atopic dermatitis, even though both respond to similar anti-inflammatory management.

Food Allergy and the Role of Dietary Modification

When Food Allergy Genuinely Contributes to Disease Activity

A subset of children with moderate to severe atopic dermatitis, particularly those with early-onset disease and elevated allergen-specific immunoglobulin E levels, have a genuine food allergy that measurably contributes to disease flares, most commonly to egg, milk, peanut, wheat, or soy, and in this specific, carefully identified subset, targeted elimination of the confirmed trigger food can produce meaningful clinical improvement. Identifying this subset accurately, rather than assuming food allergy is a universal driver of atopic dermatitis, is essential, since the majority of patients with atopic dermatitis do not have a clinically significant food trigger despite the historical and persistent lay association between the two conditions.

The Risks of Empiric, Unsupervised Elimination Diets

Empiric elimination of multiple food groups without confirmed allergy, a common practice among worried caregivers acting on unverified online information, carries genuine risk, including nutritional deficiency in growing children and, counterintuitively, an increased risk of subsequently developing a true immunoglobulin E-mediated food allergy upon reintroduction after a period of avoidance, a phenomenon attributed to loss of oral tolerance during the elimination period. For this reason, dietary modification for suspected food-triggered atopic dermatitis should be pursued only after appropriate allergy evaluation confirms a specific trigger, and should involve structured, supervised reintroduction protocols rather than indefinite, unsupervised avoidance of multiple food groups based on parental suspicion alone.

CAUTION: Empiric, unsupervised elimination of multiple food groups in a child with atopic dermatitis carries real nutritional and allergic risk and should not be undertaken without confirmed allergy testing and, ideally, allergy and immunology involvement.

Clinical Case: Escalating Care in Refractory Pediatric Disease

A 4-year-old boy with a history of atopic dermatitis since infancy presents with his mother for worsening flexural dermatitis despite consistent use of a mid-potency topical corticosteroid and daily emollient application for the past six weeks. His mother reports he continues to scratch through the night, waking multiple times, and that the affected skin in both antecubital fossae has become progressively thicker and darker over the past month. He has a maternal history of asthma and his own history of mild seasonal allergic rhinitis.

Applying the structured approach to apparent treatment failure introduced in the diagnostic-approach chapter, the clinician first confirms adherence and technique, verifying adequate quantity applied using the fingertip unit method and correct application to the affected flexural areas twice daily, and confirms that his mother has not been avoiding treatment out of steroid-related concern, a factor identified explicitly in the patient-education discussion in this chapter as a common and correctable barrier. Adherence and technique are confirmed adequate, indicating true escalation rather than an adherence gap, consistent with moderate disease inadequately controlled by optimized topical therapy alone. The progressive lichenification is recognized as a direct consequence of the ongoing itch-scratch cycle described in the pathophysiology section of this chapter, reinforcing that breaking the cycle, rather than further increasing topical corticosteroid potency alone, is the appropriate next step.

Following the Management Pivot established in the Rhythm Layer callout earlier in this chapter, the family and clinician discuss escalation options; given his age, his mother's asthma history suggesting a strong atopic predisposition, and the disproportionate sleep disruption driving both his and his family's distress, the family elects to pursue systemic therapy after appropriate specialist referral, with interleukin-4 receptor alpha blockade discussed as an option given its pediatric approval for his age range and its combination of anti-inflammatory efficacy and rapid pruritus relief that would be expected to interrupt the itch-scratch cycle more effectively than continued topical escalation alone. The family is also counseled on ongoing screening for asthma and allergic rhinitis symptoms given his family history and the atopic march model discussed earlier in this chapter, and a coordinated follow-up plan with allergy and immunology is established alongside continued dermatologic care.

KEY POINT: Progressive lichenification despite adequate topical therapy reflects an unbroken itch-scratch cycle and should prompt consideration of systemic therapy targeting the underlying inflammatory and pruritic drivers, rather than further escalation of topical corticosteroid potency alone.

At three-month follow-up after initiating systemic therapy, his mother reports substantially reduced nighttime scratching within the first two weeks of treatment, well before the flexural lichenification itself had visibly begun to soften, illustrating the rapid, itch-specific benefit of interleukin-4 receptor alpha blockade discussed earlier in this chapter. His topical corticosteroid use has been tapered to an as-needed basis for isolated breakthrough areas, and foundational emollient use has continued unchanged throughout, reinforcing the point made earlier in this chapter that foundational skin care remains the constant base of therapy regardless of what systemic or topical anti-inflammatory agent is layered on top of it. His mother also reports she and her son are both sleeping through the night for the first time in over a year, a functional outcome that the family identifies as the most meaningful measure of treatment success, more so than the residual mild hyperpigmentation still visible in both antecubital fossae, which is expected to fade gradually over the following months as the underlying inflammation continues to resolve.

THE MORPHOLOGY-TO-MANAGEMENT SYSTEM — The Eczematous Disease Family

Pattern Introduced This Chapter: The flexural lichenified plaque, and its discrimination from allergic contact dermatitis, nummular eczema, and scabies.

Cross-Cutting Anchor: Pruritus intensity disproportionate to visible erythema, combined with flexural distribution and a personal or family atopic history, is the recurring anchor for atopic dermatitis across every age group discussed in this chapter.

Summary and Key Concepts

Atopic dermatitis arises from mutually reinforcing barrier dysfunction, type 2 immune dysregulation, and a self-perpetuating itch-scratch cycle, and effective management addresses all three mechanisms together.

Clinical presentation shifts predictably across the lifespan, from weeping facial and extensor involvement in infancy to flexural, lichenified disease in childhood and beyond.

Trap Logic discrimination from nummular eczema, allergic contact dermatitis, and scabies depends on configuration, distribution, and specific exposure or contact history rather than gestalt impression alone.

Treatment follows a stepwise escalation from foundational skin care and topical anti-inflammatory therapy through phototherapy to systemic biologic or targeted therapy, guided by an explicit reassessment interval.

Eczema herpeticum and secondary bacterial infection are recognizable, treatable complications that must be distinguished promptly from a routine disease flare.

CHAPTER 6: CONTACT DERMATITIS, LICHEN PLANUS, AND LICHENOID DERMATOSES

Learning Objectives

1. Distinguish irritant contact dermatitis from allergic contact dermatitis based on mechanism, morphology, and time course.
2. Apply patch testing appropriately to identify a causative allergen in suspected allergic contact dermatitis.
3. Recognize the cutaneous, oral, and nail manifestations of lichen planus and relate them to the disease's characteristic histopathology.
4. Distinguish lichen planus from lichenoid drug eruptions and other lichenoid mimics using Trap Logic discriminating features.
5. Apply an evidence-based, site-adapted management framework to both contact dermatitis and lichen planus.

Contact Dermatitis: Definition, Classification, and Epidemiology

Irritant Versus Allergic Contact Dermatitis

Contact dermatitis is an eczematous reaction produced by direct cutaneous exposure to an external substance, and it is divided into two mechanistically distinct categories that nonetheless produce overlapping clinical appearances. Irritant contact dermatitis results from direct cytotoxic or barrier-disrupting chemical injury that can affect any exposed individual given sufficient concentration and duration of exposure, without requiring prior sensitization, whereas allergic contact dermatitis is a delayed-type, cell-mediated hypersensitivity reaction that develops only in individuals previously sensitized to a specific allergen and therefore affects only a susceptible subset of the exposed population. This mechanistic distinction, immunologically nonspecific chemical injury versus antigen-specific memory T-cell activation, is what accounts for essentially every clinically important difference between the two conditions discussed throughout this chapter.

Epidemiology and Occupational Burden

Both forms of contact dermatitis are substantially underreported in occupational surveillance data, since many affected workers manage symptoms with over-the-counter remedies or simply endure intermittent flares without seeking formal medical evaluation, particularly early in the disease course before symptoms become severe or persistent enough to prompt a clinical visit, meaning the true occupational and population burden of both irritant and allergic contact dermatitis is very likely substantially higher than formally reported prevalence figures suggest.

Irritant contact dermatitis accounts for the large majority of occupational contact dermatitis cases overall, reflecting cumulative exposure to water, detergents, and solvents in occupations such as healthcare, food service, hairdressing, and cleaning, while allergic contact dermatitis, though less common in aggregate, carries disproportionate diagnostic and management complexity given the need to identify a specific causative allergen among thousands of potential contactants encountered in modern personal care products, occupational materials, and clothing. Both forms carry substantial occupational and economic burden, frequently affecting hand function specifically and, in severe or poorly managed cases, forcing occupational changes for affected workers in high-exposure fields.

Common Allergens and Exposure Contexts

Nickel remains the most common contact allergen identified on patch testing across most studied populations, encountered in jewelry, clothing fasteners, and certain electronic devices, and disproportionately affects individuals with pierced ears or other body piercings given the direct, prolonged metal-skin contact this practice produces. Fragrance mixes and preservatives such as methylisothiazolinone, found broadly across personal care products, cosmetics, and household cleaning products, represent another major allergen category, and plant-derived allergens, poison ivy, oak, and sumac chief among them in regions where these plants are endemic, produce a distinctive linear or geometric pattern of allergic contact dermatitis reflecting direct plant contact, discussed further later in this chapter.

Feature	Irritant Contact Dermatitis	Allergic Contact Dermatitis
Mechanism	Direct cytotoxic/barrier injury, no sensitization required	Delayed-type (type IV) hypersensitivity, requires prior sensitization
Onset	Can occur on first exposure, dose- and duration-dependent	Typically 24-72 hours after re-exposure in a sensitized individual
Distribution	Confined to area of direct contact, often sharply demarcated	May extend beyond direct contact area; can spread via hand transfer
Patch Test Result	Typically negative (unless testing the irritant itself at high concentration)	Positive to the specific causative allergen

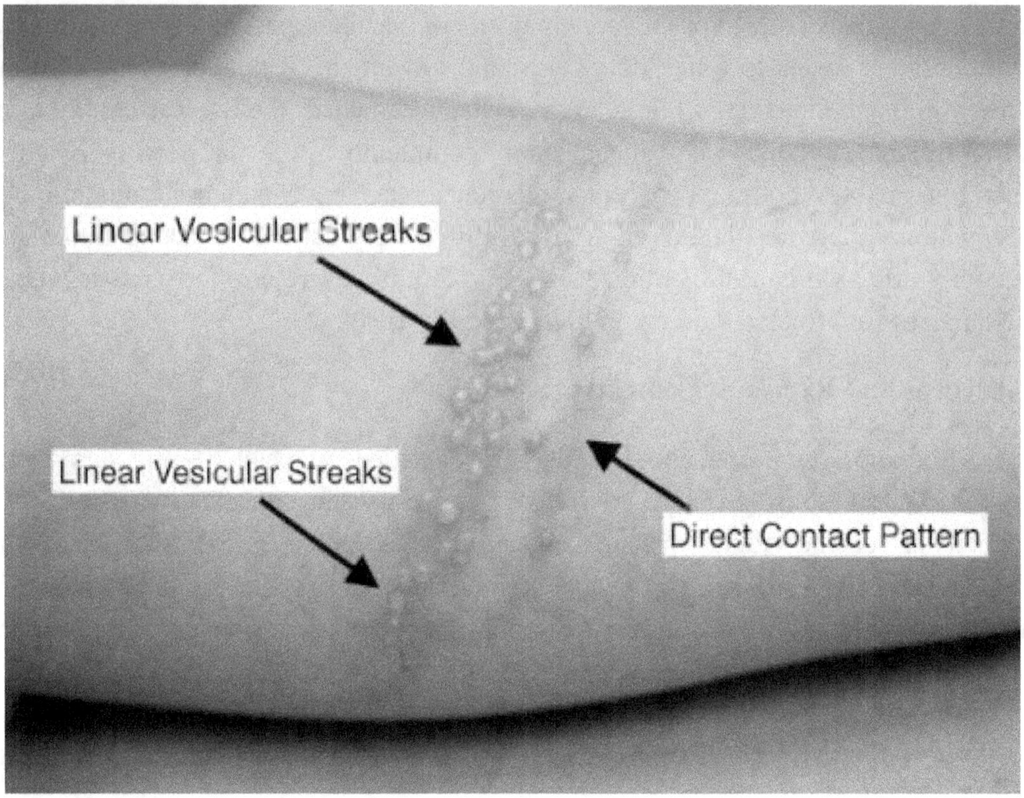

Contact Dermatitis: Pathophysiology, Presentation, and Patch Testing

Type IV Hypersensitivity Mechanism

Allergic contact dermatitis follows the two-phase sensitization and elicitation sequence introduced in the first chapter of this book: during sensitization, Langerhans cells process the allergen, typically a small molecule termed a hapten that must first bind a cutaneous protein to become immunogenic, and migrate to regional lymph nodes to prime allergen-specific T cells, a process requiring ten to fourteen days and producing no clinical symptoms at the time. Upon subsequent re-exposure, memory T cells resident within the skin or recruited from circulation rapidly recognize the allergen and orchestrate an inflammatory response within twenty-four to seventy-two hours, explaining the characteristic delayed onset relative to exposure that is a key historical clue distinguishing allergic from irritant contact dermatitis, the latter of which can produce symptoms within minutes to hours of a sufficiently concentrated exposure.

Clinical Presentation and Morphologic Clues to Causation

Acute allergic contact dermatitis presents with erythema, edema, and often vesiculation confined initially to the site of contact, frequently with a sharply geometric or linear border that directly reflects the shape of the causative contact, a shirt collar, a watch band, or a plant brushing against skin, an important configurational clue introduced in the diagnostic-language chapter of this book. Chronic, repeated exposure produces a more lichenified, less acutely inflamed pattern that can be more difficult to attribute to a specific allergen without a careful, structured exposure history, since the geometric clarity of acute disease is often lost with chronicity. Irritant contact dermatitis, by contrast, tends to present with more uniform erythema, dryness, and fissuring confined strictly to the area of direct chemical contact, most classically on the hands of individuals with frequent occupational wet work.

Patch Testing Technique and Interpretation

Patch testing applies small quantities of standardized allergens to the back under occlusion for forty-eight hours, with readings performed at removal and again forty-eight to ninety-six hours later, since some genuine allergic reactions do not peak until the delayed reading, and relying on the immediate reading alone risks missing clinically relevant positive results. A positive patch test result must be interpreted in the context of the patient's actual exposure history to establish clinical relevance, since a positive reaction to an allergen with no plausible exposure in the patient's environment is of uncertain significance, while a positive reaction to an allergen the patient is regularly exposed to strongly supports that allergen as the cause of the presenting dermatitis. Patch testing should be performed on skin free of active dermatitis and generally requires discontinuation of oral immunosuppressive therapy and, at the testing site, topical corticosteroids for a defined period beforehand to avoid a false-negative result from suppressed local immune reactivity.

KEY POINT: A positive patch test result establishes sensitization to an allergen but requires correlation with the patient's actual exposure history to establish clinical relevance to the presenting dermatitis.

Standardized allergen screening series, comprising the allergens most frequently identified across large patch test registries, capture a substantial majority of clinically relevant contact allergens, but supplemental, occupation- or exposure-specific series, for example a hairdressing series or a series targeted to a specific industrial exposure, meaningfully increase diagnostic yield in patients whose history suggests a specialized exposure not well represented on the standard screening series alone, illustrating why a detailed occupational and product-use history, obtained before testing rather than after, should directly inform which supplemental series are included.

THE MORPHOLOGY-TO-MANAGEMENT SYSTEM — The Geometric Contact Dermatitis Arc

---

The Pattern: Erythematous, often vesicular dermatitis with a sharply geometric, linear, or otherwise unnaturally regular border corresponding to a specific external contact.

Presentation Variance: In richly pigmented skin, acute allergic contact dermatitis may show less obvious erythema and more prominent edema and post-inflammatory hyperpigmentation that can persist for months after the acute reaction resolves, occasionally leading to underrecognition of an acute allergic reaction at the time it is most clinically active and most identifiable by its geometric configuration.

Trap Logic: Nummular eczema and atopic dermatitis, discussed in the previous chapter, lack the sharply geometric, contact-pattern border characteristic of allergic contact dermatitis and instead favor characteristic flexural or discoid distributions unrelated to a specific external contact shape; cellulitis can mimic acute contact dermatitis but typically presents with systemic symptoms, warmth, and tenderness out of proportion to a well-demarcated geometric pattern, and progresses over hours to a day rather than presenting with the sharply bordered configuration established at onset.

Management Pivot: Acute allergic contact dermatitis is managed with allergen avoidance once identified, a potent topical corticosteroid matched to site and severity as introduced in the therapeutics chapter, and, for widespread or facial involvement, a short tapering course of systemic corticosteroid may be considered given the self-limited nature of a single identified exposure; irritant contact dermatitis is managed primarily through irritant avoidance and barrier protection, with topical corticosteroids offering more modest benefit than in the allergic form given the different underlying mechanism.

Pattern Anchor: A sharply geometric or linear border that does not correspond to any natural anatomic distribution is the anchor finding that should immediately prompt a directed contact-exposure history.

Lichen Planus: Definition, Epidemiology, and Pathophysiology

Definition and the Lichenoid Reaction Pattern

Lichen planus is an idiopathic, cell-mediated inflammatory disease producing the characteristic lichenoid tissue reaction, a pattern of dense, band-like lymphocytic infiltration at the dermoepidermal junction associated with basal keratinocyte damage, that can affect the skin, oral and genital mucosa, nails, and scalp, either in isolation or in combination. The term lichenoid describes both the histopathologic pattern, discussed later in this chapter, and the broader category of clinically similar eruptions, including lichenoid drug eruptions, that share this same fundamental tissue reaction despite differing underlying triggers, making lichen planus the prototype of a reaction pattern rather than a single etiologically uniform disease.

Epidemiology and Associations

Lichen planus most commonly affects middle-aged adults, with a modest female predominance for the mucosal forms of the disease, and has been epidemiologically associated with hepatitis C virus infection in several studied populations, though the strength of this association varies substantially by geographic region and studied population, warranting consideration of hepatitis C screening in appropriate clinical and epidemiologic contexts rather than as a universal reflexive test in every patient diagnosed with lichen planus.

Pathophysiology

Lichen planus reflects a cell-mediated cytotoxic immune response directed against basal keratinocytes, in which CD8-positive cytotoxic T cells, recruited and activated following an incompletely understood triggering event, an altered self-antigen, a viral infection, or a drug exposure, recognize and destroy basal keratinocytes, producing the characteristic band-like lymphocytic infiltrate and basal cell damage seen histologically. This cytotoxic, keratinocyte-directed mechanism, fundamentally different from the type 2 immune and barrier-driven mechanism of atopic dermatitis discussed in the previous chapter, or the type IV hypersensitivity mechanism of allergic contact dermatitis discussed earlier in this chapter, explains why lichen planus produces its own distinct clinical morphology, discussed next, rather than an eczematous or vesiculobullous presentation.

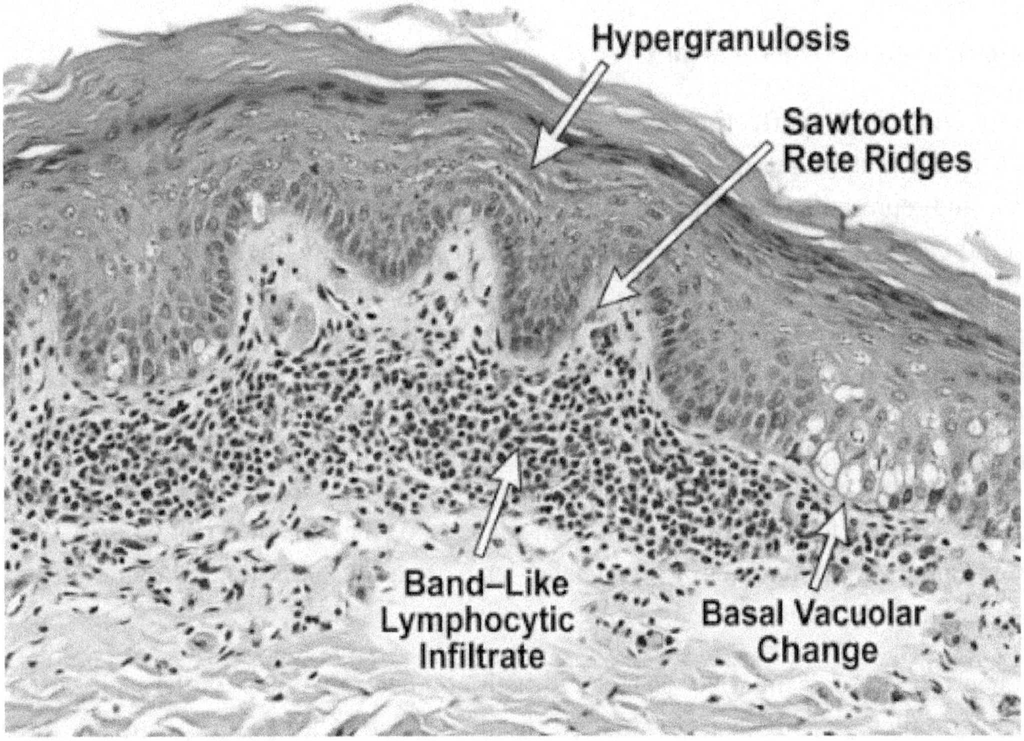

Lichen Planus: Clinical Presentation and Variants

Classic Cutaneous Presentation

Classic cutaneous lichen planus presents with the traditionally taught six Ps, purple, polygonal, planar (flat-topped), pruritic papules and plaques, most often on the flexor wrists, forearms, and shins, frequently demonstrating fine, lace-like white lines on the papule surface termed Wickham striae, a finding with substantial diagnostic value best appreciated under a hand lens or dermoscope. Koebnerization, the same phenomenon of new lesions arising at sites of mechanical trauma introduced in the psoriasis chapter, is characteristic of lichen planus as well, and linear lesions along a scratch mark are a useful supporting clue when the diagnosis is otherwise uncertain.

Oral, Genital, and Nail Involvement

Oral lichen planus, occurring either in isolation or accompanying cutaneous disease, most commonly presents as a reticular, lace-like white pattern on the buccal mucosa, termed Wickham striae in this context as well, though erosive oral lichen planus, producing painful, persistent mucosal erosions, carries additional management complexity and a small but clinically relevant risk of malignant transformation to squamous cell carcinoma warranting longitudinal monitoring. Genital lichen planus can similarly present with reticular or erosive patterns and requires the same monitoring considerations as erosive oral disease.

Nail involvement produces longitudinal ridging, thinning, and, in severe cases, a permanent scarring pattern termed pterygium formation, in which the proximal nail fold fuses with the underlying nail bed, underscoring the value of prompt recognition and treatment of nail lichen planus before this largely irreversible scarring develops.

Lichen Planopilaris and Other Variants

Lichen planopilaris, a variant affecting the scalp, produces a scarring alopecia with perifollicular erythema and scale concentrated at the periphery of expanding areas of hair loss, discussed further in the chapter on hair disorders, and represents one of the more diagnostically and therapeutically challenging lichen planus variants given the largely irreversible nature of established scarring alopecia. Hypertrophic lichen planus produces thick, verrucous, intensely pruritic plaques, most often on the shins, that can resemble other hypertrophic or verrucous conditions and may require biopsy to confirm given this diagnostic overlap, while lichen planus pigmentosus produces macular hyperpigmentation, more common in richly pigmented skin, without the classic papular morphology, illustrating that presentation variance in this disease can extend to fundamentally altering the primary lesion morphology itself rather than only its color.

CLINICAL PEARL: Wickham striae, fine white lace-like lines on the surface of a violaceous, flat-topped papule, are best appreciated with a hand lens or dermoscope and provide strong supporting evidence for lichen planus when present.

Because lichen planus can involve so many distinct anatomic sites with such different clinical appearances, a complete lichen planus evaluation should include a directed inspection of the oral mucosa, nails, scalp, and genital skin even when the presenting complaint is limited to a single visible cutaneous site, since involvement at an additional site not volunteered by the patient can materially change both prognosis and the surveillance plan established for that individual patient.

Lichenoid Drug Eruptions and Differential Diagnosis

Distinguishing Lichen Planus From a Lichenoid Drug Eruption

Lichenoid drug eruptions produce a clinical and histologic pattern that can closely resemble idiopathic lichen planus, and distinguishing between the two depends heavily on a careful medication history correlated with symptom onset, since lichenoid drug eruptions typically develop weeks to months, sometimes considerably longer, after starting the causative medication, a broader and more variable latency than the classic drug-eruption timeline discussed in the diagnostic-approach chapter. Antihypertensive agents, particularly certain thiazide diuretics and beta-blockers, antimalarials, and certain nonsteroidal anti-inflammatory drugs are among the more commonly implicated classes, and lichenoid drug eruptions often show a more photodistributed pattern and less prominent Wickham striae and oral involvement than idiopathic lichen planus, though overlap is substantial enough that a trial of discontinuing a suspected culprit medication, where clinically feasible, is often the most informative diagnostic step.

Other Lichenoid Mimics

Lichen simplex chronicus, a localized area of thickened, lichenified skin driven by chronic mechanical rubbing and scratching rather than a primary lichenoid immune process, can be distinguished by its typically solitary or limited distribution at an easily reached site and a history of chronic localized itching and rubbing rather than the widespread, symmetric, papular eruption of true lichen planus. Lupus erythematosus can occasionally present with an overlapping lichenoid pattern, and distinguishing the two when clinical overlap exists may require biopsy with direct immunofluorescence, discussed further in the chapter on connective tissue disease, since routine histology alone can be insufficient to separate the two conditions in ambiguous cases.

CAUTION: A lichenoid eruption developing after starting a new medication, even many weeks or months earlier, should prompt careful medication reconciliation and consideration of discontinuing a plausible culprit agent before committing to a diagnosis of idiopathic lichen planus.

Feature	Idiopathic Lichen Planus	Lichenoid Drug Eruption
Latency to Medication	Not applicable	Weeks to months, occasionally longer, after starting culprit agent
Wickham Striae	Frequently prominent	Often less prominent or absent
Oral Involvement	Common	Less common
Photodistribution	Not characteristic	Often more pronounced in sun-exposed areas
Resolution	Follows own chronic course	Often resolves over weeks to months after discontinuing culprit agent

Because this table's distinguishing features overlap substantially rather than providing absolute discrimination, a carefully structured medication history remains the single most valuable diagnostic tool for separating these two entities, reinforcing the broader principle from the diagnostic-approach chapter that history frequently carries as much diagnostic weight as morphology itself.

Management and Treatment

Topical and Localized Therapy

Limited cutaneous lichen planus is managed first-line with a potent topical corticosteroid, following the site- and potency-matching principles introduced in the therapeutics chapter, and intralesional corticosteroid injection is a useful option for hypertrophic lichen planus plaques that respond poorly to topical therapy alone given their thickness. Oral lichen planus, particularly the erosive form, is managed with topical corticosteroid preparations formulated for mucosal use or with topical calcineurin inhibitors, and coordinated management with oral medicine or dentistry is valuable both for optimizing topical therapy technique at this challenging anatomic site and for establishing the longitudinal surveillance appropriate given the malignant transformation risk discussed earlier in this chapter.

Systemic Therapy for Widespread or Refractory Disease

Widespread cutaneous lichen planus, or disease refractory to topical therapy, may warrant a short course of systemic corticosteroid or, for more chronic or recurrent disease, other systemic immunomodulatory agents such as those introduced in the therapeutics chapter, selected based on disease severity, site involvement, and patient-specific comorbidity and risk profile. Narrowband ultraviolet B phototherapy, discussed in the therapeutics chapter, is also an effective option for widespread cutaneous disease and avoids the systemic immunosuppression associated with oral agents, making it a reasonable intermediate option between topical therapy and systemic immunomodulation for appropriately selected patients.

Management of Allergic Contact Dermatitis: Allergen Avoidance as Definitive Therapy

Unlike lichen planus, where the underlying trigger is often unidentifiable or unmodifiable, allergic contact dermatitis has a genuinely curative management strategy once the causative allergen is identified through patch testing: strict avoidance of that specific allergen, supported by patient education on the many product categories and material sources in which it may be encountered, since a single identified allergen such as a specific preservative may appear under multiple different ingredient names across personal care products, cosmetics, and household items. Patients should be provided with a written list of the specific allergen and its common synonyms and sources, since without this structured guidance, avoidance based on memory alone is frequently incomplete and leads to ongoing, unexplained low-grade dermatitis from unrecognized cross-exposure.

Special Presentations Across the Lifespan and Body Site

Diaper Dermatitis as a Prototypical Irritant Contact Reaction

Irritant diaper dermatitis, among the most common dermatologic presentations in infancy, illustrates the irritant mechanism introduced earlier in this chapter with particular clarity: prolonged occlusion combined with contact between skin and urine and stool produces direct chemical and enzymatic irritation, characteristically sparing the deep inguinal folds where the diaper itself, rather than its contents, is in direct contact, a distribution pattern that itself supports the irritant rather than allergic mechanism given the absence of a specific sensitizing allergen. Secondary candidal infection is common in this setting given the warm, moist, occluded environment favorable to yeast overgrowth, and is suggested by satellite pustules extending beyond the main area of erythema and by involvement of the inguinal folds that irritant dermatitis characteristically spares, a distinction with direct treatment implications since candidal superinfection requires topical antifungal therapy in addition to standard irritant dermatitis management.

Eyelid and Facial Allergic Contact Dermatitis

The eyelid represents a site of particularly high percutaneous absorption, as introduced in the therapeutics chapter, and is disproportionately affected by allergic contact dermatitis relative to its actual surface area of direct exposure, since patients frequently transfer allergens to the eyelid via the hands, from nail polish, hair products, or other allergens applied elsewhere on the body, without the eyelid itself ever directly contacting the causative product. This connection-by-transfer pattern means that patch testing for eyelid dermatitis must consider the patient's full range of product exposure, including products applied to the hands, hair, and face generally, rather than restricting consideration to products applied directly to the eyelid or periorbital area.

Systemic Contact Dermatitis

In a subset of previously sensitized patients, systemic exposure to a previously topically sensitizing allergen, through diet, medication, or other systemic route, can provoke a widespread dermatitis flare, a phenomenon termed systemic contact dermatitis, classically described with nickel-containing foods in nickel-sensitized individuals and with certain systemic medications structurally related to a previously topically sensitizing allergen. Recognizing this possibility is important in patients with a confirmed patch test allergy who continue to experience unexplained widespread flares despite apparently successful avoidance of direct topical contact with the identified allergen, since the explanation in this circumstance may lie in a systemic rather than purely topical exposure route.

CLINICAL PEARL: Diaper dermatitis sparing the deep inguinal folds supports an irritant mechanism; involvement of those folds, or satellite pustules beyond the main affected area, should raise suspicion for secondary candidal infection requiring additional antifungal therapy.

Complications, Special Populations, and Patient Education

Malignant Transformation Risk in Erosive Mucosal Disease

Erosive oral and genital lichen planus carry a small but well-documented risk of malignant transformation to squamous cell carcinoma over years of chronic disease activity, and patients with erosive mucosal lichen planus warrant longitudinal surveillance, generally through periodic oral medicine or dermatology examination, with biopsy of any area demonstrating induration, ulceration that fails to heal, or other atypical features that would be unusual for the patient's baseline erosive disease pattern.

Tobacco and alcohol use independently increase squamous cell carcinoma risk in the oral cavity and act synergistically with the chronic mucosal inflammation of erosive lichen planus, making tobacco cessation counseling a directly relevant preventive intervention for these patients rather than a generic health maintenance recommendation disconnected from their dermatologic disease. Patients should also be counseled to promptly report any new area of persistent ulceration, induration, or a mucosal texture change distinct from their established baseline pattern, since self-monitoring between scheduled surveillance visits meaningfully shortens the interval to biopsy and diagnosis should malignant transformation begin to occur.

Occupational Considerations in Contact Dermatitis

Occupational contact dermatitis, whether irritant or allergic, frequently requires workplace modification alongside medical management, including protective equipment appropriate to the specific irritant or allergen identified, barrier creams for irritant-predominant occupational exposure, and, in refractory cases affecting hand function significantly, formal occupational health involvement to evaluate reasonable accommodation or, in the most severe and refractory cases, occupational change, a discussion that should be approached collaboratively and with attention to the substantial economic and psychosocial impact such a change can carry for an affected worker.

Patient Education Across Both Conditions

Patients with allergic contact dermatitis benefit from explicit education that positive patch test results represent lifelong sensitization, since the immunologic memory underlying allergic contact dermatitis does not resolve over time even after the acute dermatitis itself clears, meaning avoidance must be sustained indefinitely rather than only during an active flare. Patients with lichen planus benefit from education that the disease, while sometimes self-limited over one to two years for cutaneous disease, can follow a more chronic course for mucosal and nail variants, and that residual post-inflammatory hyperpigmentation, particularly prominent in richly pigmented skin, may persist well after active inflammation has resolved and should not be mistaken for ongoing disease activity requiring treatment escalation.

Written, take-home educational materials listing allergen synonyms and common product sources, discussed earlier in this chapter's management section, meaningfully improve avoidance success compared with verbal counseling alone, since patients cannot reasonably be expected to memorize the full range of product categories and ingredient synonyms in which a single chemical allergen may appear, and providing this information in a durable, referenceable format allows patients to check product labels confidently at the point of purchase rather than relying on memory of a single clinical conversation.

Coordination between dermatology and dentistry or oral medicine, and between dermatology and gynecology or urology where genital involvement is present, is valuable both for optimizing site-specific topical therapy technique and for sharing surveillance responsibility across specialties rather than assuming any single clinician is tracking the full multi-site disease course.

Longitudinal Follow-Up Planning

Both conditions benefit from a structured follow-up plan tailored to their distinct natural histories: allergic contact dermatitis follow-up should confirm both symptomatic improvement and, where feasible, objective confirmation that allergen avoidance has been successfully implemented, since incomplete avoidance despite a correctly identified allergen is a common and correctable cause of persistent symptoms, while lichen planus follow-up, particularly for erosive mucosal or nail variants, should be structured around the surveillance intervals appropriate to the malignant transformation and scarring risks discussed earlier in this chapter rather than around symptomatic improvement alone.

Clinical Case: Identifying an Occult Allergen in Chronic Hand Dermatitis

A 38-year-old hairdresser presents with an eighteen-month history of recurrent, itchy, fissured dermatitis on both hands, previously treated intermittently with topical corticosteroids with only partial and temporary improvement. She reports the dermatitis worsens noticeably during the work week and improves somewhat, though never completely, during vacations. She wears gloves inconsistently at work given the fine finger dexterity her job requires.

Applying the diagnostic framework from this chapter, the temporal pattern, worsening with work exposure and partial improvement away from work, raises concern for an occupationally acquired contact dermatitis, though the incomplete resolution during time away from work suggests either an allergic component with a sensitization persisting beyond active workplace exposure, ongoing low-level exposure from products used outside of work, or a superimposed irritant component from the cumulative wet work and chemical exposure inherent to her occupation, potentially all three occurring simultaneously. Patch testing is performed using a comprehensive series including allergens relevant to hairdressing-specific exposures, and testing reveals a positive reaction to para-phenylenediamine, a common component of permanent hair dye, confirmed as clinically relevant given her direct, frequent occupational exposure to this specific chemical.

Following the management framework from this chapter, she is counseled on strict glove use, specifically nitrile rather than latex gloves given adequate barrier properties against this allergen, for all hair coloring procedures, and provided with a written list of para-phenylenediamine synonyms to check on product labels both at work and in any personal hair coloring products she may use. Given her substantial occupational exposure and the functional impact on her livelihood, coordinated occupational health involvement is arranged to evaluate additional workplace protective measures, and a topical corticosteroid is continued for residual dermatitis during the interval before consistent allergen avoidance produces full clinical improvement, with the family informed that ongoing, low-grade irritant contribution from her overall wet-work exposure may mean some background dryness persists even once the allergic component is fully controlled.

CLINICAL PEARL: Occupational hand dermatitis that improves but does not fully resolve away from work, combined with inconsistent protective equipment use, should prompt patch testing with an occupation-specific allergen series rather than continued empiric topical treatment alone.

Clinical Case: Distinguishing Lichen Planus From a Lichenoid Drug Eruption

A 58-year-old man presents with a four-month history of intensely pruritic, violaceous, flat-topped papules on his volar wrists and shins, with fine white lines visible on several lesions under close inspection. He was started on hydrochlorothiazide for hypertension approximately five months before symptom onset, and this medication has not been changed since. He has no oral or genital symptoms and no nail changes on examination.

Applying the differential framework from this chapter, the classic morphology, violaceous, polygonal, flat-topped papules with Wickham striae, favors idiopathic lichen planus over a lichenoid drug eruption, which would more typically show a less prominent Wickham striae pattern and, often, a more photodistributed component, though the temporal relationship to his antihypertensive medication, started approximately one month before symptom onset, falls within the broad and variable latency window discussed earlier in this chapter for lichenoid drug eruptions and cannot be dismissed on temporal grounds alone. Given the ambiguity, and after discussion with the patient's primary care clinician regarding alternative antihypertensive options, a trial substitution to a different antihypertensive class is undertaken as both a diagnostic and therapeutic maneuver, while a potent topical corticosteroid is started concurrently for symptomatic relief given the significant pruritus he is experiencing.

At eight-week follow-up after the medication substitution, his lesions have substantially improved beyond what would be expected from topical therapy alone over that interval, supporting a lichenoid drug eruption related to the thiazide diuretic rather than idiopathic lichen planus, a distinction with meaningful prognostic value for the patient since a confirmed drug-related lichenoid eruption would not be expected to recur once the causative medication is permanently avoided, whereas idiopathic lichen planus can follow a more prolonged or recurrent course. He is counseled to avoid this specific medication class going forward and to inform future prescribers of this reaction, and given the absence of oral, genital, or nail involvement throughout his course, no additional site-specific surveillance beyond routine follow-up is required.

KEY POINT: When a lichenoid eruption's temporal relationship to a plausible culprit medication is ambiguous, a trial substitution to an alternative medication class, performed in coordination with the prescribing clinician, can serve as both a diagnostic and therapeutic maneuver.

THE MORPHOLOGY-TO-MANAGEMENT SYSTEM — Contact and Lichenoid Reaction Patterns

---

Patterns Introduced This Chapter: The geometric contact dermatitis arc, and the classic violaceous, polygonal, flat-topped papule of lichen planus with its oral, nail, and scalp variants.

Cross-Cutting Anchor: A sharply geometric or linear lesion border points to an external contact cause, while a symmetric, widespread, violaceous papular eruption with Wickham striae points to a lichenoid immune process; distinguishing shape-driven from immune-driven distribution is the recurring anchor discrimination introduced in this chapter.

Summary and Key Concepts

Irritant and allergic contact dermatitis share an eczematous appearance but differ fundamentally in mechanism, time course, and management, with allergen avoidance offering genuinely curative potential once patch testing identifies the causative allergen.

A sharply geometric or linear lesion border is a key configurational clue pointing toward an external contact cause and should prompt a directed exposure history.

Lichen planus reflects a cytotoxic, keratinocyte-directed immune process producing violaceous, polygonal, flat-topped papules with Wickham striae, and can involve oral, genital, nail, and scalp sites with distinct management and surveillance implications.

Lichenoid drug eruptions closely mimic idiopathic lichen planus and require careful medication reconciliation, since discontinuing a culprit medication is often the most informative diagnostic and therapeutic step.

Erosive oral and genital lichen planus carry a small but clinically meaningful malignant transformation risk requiring longitudinal surveillance beyond symptomatic management alone.

CHAPTER 7: ACNE, ROSACEA, AND SEBORRHEIC DERMATITIS

Learning Objectives

1. Explain the four-factor pathophysiologic model of acne vulgaris and connect each factor to a specific therapeutic target.
2. Grade acne severity and select an evidence-based, antibiotic-sparing treatment regimen matched to that severity.
3. Distinguish the clinical subtypes of rosacea and differentiate rosacea from acne vulgaris and other facial dermatoses using Trap Logic discriminating features.
4. Recognize and manage ocular rosacea and rhinophyma as distinct disease manifestations requiring their own treatment approach.
5. Apply an evidence-based management framework to seborrheic dermatitis across infantile, pediatric, and adult presentations.

Acne Vulgaris: Definition, Epidemiology, and Pathophysiology

Definition and the Four-Factor Model

Acne vulgaris is a chronic inflammatory disease of the pilosebaceous unit, introduced in the first chapter of this book, arising from the interaction of four interconnected pathophysiologic factors: abnormal follicular keratinization producing a microcomedone, increased sebum production under androgenic stimulation, proliferation of Cutibacterium acnes within the sebum-rich follicular environment, and a resulting inflammatory response. Understanding acne as a four-factor model rather than a single-cause disease is what allows rational, mechanism-matched combination therapy, discussed later in this chapter, since an effective regimen typically must address more than one of these factors simultaneously to achieve durable control.

Epidemiology and Natural History

Acne affects the substantial majority of adolescents to some degree, making it one of the most common conditions encountered in general medical and dermatologic practice, with onset typically coinciding with the androgenic surge of puberty and a natural history that for many patients improves through the third decade of life, though a meaningful proportion of adults, women in particular, experience persistent or new-onset disease well beyond adolescence. Adult-onset and persistent acne in women frequently demonstrates a distinct distribution favoring the lower face, jawline, and neck, and often follows a cyclical pattern linked to the menstrual cycle, a pattern that should prompt consideration of an underlying hormonal contribution discussed later in this chapter.

Follicular Keratinization and Comedone Formation

The earliest event in acne pathogenesis is abnormal desquamation of follicular keratinocytes, which fail to shed normally and instead accumulate within the follicular canal along with sebum, forming a microscopic plug termed a microcomedone that is the precursor lesion to every subsequent visible acne lesion. This retained material provides both the anaerobic, lipid-rich environment favorable to Cutibacterium acnes proliferation and the physical obstruction that, once inflammation develops, cannot decompress normally, and this obstruction-plus-inflammation combination is what produces the eventual follicular rupture responsible for the deeper inflammatory lesions and resulting scarring discussed later in this chapter.

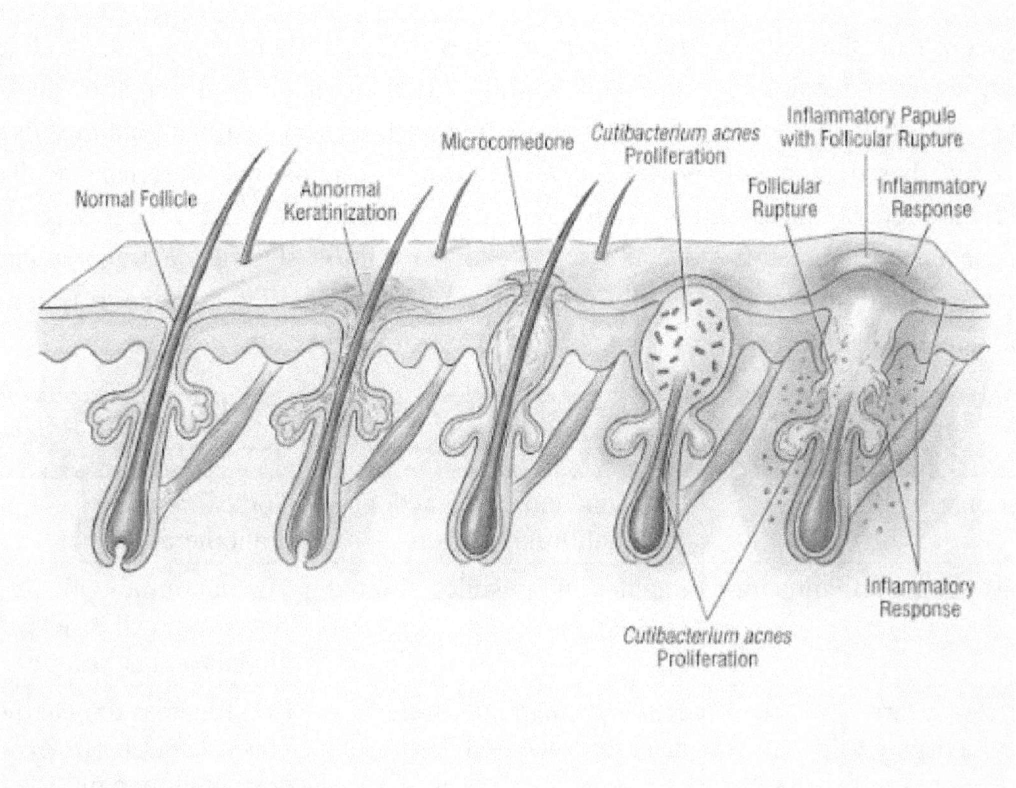

Acne Vulgaris: Clinical Presentation and Grading

Comedonal, Inflammatory, and Nodulocystic Lesions

Comedonal acne presents as open comedones, blackheads, in which the follicular plug is visible at the skin surface and darkened by oxidized melanin rather than dirt, a common patient misconception worth correcting during counseling, and closed comedones, whiteheads, in which the plug remains covered by a thin layer of epidermis. Inflammatory acne presents as erythematous papules and pustules reflecting the inflammatory response to follicular rupture described earlier in this chapter, while nodulocystic acne, the most severe presentation, produces deep, painful, often interconnected inflammatory nodules and pseudocysts with substantial risk of permanent scarring, warranting the more aggressive treatment approach discussed later in this chapter.

Distribution and Grading Severity

Acne characteristically affects the face, chest, and back, the anatomic sites of highest sebaceous gland density introduced in the first chapter of this book, and severity grading, whether by a formal validated instrument or a practical bedside assessment of predominant lesion type and lesion count, should guide treatment selection according to the escalation framework discussed later in this chapter: comedonal-predominant disease, inflammatory papulopustular disease of mild to moderate extent, and nodulocystic or scarring disease each warrant a different starting point on the treatment ladder rather than a uniform initial approach.

Acne Scarring

Scarring develops from the tissue destruction associated with deep inflammatory and nodulocystic lesions and is classified into icepick, boxcar, and rolling morphologies based on scar depth and edge characteristics, a classification with direct relevance to procedural scar treatment options discussed in the chapter on office-based dermatologic procedures. Because scarring risk correlates with both lesion severity and duration of inadequately controlled disease, early, adequately aggressive treatment of moderate to severe inflammatory acne is itself a scar-prevention strategy, a framing that should be communicated explicitly to patients and, in pediatric cases, their families to support timely rather than delayed treatment escalation.

Severity Category	Predominant Lesion Type	Typical Starting Treatment Tier
Comedonal	Open and closed comedones, minimal inflammation	Topical retinoid monotherapy
Mild-Moderate Inflammatory	Papules and pustules, limited nodules	Topical retinoid plus benzoyl peroxide, with or without topical/oral antibiotic
Moderate-Severe Inflammatory	Extensive papulopustular disease, some nodules	Combination topical therapy plus oral antibiotic or hormonal therapy
Nodulocystic/Scarring	Deep nodules, cysts, active scarring	Oral isotretinoin

Acne Vulgaris: Management and Treatment

Topical Therapy: Retinoids and Benzoyl Peroxide

Topical retinoids normalize follicular keratinization, directly addressing the earliest pathogenic step described earlier in this chapter, and serve as the foundation of nearly every acne regimen regardless of severity, including as maintenance therapy after successful treatment of more severe disease. Benzoyl peroxide provides direct antimicrobial activity against Cutibacterium acnes without any associated resistance risk, as introduced in the therapeutics chapter, making the combination of a topical retinoid with benzoyl peroxide a rational, first-line, antibiotic-sparing regimen that addresses both follicular keratinization and bacterial proliferation simultaneously.

Antibiotic Stewardship in Acne Management

Topical or oral antibiotics may be added for moderate inflammatory disease, but the stewardship principles introduced in the therapeutics chapter apply with particular force in acne: oral antibiotic courses should be limited to the shortest duration consistent with clinical response, generally no more than three to four months, with benzoyl peroxide co-prescribed to reduce resistance development, and a non-antibiotic maintenance regimen, typically a topical retinoid with or without benzoyl peroxide, established before the antibiotic course concludes rather than after disease has already begun to relapse.

Hormonal Therapy and Isotretinoin

Hormonal therapy, combined oral contraceptives or spironolactone, is a valuable option for women with acne demonstrating the jawline-predominant, cyclical pattern discussed earlier in this chapter, particularly when other signs of androgen excess are present, and can be used alone or in combination with topical therapy depending on severity. Oral isotretinoin, introduced in the therapeutics chapter, remains the most effective available therapy for severe nodulocystic or scarring acne and for inflammatory acne refractory to combination topical and oral antibiotic therapy, addressing all four pathogenic factors simultaneously and often producing durable, long-term remission after a single completed course, but requires the strict pregnancy prevention protocol, baseline and interval lipid and hepatic monitoring, and mucocutaneous dryness counseling detailed in the therapeutics chapter.

EVIDENCE: Combining a topical retinoid with benzoyl peroxide, rather than either agent alone, addresses two of the four acne pathogenic factors simultaneously and represents a rational, antibiotic-sparing first-line regimen for mild to moderate inflammatory acne.

Fixed-dose combination products incorporating a topical retinoid, benzoyl peroxide, and, where appropriate, a topical antibiotic into a single formulation can meaningfully improve adherence compared with prescribing each component separately, since a simplified regimen with fewer individual steps and application times reduces the cumulative adherence burden discussed in the therapeutics chapter, and this practical consideration should factor into regimen selection alongside the purely pharmacologic rationale for combination therapy.

Rosacea: Definition, Classification, and Pathophysiology

Definition and Clinical Subtypes

Rosacea is a chronic inflammatory facial dermatosis distinct from acne despite frequent lay conflation of the two conditions, classified into four principal subtypes that can occur individually or in combination: erythematotelangiectatic rosacea, dominated by persistent facial erythema and visible telangiectasias; papulopustular rosacea, presenting with inflammatory papules and pustules without the comedones characteristic of acne; phymatous rosacea, producing progressive sebaceous gland and connective tissue hypertrophy most classically affecting the nose as rhinophyma; and ocular rosacea, affecting the eyes and periocular tissue, discussed in detail later in this chapter given its distinct management implications.

Pathophysiology: Vascular, Immune, and Neurovascular Mechanisms

Rosacea pathophysiology involves dysregulated innate immune signaling, particularly abnormal cathelicidin peptide processing that produces proinflammatory fragments, combined with neurovascular dysregulation that produces exaggerated flushing responses to triggers that would not provoke a comparable response in unaffected skin, and increased density of the skin mite Demodex folliculorum, whose precise causal role remains an area of active investigation rather than firmly established. This combination of innate immune dysregulation and neurovascular hyperreactivity, fundamentally distinct from the follicular, androgen-driven mechanism of acne discussed earlier in this chapter, explains why rosacea treatment targets inflammation and vascular reactivity rather than follicular keratinization or sebum production.

Common Triggers

Common rosacea triggers, identified through patient-reported flare patterns, include ultraviolet exposure, heat, spicy food, alcohol, and emotional stress, each believed to act through the neurovascular hyperreactivity mechanism described above rather than through a specific immunologic sensitization analogous to the contact allergens discussed in the previous chapter, and trigger identification through a structured patient-maintained flare diary is a valuable, low-risk component of management discussed further later in this chapter.

KEY POINT: Rosacea and acne are mechanistically distinct diseases despite frequent lay conflation; rosacea lacks comedones and reflects innate immune and neurovascular dysregulation rather than the androgen-driven, follicular process underlying acne.

Rosacea onset typically occurs later than the puberty-associated onset of acne, most commonly presenting in the third through fifth decades of life, and this age-of-onset distinction, combined with the comedone-based discrimination emphasized throughout this chapter, provides an additional layer of diagnostic support in cases where morphology alone leaves some residual ambiguity, particularly in an adult patient with a remote adolescent acne history that could otherwise confound the clinical picture.

Rosacea: Clinical Presentation and Differential Diagnosis

Ocular Rosacea

Ocular rosacea can occur with or without notable cutaneous disease and presents with blepharitis, conjunctival injection, foreign-body sensation, and, in more severe cases, keratitis that can threaten vision if inadequately treated, making prompt recognition and, for significant or refractory cases, ophthalmologic referral an important component of comprehensive rosacea care rather than a peripheral consideration. Patients presenting with facial rosacea should be specifically asked about ocular symptoms, since patients frequently do not volunteer eye complaints as related to their skin diagnosis without being asked directly.

Rhinophyma

Rhinophyma, progressive sebaceous and connective tissue hypertrophy of the nose, develops in a subset of patients with long-standing phymatous rosacea, more commonly in men, and represents a largely irreversible structural change once fully established that responds poorly to medical therapy alone, generally requiring procedural intervention, discussed in the office-based procedures chapter, for meaningful cosmetic and functional improvement, underscoring the value of controlling inflammatory rosacea early before phymatous change becomes established and irreversible.

Differential Diagnosis

Papulopustular rosacea is distinguished from acne vulgaris by the complete absence of comedones, a discriminating feature emphasized throughout this chapter, and by its later, more centrofacial-predominant onset relative to the puberty-associated onset of typical acne. Perioral dermatitis, a related papulopustular eruption concentrated around the mouth with a characteristic clear zone immediately adjacent to the vermilion border, can mimic rosacea but has a distinct association with topical corticosteroid overuse on the face, and seborrheic dermatitis, discussed later in this chapter, can coexist with or be mistaken for erythematotelangiectatic rosacea given overlapping facial erythema, though seborrheic dermatitis characteristically produces greasy scale absent in rosacea.

THE MORPHOLOGY-TO-MANAGEMENT SYSTEM — Centrofacial Erythema and Papulopustular Eruption Arc

The Pattern: Persistent centrofacial erythema, telangiectasias, and inflammatory papules or pustules without comedones, often with a history of flushing triggered by heat, alcohol, or spicy food.

Presentation Variance: Background erythema and telangiectasias are frequently more difficult to appreciate in richly pigmented skin, where papulopustular lesions and, in more advanced cases, phymatous change may be the more clinically apparent presenting features, and this variance has been implicated in delayed rosacea diagnosis in patients with darker skin tones, who are sometimes incorrectly presumed not to develop the condition at all.

Trap Logic: Acne vulgaris is excluded by the complete absence of comedones and by the more centrofacial, later-onset presentation of rosacea; perioral dermatitis is distinguished by its characteristic sparing of the immediate perioral vermilion border and its association with topical corticosteroid overuse; seborrheic dermatitis is distinguished by greasy, yellowish scale, absent in rosacea, favoring the nasolabial folds, eyebrows, and scalp margin.

Management Pivot: Erythematotelangiectatic rosacea is managed with trigger avoidance, daily broad-spectrum photoprotection, and, for persistent erythema, topical alpha-adrenergic agonists; papulopustular rosacea adds a topical anti-inflammatory agent such as topical metronidazole, azelaic acid, or ivermectin, with oral antibiotics reserved for more extensive or refractory disease using anti-inflammatory rather than antimicrobial dosing strategies where available; phymatous change requires procedural referral once established.

Pattern Anchor: Absence of comedones combined with a trigger-responsive flushing history is the anchor combination that most reliably distinguishes rosacea from acne vulgaris at the bedside.

Rosacea: Management and Treatment

Trigger Avoidance and Photoprotection

Daily broad-spectrum photoprotection is a foundational element of rosacea management given the disease's photosensitivity and the role of ultraviolet exposure as a common flare trigger discussed earlier in this chapter, and a structured, patient-maintained trigger diary, tracking food, beverage, temperature, and stress exposures against symptom flares, can identify individually relevant triggers that, once avoided, meaningfully reduce flare frequency without any pharmacologic intervention.

Topical and Oral Anti-Inflammatory Therapy

Topical metronidazole, azelaic acid, and ivermectin each provide anti-inflammatory benefit for papulopustular rosacea through mechanisms distinct from the antimicrobial mechanisms these same or related agents provide in other contexts, and topical alpha-adrenergic agonists, brimonidine or oxymetazoline, provide temporary vasoconstriction that reduces visible erythema for erythematotelangiectatic disease, though effects are temporary and require ongoing daily application rather than producing durable disease modification. Oral antibiotics, most often from the tetracycline class, are used at anti-inflammatory rather than antimicrobial dosing for more extensive papulopustular disease, an important stewardship-consistent distinction from the antimicrobial dosing used for infectious indications.

Procedural Options for Vascular and Phymatous Disease

Persistent telangiectasias unresponsive to topical vasoconstrictor therapy can be treated with vascular laser or light-based therapy, discussed in the office-based procedures chapter, and established rhinophyma generally requires ablative or excisional procedural correction for meaningful improvement, since medical therapy alone does not reverse the connective tissue and sebaceous hypertrophy once fully developed, reinforcing the earlier point in this chapter that early control of inflammatory rosacea is itself a strategy to prevent this largely irreversible phymatous progression.

Seborrheic Dermatitis: Pathophysiology, Presentation, and Management

Pathophysiology and the Role of Malassezia

Seborrheic dermatitis reflects an inflammatory response to Malassezia yeast species, normal skin flora that become pathogenic through their lipase activity, which breaks down sebum triglycerides into free fatty acids that irritate the skin and provoke an inflammatory response in susceptible individuals, explaining the disease's characteristic concentration in sebaceous gland-dense areas, the scalp, face, and central chest, introduced in the first chapter of this book. This mechanism also explains the infantile presentation discussed in the first chapter, driven by transiently hyperfunctional neonatal sebaceous glands under maternal androgenic influence, which resolves as that hormonal influence wanes over the following months.

Clinical Presentation Across the Age Spectrum

Infantile seborrheic dermatitis, commonly termed cradle cap when affecting the scalp, presents with greasy, yellowish scale that is generally not pruritic and resolves spontaneously over the first several months of life without necessarily requiring treatment beyond gentle mechanical removal with a soft brush and emollient. Adult seborrheic dermatitis presents as ill-defined, greasy, yellowish, scaling patches concentrated on the scalp, eyebrows, nasolabial folds, and central chest, often with a waxing and waning course influenced by stress, seasonal change, and immune status, and, as discussed in the psoriasis chapter, must be distinguished from scalp psoriasis based on scale character and distribution relative to the hairline.

Management Across Presentations

Adult scalp disease is managed first-line with an antifungal shampoo targeting Malassezia, ketoconazole or selenium sulfide among the most commonly used options, used regularly rather than only during active flares to maintain control given the disease's chronic, relapsing nature, with a low-potency topical corticosteroid or topical calcineurin inhibitor added for more inflamed facial or truncal involvement given the atrophy risk discussed in the therapeutics chapter at these thinner-skinned sites. Disease that is unusually severe, extensive, or refractory to standard therapy, particularly in an adult without a clear alternative explanation, should prompt consideration of an underlying immunosuppressed state, since severe seborrheic dermatitis is a recognized cutaneous marker of HIV infection and other immunocompromising conditions.

CAUTION: Unusually severe, extensive, or treatment-refractory seborrheic dermatitis in an adult, particularly without another clear explanation, should prompt consideration of an underlying immunocompromised state, since this pattern is a recognized cutaneous marker of HIV infection.

Seborrheic dermatitis also demonstrates a well-documented association with Parkinson disease, believed to reflect autonomic dysfunction affecting sebaceous gland activity rather than a shared primary pathophysiologic mechanism, and while this association does not warrant reflexive neurologic evaluation in every adult presenting with routine seborrheic dermatitis, awareness of the association is clinically useful in a patient who additionally demonstrates other early signs suggestive of parkinsonism, where the coexistence of both findings may prompt earlier neurologic referral than either finding would in isolation.

Post-Inflammatory Hyperpigmentation and Presentation Variance

Post-Inflammatory Hyperpigmentation as a Primary Treatment Concern

Post-inflammatory hyperpigmentation following resolved acne lesions is substantially more common and more prominent in richly pigmented skin, and for many patients in this population, the residual pigmentary change, rather than active inflammatory lesions themselves, becomes the primary presenting concern and the dominant driver of perceived treatment success or failure, a distinction clinicians should explicitly ask about rather than assuming that resolution of active inflammatory lesions alone constitutes a complete treatment response from the patient's perspective. Treatment approaches that minimize inflammatory lesion duration and severity, through the early, adequately aggressive therapy discussed earlier in this chapter, are the most effective available strategy for limiting the severity and extent of subsequent post-inflammatory hyperpigmentation, since the pigmentary change is a direct downstream consequence of the inflammatory process itself rather than an independent phenomenon requiring separate primary treatment.

Treating Post-Inflammatory Hyperpigmentation Directly

Once present, post-inflammatory hyperpigmentation can be addressed with topical agents that reduce melanin synthesis or promote epidermal turnover, including azelaic acid, which carries the additional benefit of anti-inflammatory and antimicrobial activity relevant to concurrent acne treatment discussed earlier in this chapter, and topical retinoids, already a foundational component of most acne regimens, which accelerate epidermal turnover and can hasten resolution of pigmentary change as a secondary benefit beyond their primary comedolytic effect. Patients should be counseled that post-inflammatory hyperpigmentation typically fades gradually over several months to a year even without specific pigment-targeted therapy, and that aggressive procedural intervention is rarely necessary or appropriate as an initial approach given this expected natural resolution.

Scar and Pigmentation Risk From Aggressive Extraction and Manipulation

Patient counseling regarding acne lesion manipulation, picking, squeezing, or aggressive at-home extraction, should explicitly address the elevated scarring and post-inflammatory hyperpigmentation risk this behavior carries, particularly in patients with richly pigmented skin where both complications are more pronounced, reframing this common behavior not as a hygiene failure but as a specific, modifiable risk factor for the two complications patients most want to avoid, an framing that in practice improves counseling receptiveness compared with a generic instruction simply to stop picking.

PATIENT EDUCATION: Post-inflammatory hyperpigmentation following acne typically fades gradually over several months to a year without requiring aggressive treatment; early, adequately effective control of active inflammatory lesions is the most reliable strategy for limiting its severity and extent.

Hormonal Contributors and Adjunctive Considerations in Acne

Recognizing an Underlying Hyperandrogenic Contribution

Adult women presenting with the jawline-predominant, cyclical acne pattern introduced earlier in this chapter should be evaluated for additional signs of androgen excess, including irregular menses, hirsutism, and androgenic alopecia, since polycystic ovary syndrome and, less commonly, other hyperandrogenic states can present with acne as a prominent or presenting feature, and identifying an underlying hyperandrogenic contribution both informs treatment selection toward the hormonal therapies discussed earlier in this chapter and prompts appropriate additional evaluation and, where indicated, gynecologic or endocrinologic referral for the broader hyperandrogenic condition itself rather than treating the cutaneous manifestation in isolation.

Diet and Acne: What the Evidence Supports

Emerging evidence suggests a modest association between high-glycemic-index diets and dairy consumption and acne severity in some patients, though this association is considerably weaker and less consistent than the historical, now largely discredited belief that specific foods such as chocolate directly cause acne, and dietary modification should be discussed as a potential adjunctive consideration for interested patients rather than presented as a primary or required treatment strategy, since the evidence does not support dietary change alone as an adequate substitute for the topical and systemic therapies discussed throughout this chapter.

KEY POINT: Jawline-predominant, cyclical acne in an adult woman, particularly with additional signs of androgen excess, should prompt evaluation for an underlying hyperandrogenic contribution such as polycystic ovary syndrome rather than escalation of standard topical acne therapy alone.

Complications, Special Populations, and Patient Education

Demodex and Adjunctive Rosacea Considerations

While the precise causal contribution of Demodex folliculorum density to rosacea remains an area of ongoing investigation, as noted earlier in this chapter, topical ivermectin's dual anti-inflammatory and anti-parasitic mechanism has made it a particularly useful option for papulopustular rosacea regardless of the ultimate resolution of this mechanistic question, since its clinical efficacy has been well demonstrated independent of the specific relative contribution of its two mechanisms of action in any individual patient. Patients frequently ask about Demodex specifically after encountering the topic through consumer health information, and providing a clear, accurate explanation of the current state of evidence, genuine association without fully established causation, helps set realistic expectations for treatment response and avoids both dismissing a legitimate area of ongoing research and overstating certainty the evidence does not yet support.

Psychosocial Impact Across All Three Conditions

Acne, rosacea, and seborrheic dermatitis each carry a substantial psychosocial burden disproportionate to their generally limited physical morbidity, given their near-universal facial involvement and visibility to others, and screening for depression, anxiety, and social withdrawal should be incorporated into routine care for each condition, particularly for adolescents with moderate to severe acne and adults with visible rosacea, populations in which this psychosocial burden is well documented and frequently underrecognized by clinicians focused primarily on physical severity grading.

Rosacea and Seborrheic Dermatitis in Special Populations

Rosacea management during pregnancy similarly follows the pregnancy-specific safety framework introduced in the therapeutics chapter, with topical azelaic acid generally favored given its established safety profile while systemic tetracycline-class antibiotics are avoided given known effects on fetal bone and teeth development. Seborrheic dermatitis in infants, discussed earlier in this chapter as cradle cap, requires reassurance and gentle mechanical scale removal as first-line management, with escalation to antifungal or low-potency anti-inflammatory therapy reserved for more extensive or persistent presentations rather than applied routinely to the typical, self-limited infantile pattern.

Special Populations: Pregnancy and Adolescents

Acne treatment during pregnancy requires the pregnancy-specific safety framework introduced in the therapeutics chapter, with topical benzoyl peroxide and azelaic acid generally considered reasonable options while oral isotretinoin and topical retinoids are avoided given teratogenicity concerns, and hormonal therapy options are reconsidered given pregnancy's own hormonal state. Adolescent patients and their families benefit from explicit counseling that acne is not caused by poor hygiene or diet in the way often assumed, a persistent misconception that can drive both excessive, barrier-damaging skin cleansing and unwarranted guilt, and that consistent, correctly applied therapy over weeks to months, rather than an immediately visible response, is the expected and appropriate treatment course.

Patient Education on Expected Time Course

All three conditions discussed in this chapter require sustained treatment over weeks to months before maximal benefit is achieved, and setting this expectation explicitly at the time treatment is initiated is one of the most effective available strategies for preventing premature treatment discontinuation, directly applying the adherence principles introduced in the therapeutics chapter to this specific and common category of chronic facial dermatoses.

A brief, structured explanation of why improvement takes weeks rather than days, connecting the expected time course to the underlying pathophysiologic mechanism being targeted, follicular turnover for acne, or reduction of chronic inflammatory infiltrate for rosacea and seborrheic dermatitis, helps patients understand that a lack of immediate visible improvement does not indicate the chosen therapy is ineffective, and this mechanistic framing has been shown in practice to improve treatment persistence compared with a generic instruction to simply continue the medication as directed.

Clinical Case: Distinguishing Rosacea From Acne in an Adult

A 42-year-old woman presents with a two-year history of facial redness and intermittent breakouts that she has been treating with an over-the-counter acne wash and benzoyl peroxide gel without significant improvement. She reports her face flushes noticeably after drinking wine or being in a hot room, and on examination there is persistent erythema and visible telangiectasias over the cheeks and nose, with several inflammatory papules but no visible comedones anywhere on careful inspection.

Applying the Trap Logic discrimination established in the Rhythm Layer callout earlier in this chapter, the complete absence of comedones despite a two-year disease course argues strongly against acne vulgaris, since comedones would be expected to be present at least intermittently over that duration if acne were the correct diagnosis, and the trigger-responsive flushing history, combined with background telangiectasias, supports papulopustular rosacea instead. Her benzoyl peroxide-based acne regimen is discontinued, since this therapy is directed at a pathogenic mechanism, follicular keratinization and bacterial proliferation, that is not operative in her actual disease process and may in fact be contributing to irritation and worsened erythema given her already inflamed, sensitive skin.

She is started on topical ivermectin for her papulopustular lesions, counseled on daily broad-spectrum photoprotection and encouraged to maintain a trigger diary tracking her wine and heat-associated flares, and asked specifically about ocular symptoms, which she confirms she has noticed as intermittent eye irritation she had not previously connected to her skin complaint. She is referred for ophthalmologic evaluation given this finding, and at eight-week dermatologic follow-up her papulopustular lesions have substantially improved, though her background erythema and telangiectasias remain largely unchanged, as expected given that topical anti-inflammatory therapy addresses the inflammatory component of rosacea more effectively than the vascular component, for which she is offered a topical alpha-adrenergic agonist and, if desired, subsequent referral for vascular laser therapy.

CLINICAL PEARL: A treatment-refractory presumed acne diagnosis in an adult that has never demonstrated a single comedone should prompt reconsideration of rosacea, since continued acne-directed therapy in a patient with rosacea can worsen the underlying facial inflammation and erythema.

Clinical Case: Severe Nodulocystic Acne and Early Isotretinoin Consideration

A 17-year-old boy presents with a two-year history of progressively worsening facial and truncal acne, now characterized by numerous deep, painful, interconnected nodules across his cheeks, jawline, and back, with visible early scarring already present on both cheeks. He has completed two separate three-month courses of oral antibiotics combined with topical retinoid and benzoyl peroxide therapy over the past year, with only partial and temporary improvement each time, and his nodules have recurred within weeks of completing each antibiotic course.

Applying the severity-based treatment framework from this chapter, his presentation, nodulocystic morphology with active scarring already present, meets the threshold for oral isotretinoin consideration discussed earlier in this chapter, and his history of two prior antibiotic courses with recurrence shortly after each course ended demonstrates that his disease is not adequately controlled by combination topical and oral antibiotic therapy, satisfying the treatment-failure criterion that supports escalation to isotretinoin rather than a third antibiotic course, which would raise further antibiotic stewardship concerns given the pattern already established. Given the visible scarring already present, earlier rather than delayed escalation is explicitly framed to the patient and his family as a scar-prevention strategy, directly applying the principle introduced earlier in this chapter that scarring risk correlates with both severity and duration of inadequately controlled disease.

Baseline laboratory testing, including a lipid panel and hepatic function panel, is obtained per the monitoring framework introduced in the therapeutics chapter, and given his age and the mandatory pregnancy prevention protocol requirements for isotretinoin, his treating clinician confirms he is not currently or anticipated to become a reproductive partner requiring pregnancy prevention counseling directed at a partner, though comprehensive counseling regarding the medication's teratogenicity, mucocutaneous dryness, and required monitoring intervals is still provided in full. He is started on oral isotretinoin at a weight-based dose with monthly follow-up for laboratory monitoring and clinical reassessment, and his family is counseled that meaningful improvement typically requires two to three months to become apparent, with many patients achieving durable remission after a single completed course lasting four to six months, an important expectation-setting step given his prior experience of rapid relapse after shorter antibiotic courses.

KEY POINT: Recurrence of nodulocystic acne shortly after each of two completed antibiotic courses, with active scarring already present, supports escalation to oral isotretinoin rather than a third antibiotic course, both for stewardship reasons and because earlier escalation itself functions as a scar-prevention strategy.

THE MORPHOLOGY-TO-MANAGEMENT SYSTEM — Facial Dermatoses: Acne, Rosacea, and Seborrheic Dermatitis

---

Pattern Introduced This Chapter: Centrofacial erythema and papulopustular eruption without comedones (rosacea), discriminated from acne, perioral dermatitis, and seborrheic dermatitis.

Cross-Cutting Anchor: The presence or absence of comedones is the single fastest anchor discriminating acne from rosacea and perioral dermatitis, while greasy, yellow scale in a sebaceous-gland-dense distribution is the anchor for seborrheic dermatitis.

Summary and Key Concepts

Acne vulgaris arises from four interconnected factors, follicular keratinization, sebum production, Cutibacterium acnes proliferation, and inflammation, and effective treatment typically must address more than one factor simultaneously.

Antibiotic stewardship principles apply with particular force in acne management, limiting oral antibiotic courses to three to four months with early transition to non-antibiotic maintenance therapy.

Rosacea is mechanistically distinct from acne, reflecting innate immune dysregulation and neurovascular hyperreactivity, and is reliably distinguished from acne by the complete absence of comedones.

Ocular rosacea and rhinophyma are distinct disease manifestations requiring their own recognition, referral, and treatment pathways beyond standard cutaneous rosacea management.

Seborrheic dermatitis reflects an inflammatory response to Malassezia yeast and is managed with antifungal shampoo and, for inflamed sites, low-potency topical anti-inflammatory therapy, with unusually severe adult disease warranting consideration of underlying immunosuppression.

CHAPTER 8: BACTERIAL SKIN AND SOFT TISSUE INFECTIONS

Learning Objectives

1. Distinguish impetigo, folliculitis, cellulitis, and erysipelas based on depth of infection, morphology, and causative organism.
2. Recognize the clinical features that distinguish cellulitis from its principal noninfectious mimics.
3. Identify the red flag findings that should prompt urgent evaluation for necrotizing soft tissue infection.
4. Select empiric antibiotic therapy for common bacterial skin and soft tissue infections informed by local resistance patterns and severity.
5. Recognize staphylococcal and streptococcal toxin-mediated syndromes and distinguish them from primary infectious processes.

Impetigo and Superficial Bacterial Infections

Nonbullous Impetigo

Nonbullous impetigo, the more common form, is caused by Staphylococcus aureus, Streptococcus pyogenes, or a combination of both, and begins as small vesicles or pustules that rapidly rupture to form the characteristic honey-colored crust introduced in the first chapter of this book, most often affecting the face and extremities of children, with lesions spreading readily to adjacent skin and to close contacts through direct contact with infected exudate given the disease's high contagiousness. This crust morphology directly reflects the superficial, intraepidermal location of the infection, which does not extend into the dermis and therefore does not typically produce the surrounding warmth, induration, or systemic symptoms characteristic of the deeper infections discussed later in this chapter.

Bullous Impetigo

Bullous impetigo, caused specifically by strains of Staphylococcus aureus that produce exfoliative toxins targeting desmoglein 1, a desmosomal protein also relevant to the pemphigus foliaceus discussed in the chapter on immunobullous disease, produces flaccid, fragile bullae that rupture easily to leave a thin, collarette-like scale rather than the thick honey-colored crust of the nonbullous form, reflecting a distinct toxin-mediated mechanism of superficial epidermal splitting rather than simple exudate desiccation. Because the exfoliative toxin acts locally at the site of bacterial colonization in bullous impetigo, the disease remains localized in most affected patients, in contrast to the disseminated toxin effect of staphylococcal scalded skin syndrome discussed later in this chapter, in which the same toxin class acts systemically following hematogenous spread rather than local secretion alone.

Ecthyma

Ecthyma represents a deeper variant of impetigo in which infection extends through the epidermis into the superficial dermis, producing a punched-out ulceration with an overlying adherent crust rather than the epidermis-confined crust of simple impetigo, and, unlike impetigo, ecthyma characteristically heals with scarring given this deeper dermal involvement, a distinction that should prompt more assertive treatment and closer follow-up than uncomplicated impetigo would otherwise warrant.

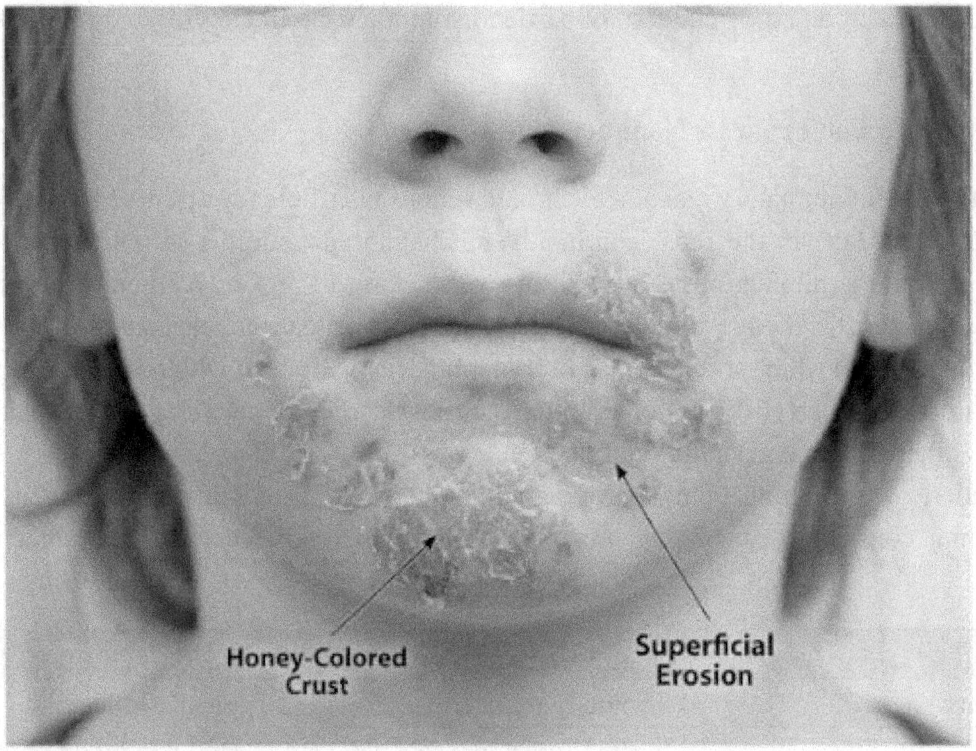

Cellulitis and Erysipelas

Erysipelas: Superficial Dermal and Lymphatic Infection

Erysipelas is a superficial infection involving the upper dermis and superficial lymphatics, most often caused by Streptococcus pyogenes, producing a sharply demarcated, raised, bright erythematous plaque with a distinct border that is readily palpable as a clear edge separating involved from uninvolved skin, a morphologic feature directly reflecting the infection's confinement to the superficial dermis and lymphatics, in contrast to the poorly demarcated border of cellulitis discussed next. Erysipelas classically affects the face or lower extremities and is frequently accompanied by fever and systemic symptoms that can precede the visible skin findings, an important historical clue when the cutaneous findings are still evolving at initial presentation.

Cellulitis: Deeper Dermal and Subcutaneous Infection

Cellulitis extends more deeply into the dermis and subcutaneous tissue, most often caused by Streptococcus pyogenes or Staphylococcus aureus, and produces a poorly demarcated area of erythema, warmth, tenderness, and edema without the sharp, raised border of erysipelas, reflecting the less lymphatic-confined, deeper tissue plane of infection. Cellulitis typically arises at a site of disrupted skin barrier, an area of tinea pedis-associated fissuring, a chronic wound, or an insect bite, and the lower extremity is the most commonly affected site given the combination of dependent edema, which impairs local immune clearance, and the frequency of barrier disruption from tinea pedis and venous stasis changes at this location.

Distinguishing Infection From Its Noninfectious Mimics

Stasis dermatitis, an inflammatory reaction to chronic venous insufficiency discussed further in the chapter on pigmentary disorders, is the most commonly misdiagnosed cellulitis mimic, typically presenting bilaterally with a more indolent onset over weeks and lacking the fever, marked tenderness, and rapid progression characteristic of true infection, and this distinction carries substantial clinical importance given the frequency with which stasis dermatitis is inappropriately treated with repeated antibiotic courses. Deep vein thrombosis can also mimic cellulitis with unilateral leg swelling and erythema, though it typically lacks the warmth and sharply defined tenderness of infection and instead presents with a more diffusely tender, swollen limb, and appropriate imaging should be pursued when this diagnosis is genuinely being considered rather than assumed to have been excluded by treating empirically for cellulitis.

Feature	Cellulitis/Erysipelas	Stasis Dermatitis
Laterality	Typically unilateral	Typically bilateral
Onset	Acute, over hours to a day or two	Chronic, indolent, over weeks to months
Systemic Symptoms	Fever and malaise common	Absent
Tenderness	Marked	Mild or absent

THE MORPHOLOGY-TO-MANAGEMENT SYSTEM — Acute Unilateral Lower Extremity Erythema Arc

The Pattern: Acute, unilateral erythema, warmth, tenderness, and edema of the lower extremity, with or without accompanying fever.

Presentation Variance: Erythema can be substantially more difficult to detect visually in richly pigmented skin, and warmth, tenderness, and edema, findings that do not depend on color perception, should be weighted more heavily when assessing severity and extent in this population, since relying on visual erythema alone risks underestimating the true extent of infection and delaying appropriately extensive antibiotic coverage or, when relevant, surgical consultation.

Trap Logic: Bilateral onset, indolent progression over weeks, and absence of fever favor stasis dermatitis over cellulitis; disproportionate pain out of keeping with the visible skin findings, rapidly progressive erythema, hemorrhagic bullae, or skin anesthesia are red flag findings that should raise concern for necrotizing fasciitis rather than uncomplicated cellulitis, discussed in the chapter on dermatologic emergencies; a tender, swollen limb without the warmth and sharply defined erythema typical of infection should prompt consideration of deep vein thrombosis and appropriate imaging.

Management Pivot: Uncomplicated cellulitis without systemic toxicity is managed with empiric oral antibiotic therapy covering streptococcal species and, where clinically indicated based on purulence or risk factors, methicillin-resistant Staphylococcus aureus, with the specific agent selected according to local resistance patterns and confirmed against current guideline recommendations; systemic toxicity, rapid progression, or failure to improve after forty-eight to seventy-two hours of appropriate oral therapy warrants escalation to intravenous antibiotics and, if any red flag findings for necrotizing infection are present, emergent surgical evaluation.

Pattern Anchor: Pain disproportionate to visible skin findings is the single most important anchor finding that should override an otherwise reassuring appearance and prompt urgent evaluation for necrotizing soft tissue infection.

Folliculitis, Furuncles, and Carbuncles

Superficial Folliculitis

Folliculitis represents infection or inflammation confined to the hair follicle, presenting as small, discrete follicular pustules, most often caused by Staphylococcus aureus, though a related, non-infectious form termed pseudofolliculitis barbae, driven by ingrown curved hairs rather than infection, is common in individuals with tightly coiled hair textures in areas subject to close shaving, most classically the beard area, and requires a fundamentally different management approach, altered shaving technique and hair growth allowance rather than antibiotic therapy, underscoring the importance of correctly distinguishing infectious from mechanical folliculitis before treatment is selected.

Furuncles and Carbuncles

A furuncle represents a deeper follicular infection extending into the surrounding dermis and subcutaneous tissue, producing a tender, fluctuant nodule that frequently drains spontaneously, while a carbuncle represents coalescence of multiple adjacent furuncles into a single, larger, multi-loculated inflammatory mass with several draining sinus tracts, most often occurring at friction-prone, hair-bearing sites such as the neck, axillae, and buttocks. Recurrent furunculosis warrants evaluation for predisposing factors, including nasal Staphylococcus aureus carriage, obesity, diabetes, and, in some cases, an underlying immunodeficiency, and decolonization strategies targeting nasal carriage can meaningfully reduce recurrence in appropriately selected patients.

Hot Tub Folliculitis

A distinct folliculitis pattern caused by Pseudomonas aeruginosa, termed hot tub folliculitis, develops after exposure to inadequately chlorinated hot tubs or pools, presenting with widespread, pruritic follicular pustules concentrated in areas covered by a swimsuit, a distribution pattern that itself supports the diagnosis given the correlation with the specific exposure, and is typically self-limited, resolving without specific antimicrobial therapy in most immunocompetent patients given the generally low pathogenicity of this organism in the setting of an intact immune system and limited exposure duration.

CLINICAL PEARL: Widespread follicular pustules developing one to four days after hot tub or pool exposure, concentrated under swimwear, suggest Pseudomonas folliculitis and typically resolve without specific antimicrobial therapy in immunocompetent patients.

A shared exposure history among multiple affected individuals who used the same hot tub or pool within the preceding several days provides strong supporting evidence for this diagnosis and should be specifically elicited whenever a cluster of similar follicular eruptions is encountered, since this epidemiologic pattern is rarely seen with the staphylococcal folliculitis discussed earlier in this section.

Staphylococcal and Streptococcal Toxin-Mediated Syndromes

Staphylococcal Scalded Skin Syndrome

Staphylococcal scalded skin syndrome results from hematogenous dissemination of exfoliative toxin from a localized staphylococcal infection, often at an inconspicuous site such as the nasopharynx or umbilicus, producing widespread, tender erythema followed by superficial epidermal sloughing at the level of the granular layer, sparing mucous membranes, a distinction with substantial diagnostic value separating this condition from the mucosa-involving, full-epidermal-thickness detachment of the severe cutaneous adverse drug reactions discussed in the chapter on dermatologic emergencies. The disease predominantly affects infants and young children, who lack the renal clearance capacity and specific antitoxin immunity of most older children and adults, and a positive Nikolsky sign, introduced in the diagnostic-approach chapter, is characteristically present given the superficial plane of epidermal splitting.

Toxic Shock Syndrome

Toxic shock syndrome, caused by superantigen-producing strains of Staphylococcus aureus or Streptococcus pyogenes, produces a diffuse, sunburn-like erythema accompanied by fever, hypotension, and multiorgan dysfunction, classically associated with retained tampon use, though nonmenstrual cases associated with surgical wound infection, skin and soft tissue infection, or other sources of toxin-producing bacterial colonization are well recognized and should not be excluded simply based on the absence of a menstrual history. Recognition depends on the combination of the characteristic rash with systemic toxicity rather than the rash in isolation, and this condition represents a medical emergency requiring immediate source identification and removal, aggressive supportive care, and antimicrobial therapy targeting the causative organism and its toxin production.

Scarlet Fever

Scarlet fever, caused by erythrogenic toxin-producing strains of Streptococcus pyogenes, most often complicating streptococcal pharyngitis, produces a diffuse, finely papular, sandpaper-textured erythema with characteristic accentuation in skin folds, termed Pastia lines, and a strawberry tongue appearance from prominent, edematous lingual papillae, and recognition is important both for appropriate antibiotic treatment of the underlying streptococcal infection and for counseling regarding the small but recognized risk of poststreptococcal complications, including acute rheumatic fever and glomerulonephritis, if the underlying infection is inadequately treated.

CAUTION: Toxic shock syndrome should be considered in any patient with diffuse erythema, fever, and hypotension regardless of tampon use history, since nonmenstrual cases associated with a wound or other localized staphylococcal or streptococcal infection are well recognized and require the same urgent evaluation and treatment.

Desquamation of the palms and soles occurring one to two weeks after resolution of the acute erythema is a characteristic late finding common to both staphylococcal scalded skin syndrome and toxic shock syndrome, reflecting the shared toxin-mediated epidermal injury underlying both conditions, and recognizing this delayed desquamation as an expected part of the disease course, rather than a new or separate process, helps avoid unnecessary additional evaluation during the recovery phase.

Management and Antibiotic Selection

Community-Acquired Methicillin-Resistant Staphylococcus Aureus

Community-acquired methicillin-resistant Staphylococcus aureus has become a common cause of purulent skin and soft tissue infection in many regions, distinct from the healthcare-associated methicillin-resistant strains historically associated primarily with hospitalized or institutionalized patients, and typically presents as a recurrent or particularly severe furuncle or abscess in an otherwise healthy individual without traditional healthcare-associated risk factors. Local antibiogram data should directly inform empiric antibiotic selection given substantial geographic variability in community-acquired methicillin-resistant Staphylococcus aureus prevalence, and clinicians practicing in a region with a high local prevalence should maintain a correspondingly lower threshold for selecting empiric coverage active against this organism for purulent infections, consistent with the stewardship-balanced but locally calibrated approach to empiric antibiotic selection introduced in the therapeutics chapter.

Empiric Antibiotic Selection Principles

Empiric antibiotic selection for bacterial skin and soft tissue infections should be guided by the likely causative organism based on the specific clinical presentation, local antimicrobial resistance patterns, particularly the local prevalence of methicillin-resistant Staphylococcus aureus, and disease severity, applying the antibiotic stewardship principles introduced in the therapeutics chapter to favor the narrowest effective spectrum rather than broad empiric coverage in every case. Purulent infections, abscesses, furuncles, and carbuncles, are more often caused by Staphylococcus aureus, including methicillin-resistant strains in many regions, and empiric therapy should account for this local resistance pattern, while nonpurulent cellulitis and erysipelas are more often streptococcal and can frequently be treated with a narrower-spectrum agent when purulence and specific risk factors for methicillin-resistant Staphylococcus aureus are absent.

Incision and Drainage as Primary Therapy

For fluctuant abscesses, furuncles, and carbuncles, incision and drainage is the primary and most important therapeutic intervention, often sufficient on its own for adequately drained, uncomplicated lesions without systemic symptoms, with antibiotic therapy reserved as an adjunct for larger lesions, surrounding cellulitis, systemic symptoms, or specific host risk factors such as immunosuppression, since antibiotic therapy alone without adequate source control through drainage frequently fails to resolve a well-formed abscess regardless of the antibiotic agent selected.

Oral Versus Intravenous Route Selection

The oral route is appropriate and effective for the substantial majority of uncomplicated cellulitis and erysipelas presentations in patients able to tolerate oral intake and without signs of systemic toxicity, and current evidence does not support a general assumption that intravenous therapy is more effective than appropriately dosed oral therapy for uncomplicated disease, meaning the intravenous route should be reserved for patients with systemic toxicity, an inability to tolerate oral medication, rapidly progressive disease, or failure of an adequate oral regimen rather than selected by default for infections that appear moderately severe on visual inspection alone. This evidence-based preference for the oral route where clinically appropriate also reduces the cost, resource utilization, and line-associated complication risk associated with unnecessary intravenous therapy and hospitalization.

Duration of Therapy and Assessing Treatment Response

Treatment duration for uncomplicated cellulitis is generally five to ten days depending on clinical response, with current stewardship-oriented practice favoring the shorter end of this range for patients demonstrating clear improvement, and clinical improvement, reduction in erythema, warmth, and tenderness, is expected within forty-eight to seventy-two hours of appropriate therapy, since it is important to note that the visible border of erythema is often marked at the initial visit specifically to allow objective assessment of progression or improvement at follow-up, a simple, low-cost practice that meaningfully improves the accuracy of treatment response assessment compared with relying on subjective recollection of the initial extent of erythema alone.

EVIDENCE: Marking the visible border of cellulitis erythema at the initial visit provides an objective reference for assessing progression or improvement at follow-up and should be routine practice whenever cellulitis is diagnosed.

Apparent treatment failure at the forty-eight to seventy-two hour reassessment, applying the diagnostic-approach principle that inadequate response to appropriately selected therapy should prompt reconsideration rather than automatic escalation of the same agent class, should trigger review of several possibilities in a specific order: first, confirmation of adherence and correct dosing; second, reconsideration of the working diagnosis itself, since a poorly responding presumed cellulitis may in fact be one of the noninfectious mimics discussed earlier in this chapter; third, consideration of an inadequately covered organism, particularly methicillin-resistant Staphylococcus aureus if not initially covered; and only after these possibilities have been addressed, escalation to a broader-spectrum agent or the intravenous route, since reflexive broadening of antibiotic coverage without first working through this sequence frequently fails to address the actual reason for apparent treatment failure.

Erythrasma and Other Superficial Bacterial Conditions

Erythrasma

Erythrasma, caused by Corynebacterium minutissimum, presents as well-demarcated, reddish-brown, minimally scaling patches in intertriginous sites, most often the groin, axillae, and toe webs, and is frequently mistaken for a dermatophyte infection or intertriginous candidiasis given the shared intertriginous distribution, though erythrasma characteristically demonstrates the coral-red Wood lamp fluorescence introduced in the diagnostic-approach chapter, reflecting porphyrin production by the causative organism, a simple and rapid bedside test that reliably distinguishes it from its fungal mimics without requiring culture or biopsy.

Pitted Keratolysis

Pitted keratolysis, caused by several Corynebacterium and Kytococcus species that produce keratin-degrading proteases, presents with characteristic punched-out pits on the weight-bearing plantar surface, frequently associated with malodor and hyperhidrosis given the moist, occlusive footwear environment that favors bacterial proliferation, and management centers on reducing moisture through improved foot hygiene, moisture-wicking socks, and antiperspirant use, combined with a topical antibacterial agent for more symptomatic or extensive cases.

Trichomycosis

Trichomycosis, a superficial bacterial colonization of axillary or pubic hair shafts by Corynebacterium species, produces yellow, red, or black granular concretions adherent to the hair shaft itself rather than a rash on the surrounding skin, and is frequently associated with hyperhidrosis, similarly to pitted keratolysis, reinforcing that this family of superficial corynebacterial conditions shares moisture and occlusion as a common underlying predisposing factor despite their distinct individual clinical presentations.

CLINICAL PEARL: Coral-red fluorescence on Wood lamp examination reliably distinguishes erythrasma from its dermatophyte and candidal mimics at the bedside without requiring culture, biopsy, or a trial of antifungal therapy.

This family of superficial bacterial conditions is frequently underrecognized in general medical practice precisely because each is easily mistaken for a fungal process given the shared intertriginous or moisture-associated distribution, and a low threshold for Wood lamp examination or, where unavailable, empiric consideration of a topical antibacterial rather than antifungal agent when a presumed fungal infection fails to respond to appropriate antifungal therapy can meaningfully shorten time to correct diagnosis in these commonly overlooked conditions.

Bite Wound Infections

Animal Bite Wounds

Dog and cat bite wounds carry a substantial polymicrobial infection risk reflecting the diverse oral flora of the biting animal, with Pasteurella multocida a particularly important and rapidly progressive pathogen in cat bites given the organism's frequent presence in feline oral flora and the deep puncture wounds characteristic of cat bites, which inoculate bacteria deep into tissue despite a deceptively small entry wound. Cat bites in particular warrant a lower threshold for prophylactic antibiotic therapy given both this deep puncture mechanism and the rapid, aggressive infection course Pasteurella multocida can produce, often becoming clinically apparent within twelve to twenty-four hours, considerably faster than the typical time course for most other bacterial skin and soft tissue infections discussed in this chapter.

Human Bite Wounds

Human bite wounds, including the closed-fist injury sustained when a clenched fist strikes another person's teeth, a mechanism that should be specifically asked about given patient reluctance to volunteer the true circumstances of the injury, carry a particularly high infection risk from a polymicrobial mixture of aerobic and anaerobic oral flora and warrant prompt wound exploration to assess for joint or tendon sheath involvement, especially for wounds overlying the metacarpophalangeal joints, given the substantial risk of deep space infection and the functional consequences of inadequately treated tendon sheath or joint infection at this site.

General Bite Wound Management Principles

Bite wound management includes thorough irrigation and debridement, assessment of tetanus immunization status with booster administration when indicated, consideration of rabies postexposure prophylaxis based on the biting animal species, behavior, and local epidemiology, and prophylactic or therapeutic antibiotic coverage selected to address the polymicrobial flora relevant to the specific biting species, with amoxicillin-clavulanate a commonly used empiric choice given its coverage of both Pasteurella and typical oral anaerobic flora, confirmed against current guideline recommendations and local antibiogram data.

CAUTION: A hand wound presenting after an altercation should be specifically evaluated for a closed-fist human bite injury even when the patient does not volunteer this mechanism, given the substantial risk of joint or tendon sheath involvement at this specific location.

Primary wound closure of a bite wound is generally avoided for hand wounds and for wounds presenting more than several hours after injury, given the elevated infection risk discussed throughout this section, with delayed closure or healing by secondary intention favored in these higher-risk circumstances, while facial bite wounds, given both cosmetic considerations and generally excellent vascular supply at this site, are more often closed primarily after thorough irrigation, illustrating that wound closure decisions in bite injuries should be individualized to anatomic site and time since injury rather than applied uniformly.

Complications, Special Populations, and Prevention

Poststreptococcal Complications of Untreated Streptococcal Skin Infection

Untreated or inadequately treated streptococcal skin infection, impetigo in particular, carries a recognized risk of poststreptococcal glomerulonephritis, an immune complex-mediated renal complication that develops one to three weeks after the inciting skin infection and is not reliably prevented by antibiotic treatment of the underlying skin infection once the nephritogenic strain has already triggered the immune process, in contrast to poststreptococcal complications following pharyngitis, where prompt antibiotic treatment does meaningfully reduce the risk of subsequent acute rheumatic fever. This distinction is clinically important: antibiotic treatment of streptococcal impetigo remains appropriate for symptomatic and public health reasons, reducing contagious spread and hastening symptom resolution, but should not be presented to patients or families as reliably preventing poststreptococcal glomerulonephritis, since the evidence for that specific protective effect is considerably weaker than for the analogous pharyngitis-associated rheumatic fever relationship.

Complications of Inadequately Treated Infection

Inadequately treated or recurrent cellulitis can produce chronic lymphedema through cumulative lymphatic damage, which in turn predisposes to further episodes of cellulitis, creating a self-perpetuating cycle analogous in structure to the itch-scratch cycle discussed in the eczematous dermatoses chapter, and this cycle underscores the value of aggressive treatment of the first episode and of addressing modifiable predisposing factors, tinea pedis, venous insufficiency, and obesity chief among them, to reduce the risk of recurrence and the resulting cumulative lymphatic damage. Bacteremia and, rarely, endocarditis or osteomyelitis by contiguous or hematogenous spread are recognized complications of inadequately controlled skin and soft tissue infection, particularly in immunocompromised or otherwise vulnerable patients.

Special Populations: Diabetes and Immunosuppression

Patients with diabetes mellitus warrant particular attention given impaired local immune response, peripheral neuropathy that can mask the pain that would otherwise prompt earlier presentation, and the frequency of foot-based portal of entry from unrecognized minor trauma, and any foot infection in a patient with diabetes warrants careful assessment for osteomyelitis, especially with a chronic, non-healing wound, given the substantially elevated risk of contiguous bone involvement in this population. Immunosuppressed patients, whether from medication, malignancy, or another underlying condition, may present with blunted inflammatory signs despite substantial underlying infection, and a lower threshold for aggressive evaluation and empiric treatment is warranted in this population given the reduced reliability of clinical severity assessment based on visible inflammatory findings alone.

Special Populations: Neonates and Young Infants

Skin and soft tissue infections in neonates and very young infants warrant a lower threshold for hospitalization and intravenous antibiotic therapy compared with older children and adults, given both the immature immune system's reduced capacity to contain a localized infection and the correspondingly higher risk of rapid progression to bacteremia and systemic sepsis, and even a clinically limited-appearing infection in this age group should be evaluated with particular caution rather than assumed to follow the same benign course typically expected in an older, immunocompetent patient. Omphalitis, infection of the umbilical stump, deserves specific mention in this population, presenting with periumbilical erythema, induration, or purulent discharge, and warranting prompt treatment given the direct anatomic proximity to the peritoneal cavity and abdominal wall vasculature, which creates a potential pathway for rapid, serious systemic spread not present with skin infection at other neonatal sites.

Prevention and Reducing Recurrence

Prevention of recurrent bacterial skin and soft tissue infection centers on identifying and addressing modifiable predisposing factors: treating tinea pedis to eliminate a common portal of entry for lower extremity cellulitis, managing venous insufficiency and associated edema, optimizing glycemic control in patients with diabetes, and, for recurrent furunculosis, considering a staphylococcal decolonization protocol as introduced earlier in this chapter. Patient education on early recognition of infection, particularly in patients with a history of recurrent cellulitis or lymphedema, supports prompt treatment initiation before an episode progresses to the point of requiring hospitalization or intravenous therapy.

Clinical Case: Recognizing a Necrotizing Infection Red Flag

A 55-year-old man with type 2 diabetes presents with a one-day history of rapidly worsening left lower leg pain and swelling, initially attributed to a minor scrape sustained two days earlier while gardening. On examination, there is diffuse erythema and edema of the leg with poorly defined margins, and while the visible skin findings appear only moderately severe, the patient reports pain out of all proportion to what the examiner would expect from the visible findings alone, rating his pain as ten out of ten and requiring intravenous analgesia even before any wound manipulation has occurred. Vital signs reveal a mild tachycardia and low-grade fever.

Applying the Pattern Anchor established in the Rhythm Layer callout earlier in this chapter, pain disproportionate to visible skin findings is recognized immediately as the critical red flag finding that overrides the only moderately concerning visual appearance of the leg, and this finding alone, in a patient with diabetes and a portal of entry from minor trauma, is sufficient to warrant urgent surgical consultation for possible necrotizing soft tissue infection rather than continued outpatient management for presumed uncomplicated cellulitis. Laboratory testing is obtained emergently, and imaging is pursued to further evaluate for the presence of soft tissue gas or fascial plane involvement, while broad-spectrum empiric antibiotic therapy covering the polymicrobial flora typical of necrotizing infections is initiated immediately rather than delayed pending confirmatory imaging or laboratory results, consistent with the emergent nature of this diagnostic concern.

Surgical exploration confirms early necrotizing fasciitis, and prompt surgical debridement is performed, illustrating directly why the disproportionate-pain finding, easily overlooked if the examiner focuses primarily on the visual appearance of the skin, was the single most important clinical data point in this presentation. The patient's diabetes and the minor traumatic portal of entry, both discussed earlier in this chapter as predisposing factors, are documented as contributing factors, and his case reinforces the broader principle that disproportionate pain should always be actively elicited and weighted heavily, rather than passively noted, in any patient presenting with an apparent skin and soft tissue infection.

KEY POINT: Pain disproportionate to visible skin findings should trigger urgent evaluation for necrotizing soft tissue infection regardless of how reassuring the visual appearance of the skin itself may seem, and this history should be actively elicited rather than passively noted.

Clinical Case: Recurrent Furunculosis and Decolonization

A 26-year-old otherwise healthy man presents with his fourth episode of a painful furuncle over the past year, this time on his right thigh, each prior episode having required incision and drainage with resolution between episodes. He denies any known contacts with similar infections and has no history of diabetes or other predisposing systemic illness identified on prior evaluation. Physical examination confirms a fluctuant, tender nodule consistent with a furuncle, without surrounding cellulitis or systemic symptoms.

Applying the recurrent furunculosis framework introduced earlier in this chapter, incision and drainage is performed as primary therapy for this acute episode, consistent with the principle that adequate source control is the most important intervention for a fluctuant lesion regardless of antibiotic use, and a wound culture is sent given the recurrent nature of his presentation to confirm the causative organism and assess for methicillin resistance, information that will inform both this episode's antibiotic selection if needed and future decolonization planning. Given four episodes within a year, evaluation for predisposing factors is pursued, including screening for diabetes, which returns normal, and nasal swab culture for Staphylococcus aureus carriage, which returns positive, identifying his own nasal colonization as the most likely reservoir driving recurrent autoinoculation of his skin.

He is counseled on and started on a staphylococcal decolonization protocol, including intranasal mupirocin applied twice daily for five days, chlorhexidine body washes, and attention to personal hygiene measures including not sharing towels or razors and regularly laundering bedding and clothing in hot water, an approach directly targeting the nasal reservoir identified as his specific driver of recurrence rather than relying on antibiotic treatment of each individual episode alone. At six-month follow-up, he reports no further furuncle episodes, illustrating how identifying and addressing an individual patient's specific predisposing factor, in his case nasal carriage rather than diabetes or another systemic contributor, can break a pattern of recurrent infection that repeated antibiotic courses alone had failed to prevent.

CLINICAL PEARL: Recurrent furunculosis warrants nasal Staphylococcus aureus carriage screening and, when positive, a structured decolonization protocol, since treating each individual episode without addressing an identified carriage reservoir frequently fails to prevent recurrence.

THE MORPHOLOGY-TO-MANAGEMENT SYSTEM — Bacterial Skin and Soft Tissue Infection Depth Arc

Pattern Introduced This Chapter: Acute unilateral lower extremity erythema, discriminated by depth (erysipelas versus cellulitis), laterality and onset (versus stasis dermatitis), and disproportionate pain (versus necrotizing fasciitis).

Cross-Cutting Anchor: Depth of infection, epidermal (impetigo), superficial dermal/lymphatic (erysipelas), or deep dermal/subcutaneous (cellulitis), directly predicts both border character and appropriate treatment intensity, while disproportionate pain overrides all other findings as the anchor for necrotizing infection.

Summary and Key Concepts

Impetigo, erysipelas, and cellulitis represent progressively deeper bacterial infection of the skin, and border character, sharply demarcated versus poorly defined, directly reflects this depth of involvement.

Stasis dermatitis and deep vein thrombosis are the most commonly encountered noninfectious mimics of cellulitis and are distinguished by laterality, onset tempo, and the presence or absence of systemic symptoms and marked tenderness.

Pain disproportionate to visible skin findings is the single most important red flag for necrotizing soft tissue infection and should override an otherwise reassuring visual appearance.

Staphylococcal scalded skin syndrome, toxic shock syndrome, and scarlet fever are toxin-mediated syndromes distinguished from primary infection by their systemic, often distant-source-driven pathophysiology.

Empiric antibiotic selection should be guided by local resistance patterns and the specific clinical presentation, with incision and drainage remaining the primary therapy for fluctuant abscesses regardless of antibiotic selection.

CHAPTER 9: VIRAL CUTANEOUS INFECTIONS

Learning Objectives

1. Distinguish primary from recurrent herpes simplex virus infection and recognize its major clinical variants.
2. Explain the pathophysiologic relationship between varicella and herpes zoster and apply this relationship to recognition and management of each.
3. Recognize the major human papillomavirus-associated verrucae and select an appropriate treatment approach for each.
4. Distinguish molluscum contagiosum from its principal morphologic mimics.
5. Apply antiviral therapy appropriately across herpesvirus infections, including special considerations in immunocompromised and pregnant patients.

Herpes Simplex Virus Infections

Primary and Recurrent Infection

Herpes simplex virus establishes lifelong latency within sensory ganglia following primary infection, with herpes simplex virus type 1 classically associated with orofacial disease and herpes simplex virus type 2 classically associated with genital disease, though considerable overlap exists in both directions given changes in sexual practices and the fact that either viral type can infect either anatomic site. Primary infection, occurring in a host without preexisting immunity to the specific viral type, is often more severe and more likely to produce systemic symptoms than recurrent disease, since recurrent episodes benefit from partial preexisting immunity that limits both viral replication and symptom severity, explaining why a patient's first clinically apparent episode is not necessarily their true primary infection if prior subclinical primary infection has already occurred.

Clinical Presentation

Herpes simplex virus infection presents with grouped vesicles on an erythematous base, the herpetiform configuration introduced in the diagnostic-language chapter of this book, that evolve to erosions and crust over several days, typically preceded by a prodrome of localized tingling, burning, or itching that, once recognized by a patient with recurrent disease, can allow initiation of antiviral therapy before the eruption becomes fully established. Recurrent orolabial herpes, commonly termed a cold sore or fever blister, tends to recur at the same anatomic site with each episode, reflecting reactivation from the same latently infected sensory ganglion each time, while recurrent genital herpes similarly tends to localize to a consistent, though sometimes broader, anatomic distribution corresponding to the sacral ganglia harboring the latent virus.

Herpetic Whitlow and Other Variants

Herpetic whitlow, a herpes simplex virus infection of the distal finger, occurs through direct inoculation, historically common among healthcare workers before routine glove use and now more often seen in young children who autoinoculate from an oral lesion through thumb-sucking, and presents with painful grouped vesicles on the digit that can be mistaken for a bacterial paronychia, an important distinction since incision and drainage, appropriate for a bacterial paronychia, is not indicated and can worsen or prolong a herpetic whitlow. Herpes gladiatorum, a cutaneous herpes simplex virus infection transmitted through skin-to-skin contact in contact sports, most classically wrestling, presents with grouped vesicles at the site of contact and carries public health implications given the requirement in many athletic settings that affected athletes be excluded from competition until lesions have fully crusted to prevent transmission to opponents.

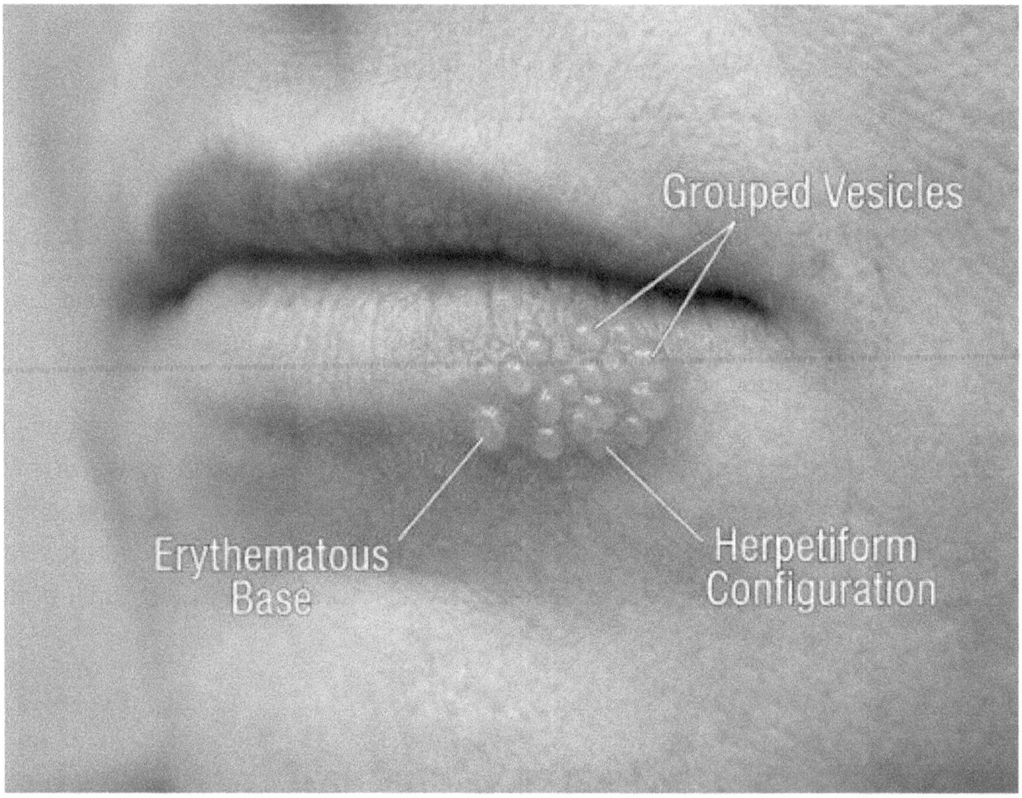

Varicella-Zoster Virus: Varicella and Herpes Zoster

Varicella (Chickenpox)

Primary varicella-zoster virus infection produces varicella, characterized by successive crops of lesions in different stages of evolution, macules progressing to papules, vesicles, and crusts, appearing over several days and producing the characteristic pattern often described as resembling a starry sky given the simultaneous presence of lesions at multiple distinct stages within the same anatomic region, a finding that itself carries diagnostic value distinguishing varicella from other vesicular eruptions that tend to present with more uniform lesion staging. Widespread varicella vaccination has substantially reduced disease incidence and severity in vaccinated populations, though breakthrough infection in vaccinated individuals can still occur, typically presenting with a milder, more limited eruption and fewer total lesions than unvaccinated primary infection.

Herpes Zoster (Shingles)

Herpes zoster results from reactivation of latent varicella-zoster virus within a single sensory ganglion, producing the sharply demarcated, unilateral, dermatomal eruption introduced in the diagnostic-language chapter of this book, most often affecting a thoracic dermatome, though ophthalmic zoster, involving the ophthalmic division of the trigeminal nerve, carries specific risk to vision and warrants urgent ophthalmologic evaluation, particularly when lesions involve the tip of the nose, a finding termed the Hutchinson sign that reflects nasociliary nerve involvement and correlates with an increased risk of ocular complications. Risk factors for zoster reactivation include advancing age, reflecting age-related decline in cell-mediated immunity to the virus, and any cause of immunosuppression, and recurrent zoster, particularly at a young age or with recurrent episodes, should prompt consideration of an underlying immunocompromising condition.

Postherpetic Neuralgia

Postherpetic neuralgia, persistent pain in the affected dermatome lasting beyond the resolution of the cutaneous eruption, represents the most common and often most functionally disabling complication of herpes zoster, with risk increasing substantially with advancing patient age, and prompt initiation of antiviral therapy within seventy-two hours of rash onset, discussed further later in this chapter, reduces both the severity of the acute eruption and, to a meaningful degree, the risk of subsequent postherpetic neuralgia, underscoring the value of rapid recognition and treatment initiation in this condition.

Feature	Herpes Simplex Virus	Varicella-Zoster Virus (Zoster)
Distribution	Localized, tends to recur at the same site	Unilateral, strictly dermatomal
Lesion Staging	Uniform within a given episode	Uniform within a given dermatome at a given time
Prodrome	Localized tingling/burning, hours to a day before	Localized pain or dysesthesia, often days before rash
Recurrence Pattern	Frequent, at the same site	Uncommon in a given dermatome; recurrent episodes at a young age warrant immune evaluation

CAUTION: Herpes zoster lesions involving the tip of the nose (a positive Hutchinson sign) indicate nasociliary nerve involvement and correlate with an increased risk of ocular complications, warranting urgent ophthalmologic evaluation regardless of whether visual symptoms are yet present.

THE MORPHOLOGY-TO-MANAGEMENT SYSTEM — The Dermatomal Vesicular Eruption Arc

---

The Pattern: A sharply demarcated, unilateral, dermatomal eruption of grouped vesicles on an erythematous base, often preceded by localized pain or dysesthesia.

Presentation Variance: Erythema underlying the vesicles can be considerably less apparent in richly pigmented skin, and post-inflammatory hyperpigmentation or, less commonly, hypopigmentation following resolution can persist for months, occasionally being mistaken for a separate or ongoing process if the patient is not counseled about this expected course at the time of initial diagnosis and treatment.

Trap Logic: Herpes simplex virus infection outside the genital or orolabial region can mimic zoster but typically lacks strict dermatomal confinement and more often recurs at the same limited site with each episode rather than following a full dermatomal distribution; contact dermatitis, discussed in an earlier chapter, can occasionally present with a linear or band-like pattern but lacks the grouped vesicular morphology and the characteristic neuropathic prodromal pain of zoster.

Management Pivot: Antiviral therapy, most commonly valacyclovir or famciclovir, should be initiated within seventy-two hours of rash onset when possible to reduce both acute severity and postherpetic neuralgia risk, with ophthalmologic referral for any ophthalmic-division involvement or Hutchinson sign, and pain management addressed proactively given the substantial burden of both acute zoster pain and potential postherpetic neuralgia.

Pattern Anchor: Strict unilateral dermatomal confinement, not crossing the midline, is the anchor finding that most reliably distinguishes herpes zoster from every other vesicular eruption discussed in this chapter.

Human Papillomavirus: Verrucae

Common, Plantar, and Flat Warts

Human papillomavirus infects keratinocytes and induces epidermal hyperproliferation, producing verrucae whose clinical appearance varies by anatomic site and infecting viral subtype: common warts present as hyperkeratotic, verrucous papules most often on the hands, plantar warts present as endophytic, inward-growing lesions on weight-bearing plantar surfaces where mechanical pressure drives the wart to grow inward rather than outward, producing a rougher, more painful lesion than its surface appearance alone might suggest, and flat warts present as minimally elevated, smooth, flesh-colored to slightly hyperpigmented papules most often on the face and dorsal hands, frequently spread by shaving or scratching given their tendency toward autoinoculation along lines of trauma.

Epidermodysplasia Verruciformis and Verruca in the Immunocompromised Host

Epidermodysplasia verruciformis, a rare inherited disorder of abnormal susceptibility to specific human papillomavirus subtypes, produces widespread, treatment-refractory flat wart-like lesions with a substantial long-term risk of malignant transformation to squamous cell carcinoma at sun-exposed sites, illustrating an extreme end of the spectrum of human papillomavirus susceptibility that, while individually rare, provides useful conceptual grounding for understanding why immunocompromised patients more broadly, including solid organ transplant recipients on chronic immunosuppression, develop more numerous, more treatment-resistant verrucae than immunocompetent patients, given the shared underlying theme of impaired cell-mediated immune surveillance against this viral family. Transplant recipients in particular warrant closer surveillance of extensive or atypical verrucae given both this increased burden and the independently elevated skin cancer risk this population carries, discussed further in the chapter on keratinocyte carcinoma.

Anogenital Warts

Anogenital warts, caused predominantly by human papillomavirus subtypes distinct from those causing cutaneous verrucae and associated with sexual transmission, present as soft, exophytic, cauliflower-like papules on the genital or perianal skin and mucosa, and their presence, particularly in a child, should prompt careful consideration of the transmission route, including the possibility of perinatal transmission in an infant or, in an older child, the need to consider and appropriately evaluate for sexual abuse, a sensitive determination requiring careful, individualized clinical judgment rather than a reflexive assumption in either direction.

Treatment Approaches

Verrucae frequently resolve spontaneously over months to years as cell-mediated immunity to the infecting viral subtype develops, and this natural history should inform a shared decision-making discussion regarding treatment, particularly in children, where observation alone is a reasonable option for asymptomatic lesions. Destructive therapies, including topical salicylic acid, cryotherapy, and, for refractory lesions, more aggressive procedural options discussed in the office-based procedures chapter, remain first-line for patients desiring active treatment, while immunotherapy approaches, including topical sensitizing agents, are reserved for refractory, extensive, or treatment-resistant disease.

PATIENT EDUCATION: Many verrucae resolve spontaneously over months to years without any treatment as the immune system develops recognition of the infecting viral subtype, and observation is a reasonable option for asymptomatic lesions, particularly in children.

Combination therapy, most often pairing a destructive modality such as cryotherapy with home application of topical salicylic acid between office visits, frequently achieves better resolution rates than either approach alone, illustrating a treatment principle analogous to the combination strategies discussed in the acne chapter, in which agents addressing complementary aspects of the underlying pathophysiology outperform escalating a single modality in isolation.

Molluscum Contagiosum

Clinical Presentation

Molluscum contagiosum, caused by a poxvirus distinct from the varicella-zoster and herpes simplex viruses discussed earlier in this chapter, produces discrete, dome-shaped, umbilicated papules with a characteristic central dell, most common in children, in whom it spreads by direct skin contact and autoinoculation, and in sexually active adults, in whom genital involvement suggests sexual transmission. As introduced in the atopic dermatitis chapter, children with atopic dermatitis experience more extensive and prolonged molluscum involvement given both the disrupted barrier and local immune dysregulation characteristic of that condition, and surrounding molluscum dermatitis, an eczematous reaction to the molluscum lesions themselves, is a common associated finding in this population that should be managed with continued appropriate anti-inflammatory therapy for the dermatitis component.

Differential Diagnosis

Molluscum contagiosum's characteristic central umbilication, best appreciated on close inspection or with dermoscopy, distinguishes it from other dome-shaped papular processes; in an immunocompromised patient, particularly one with advanced HIV infection, disseminated cutaneous cryptococcosis or other opportunistic infections can produce umbilicated papules closely mimicking molluscum contagiosum, and this mimicry should prompt biopsy for definitive diagnosis in an immunocompromised patient with an atypically extensive or treatment-refractory molluscum-like eruption rather than assuming molluscum contagiosum by morphology alone in this specific population.

Management

Molluscum contagiosum is self-limited in immunocompetent hosts, typically resolving over six to twelve months without treatment, and observation remains a reasonable first-line approach, particularly for limited, asymptomatic disease in a young child, while destructive therapies, including cryotherapy, curettage, or topical cantharidin, are appropriate options for patients or families desiring active treatment given the disease's contagiousness and cosmetic impact, with the treatment decision individualized based on lesion number, location, patient age and tolerance for a procedural approach, and family preference.

CLINICAL PEARL: The characteristic central umbilication of molluscum contagiosum, best appreciated on close inspection, is the key distinguishing feature from other dome-shaped papular eruptions and should be specifically sought whenever this diagnosis is being considered.

Topical cantharidin, a vesicant applied by the clinician and washed off by the patient several hours later at home, induces localized blister formation that removes the lesion and is generally well tolerated by children given the painless application, in contrast to cryotherapy, which causes immediate discomfort at the time of treatment, a practical consideration that often makes cantharidin the preferred initial active-treatment option specifically in young children who may not tolerate cryotherapy well.

Viral Exanthems

Measles, Rubella, and Roseola

Measles presents with a cephalocaudal-spreading, morbilliform, erythematous maculopapular eruption preceded by a prodrome of fever, cough, coryza, and conjunctivitis, with Koplik spots, small white lesions on the buccal mucosa, appearing shortly before the cutaneous eruption and carrying substantial diagnostic value when present, and recognition carries important public health implications given measles' high contagiousness and the need for prompt isolation and public health notification. Rubella produces a milder, more discrete pink maculopapular eruption with a similar cephalocaudal spread but a shorter overall course and, in contrast to measles, is particularly concerning when contracted during pregnancy given the substantial risk of congenital rubella syndrome, making rubella immunity status a relevant consideration during preconception counseling. Roseola infantum, caused by human herpesvirus 6 or 7, presents with several days of high fever in an infant, followed by resolution of fever with the near-simultaneous appearance of a diffuse, pink, macular eruption, a temporal pattern, fever resolution followed immediately by rash onset, that itself provides substantial diagnostic value.

Differentiating Viral Exanthems From Drug Eruptions

Many viral exanthems produce a morbilliform, maculopapular eruption that closely resembles the appearance of a common morbilliform drug eruption, and distinguishing the two depends heavily on the correlated clinical context introduced in the diagnostic-approach chapter: a preceding viral prodrome, fever, coryza, and conjunctivitis in the case of measles, or the specific temporal pattern of roseola, favors a viral etiology, while a temporal relationship to a new medication, particularly one started seven to fourteen days before eruption onset consistent with the classic drug-eruption timeline discussed in that earlier chapter, favors a drug cause. This distinction carries direct management significance, since a presumed viral exanthem requires no medication changes while a drug eruption requires identification and discontinuation of the causative agent, and in a patient with both a recent viral illness and a recently started medication, the two possibilities must be carefully weighed together rather than assuming either explanation reflexively.

Erythema Infectiosum and Hand-Foot-and-Mouth Disease

Erythema infectiosum, caused by parvovirus B19, produces the characteristic slapped-cheek facial erythema followed by a lacy, reticulated eruption on the extremities, and carries specific risk in pregnant patients, given the potential for fetal hydrops from parvovirus-induced suppression of fetal erythropoiesis, and in patients with chronic hemolytic anemia, in whom parvovirus infection can precipitate a transient aplastic crisis, both considerations that should prompt specific counseling and, where relevant, additional monitoring beyond the typically mild and self-limited course in an otherwise healthy child. Hand-foot-and-mouth disease, most often caused by coxsackievirus, produces oral vesicles and erosions along with vesicular or papular lesions on the palms, soles, and, in a pattern increasingly recognized with certain circulating strains, more widespread involvement including the buttocks and extremities, and is typically self-limited in children though can occasionally cause more severe systemic illness.

Diagnostic Workup for Viral Cutaneous Infections

Tzanck Smear and Direct Fluorescent Antibody Testing

A Tzanck smear, prepared by scraping the base of an unroofed vesicle and staining the sample to identify multinucleated giant keratinocytes, provides a rapid, inexpensive bedside test supporting a herpesvirus diagnosis, herpes simplex virus or varicella-zoster virus, though it cannot distinguish between the two given their shared cytopathic effect on infected keratinocytes, a limitation that should be communicated when this test is used and that direct fluorescent antibody testing, using virus-specific antibodies to distinguish herpes simplex virus from varicella-zoster virus directly from a similar vesicle scraping, can resolve when that specific distinction carries clinical significance.

Viral Culture and Polymerase Chain Reaction Testing

Polymerase chain reaction testing has largely superseded viral culture as the preferred confirmatory test for herpes simplex virus and varicella-zoster virus infection given its substantially higher sensitivity, particularly for lesions that have already begun to crust, at which point viral culture yield drops considerably as intact viral particles become less available for culture recovery, and polymerase chain reaction testing additionally allows reliable viral typing, herpes simplex virus type 1 versus type 2, information with counseling implications for a patient with a new genital herpes diagnosis given the somewhat different natural history and recurrence patterns of the two viral types at this anatomic site.

Serologic Testing and Its Limitations

Type-specific herpes simplex virus serology can identify prior infection and, in some circumstances, support a diagnosis when active lesions are not available for direct testing, but serologic testing has substantial limitations for acute diagnosis: antibody development lags behind primary infection by weeks, meaning serology can be falsely negative early in a true primary infection, and a positive result cannot by itself confirm that a current lesion represents active herpes simplex virus disease rather than an incidental finding of prior infection, underscoring why direct testing of an active lesion, by polymerase chain reaction or Tzanck smear, remains the preferred diagnostic approach whenever an active, testable lesion is available.

KEY POINT: Polymerase chain reaction testing of an active lesion is the preferred confirmatory test for herpes simplex virus and varicella-zoster virus infection, offering higher sensitivity than viral culture and, unlike a Tzanck smear, reliably distinguishing between the two viruses and, for herpes simplex virus, between viral types.

Clinical diagnosis based on the characteristic morphology, distribution, and history discussed throughout this chapter remains entirely appropriate and sufficient for most typical presentations, and laboratory confirmation should be reserved for situations where the diagnosis is genuinely uncertain, where the specific viral type or species carries meaningful management or counseling implications, or where an atypical presentation in an immunocompromised host raises concern for an alternative diagnosis, rather than applied reflexively to every classic, easily recognized presentation.

Management, Complications, and Special Populations

Symptomatic and Supportive Care

Beyond specific antiviral therapy where indicated, symptomatic management plays a substantial role across the viral cutaneous infections discussed in this chapter: oral or topical analgesics for the pain associated with herpes zoster and, when needed, herpetic whitlow; antipyretics and oral hydration for the febrile viral exanthems discussed earlier in this chapter; and, for varicella specifically, measures to reduce scratching and secondary bacterial infection given the substantial pruritus varicella lesions can produce, since secondary bacterial superinfection of scratched varicella lesions is a recognized complication that can itself require additional antibiotic therapy and, rarely, more severe invasive streptococcal or staphylococcal disease originating from this superinfected skin breach.

Antiviral Therapy Principles

Antiviral therapy for herpes simplex virus and varicella-zoster virus infections, most commonly acyclovir, valacyclovir, or famciclovir, is most effective when initiated early in the disease course, ideally within the first seventy-two hours for zoster as discussed earlier in this chapter, or at the earliest prodromal symptom for recurrent herpes simplex virus infection, and suppressive antiviral therapy is a reasonable option for patients with frequent recurrent genital or orolabial herpes simplex virus outbreaks given both symptom reduction and, for genital disease, reduction in transmission risk to sexual partners.

Immunocompromised Hosts

Immunocompromised patients, whether from HIV infection, transplant-related immunosuppression, or another cause, are at risk for more severe, more extensive, and atypical presentations of every viral infection discussed in this chapter, including disseminated or chronic ulcerative herpes simplex virus infection, disseminated varicella-zoster virus involving multiple dermatomes or visceral organs, and extensive, treatment-refractory molluscum contagiosum or verrucae, and this population warrants a lower threshold for antiviral therapy, higher doses when treatment is initiated, and closer follow-up than immunocompetent patients with analogous presentations.

Disseminated Zoster in the Immunocompromised Host

While herpes zoster in an immunocompetent host is expected to remain confined to a single dermatome as emphasized earlier in this chapter, disseminated zoster, defined as involvement extending beyond the primary and one adjacent dermatome or involvement of internal organs, occurs almost exclusively in immunocompromised patients and represents a substantially more severe disease process warranting intravenous antiviral therapy and, given the risk of visceral involvement including pneumonitis, hepatitis, and encephalitis, close inpatient monitoring rather than outpatient management. Recognizing that dermatomal confinement is itself a marker of adequate immune containment reframes disseminated disease not simply as a more extensive version of typical zoster but as a qualitatively different clinical entity reflecting a fundamentally impaired host immune response, with correspondingly different management urgency and intensity.

Neonatal Herpes Simplex Virus Infection

Neonatal herpes simplex virus infection, typically acquired during vaginal delivery from a mother with active genital herpes simplex virus infection at the time of delivery, carries substantial morbidity and mortality risk given the immature neonatal immune system's limited capacity to contain the infection, and can present with localized skin, eye, and mouth disease, central nervous system disease, or disseminated multiorgan disease, with the more severe presentations often lacking prominent cutaneous findings at initial presentation, making a high index of suspicion in an ill neonate with any maternal herpes simplex virus history essential regardless of whether cutaneous vesicles are yet apparent.

CAUTION: Neonatal herpes simplex virus infection can present with severe central nervous system or disseminated disease without prominent cutaneous findings at initial presentation, and a high index of suspicion is warranted in any ill neonate with a relevant maternal history.

Coordinated communication between obstetric, neonatal, and dermatologic teams around a mother with active or recently diagnosed genital herpes simplex virus infection at the time of delivery substantially improves early recognition and treatment of the neonate, since prompt initiation of neonatal antiviral therapy meaningfully improves outcomes across all three clinical presentations discussed above, and a shared, explicit management plan established before delivery whenever possible reduces the risk of diagnostic delay in an ill neonate presenting soon after birth.

Pregnancy, Vaccination, and Eczema Herpeticum

Herpesvirus Infection in Pregnancy

Primary genital herpes simplex virus infection acquired late in pregnancy carries a substantially higher risk of neonatal transmission than recurrent maternal infection, since the mother has not yet developed the protective antibody response that would otherwise cross the placenta and provide the neonate some degree of passive immunity, and a woman presenting with a first-episode genital herpes simplex virus infection in the third trimester requires coordinated obstetric management, including consideration of suppressive antiviral therapy approaching delivery and, in some circumstances, cesarean delivery if active lesions are present at the time of labor, to reduce the risk of the severe neonatal disease discussed earlier in this chapter. Varicella infection acquired during pregnancy carries its own distinct risk profile: infection in the first half of pregnancy carries a small but recognized risk of congenital varicella syndrome, producing limb hypoplasia, cutaneous scarring, and neurologic abnormalities in the affected fetus, while infection very close to delivery carries a risk of severe neonatal varicella given the neonate's limited passive immunity and immature immune response in this circumstance.

Vaccination as Primary Prevention

Varicella vaccination in childhood has substantially reduced the incidence and severity of primary varicella infection, as discussed earlier in this chapter, and herpes zoster vaccination in appropriate older adult populations meaningfully reduces both the incidence of zoster reactivation and the severity and duration of breakthrough cases that do occur, representing a direct, evidence-based preventive strategy against both the acute disease and the postherpetic neuralgia risk discussed earlier in this chapter. Human papillomavirus vaccination, while primarily indicated for prevention of the oncogenic viral subtypes associated with anogenital and oropharyngeal malignancy rather than the cutaneous verrucae discussed in this chapter, is a relevant preventive counseling point whenever anogenital warts are diagnosed, both for the affected patient if not previously vaccinated and as an opportunity to discuss vaccination for their sexual partners.

Eczema Herpeticum Revisited

Eczema herpeticum, introduced in the chapter on atopic dermatitis as a disseminated herpes simplex virus infection superimposed on a disrupted atopic barrier, warrants reemphasis here as the most severe cutaneous complication of herpes simplex virus infection in a susceptible host: monomorphic, punched-out vesicles or erosions spreading rapidly across a background of eczematous skin represent a dermatologic emergency requiring prompt systemic antiviral therapy, and the diagnostic threshold for initiating empiric antiviral therapy while confirmatory testing is pending should be low in any patient with atopic dermatitis presenting with a rapidly progressive vesicular or erosive eruption, given the substantial morbidity risk of treatment delay in this specific, at-risk population.

CAUTION: A first-episode genital herpes simplex virus infection identified late in pregnancy requires coordinated obstetric management given the substantially elevated neonatal transmission risk compared with recurrent maternal infection, and should prompt prompt communication with the patient's obstetric team rather than management in isolation.

Clinical Case: Recognizing Ophthalmic Zoster

A 68-year-old woman presents with a two-day history of pain and burning over the right forehead and upper eyelid, now accompanied by grouped vesicles on an erythematous base confined strictly to this distribution, with a few vesicles visible at the very tip of her nose. She reports the pain began approximately two days before any visible skin findings appeared, and she has noticed mild blurred vision in her right eye over the past day, which she had attributed to fatigue.

Applying the Pattern Anchor established in the Rhythm Layer callout earlier in this chapter, the strict, non-midline-crossing dermatomal confinement of her eruption to the ophthalmic division of the trigeminal nerve immediately confirms herpes zoster rather than another vesicular process, and the presence of vesicles at the tip of her nose, a positive Hutchinson sign discussed earlier in this chapter, together with her new visual symptoms, are recognized as red flag findings warranting urgent same-day ophthalmologic evaluation rather than routine dermatologic follow-up alone, given the substantial risk of sight-threatening ocular complications with ophthalmic zoster involving the nasociliary nerve distribution.

Oral antiviral therapy is initiated immediately given her presentation within the seventy-two hour treatment window discussed earlier in this chapter, and she is referred emergently to ophthalmology, where examination confirms early herpes zoster keratitis, allowing prompt initiation of topical ophthalmic therapy alongside her systemic antiviral treatment. Given her age, a recognized risk factor for postherpetic neuralgia discussed earlier in this chapter, pain management is proactively addressed at the initial visit rather than deferred until after acute lesion resolution, and she is counseled explicitly that some degree of dermatomal discomfort persisting beyond lesion crusting would not be unexpected given her age-related risk, with a specific follow-up plan established to reassess and escalate pain management if postherpetic neuralgia does develop.

KEY POINT: New visual symptoms accompanying a Hutchinson sign in ophthalmic zoster constitute a same-day ophthalmologic emergency and should never be deferred to routine follow-up given the risk of sight-threatening keratitis or other ocular complications.

Clinical Case: Distinguishing Herpetic Whitlow From Bacterial Paronychia

A 3-year-old boy is brought in with a two-day history of a painful, swollen right thumb, with his mother reporting he has been sucking that thumb frequently and that he had a mild cold sore on his lip approximately one week earlier that has since resolved. On examination, the distal thumb is erythematous and edematous with several small grouped vesicles on an erythematous base along the lateral nail fold, without frank purulence, and he is afebrile and otherwise well-appearing.

Applying the pattern recognition established earlier in this chapter, the grouped vesicular morphology, combined with the recent history of an oral herpes simplex virus lesion and a clear autoinoculation mechanism through thumb-sucking, strongly supports herpetic whitlow rather than a bacterial paronychia, and this distinction is communicated clearly to his mother, who had been concerned that incision and drainage, a common intervention for a bacterial paronychia, might be needed. The clinician specifically explains that incision and drainage is not indicated for herpetic whitlow and can potentially worsen or prolong the infection by disrupting the overlying skin and introducing secondary bacterial contamination, directly applying the distinction introduced earlier in this chapter between these two diagnostically similar but therapeutically divergent conditions.

A Tzanck smear performed at the bedside, per the diagnostic workup discussed in this chapter, demonstrates multinucleated giant keratinocytes consistent with a herpesvirus infection, and given his age and the visible source lesion history, herpes simplex virus rather than varicella-zoster virus is presumed as the causative agent without requiring further confirmatory testing given the straightforward clinical and epidemiologic context. Oral antiviral therapy is initiated given his young age and the discomfort he is experiencing, and his mother is counseled on measures to reduce further autoinoculation, including discouraging thumb-sucking during the active phase of both his oral and digital lesions and reinforcing hand hygiene, while being reassured that this is a self-limited infection expected to resolve over one to two weeks with appropriate supportive care.

CLINICAL PEARL: Grouped vesicles on a digit in a child with a recent oral herpes simplex virus lesion and a thumb-sucking history should suggest herpetic whitlow via autoinoculation rather than bacterial paronychia; incision and drainage is not indicated and may worsen the course.

THE MORPHOLOGY-TO-MANAGEMENT SYSTEM — Grouped Vesicular Eruptions

Pattern Introduced This Chapter: The dermatomal vesicular eruption of herpes zoster, discriminated from recurrent herpes simplex virus infection and from contact dermatitis.

Cross-Cutting Anchor: Strict, non-midline-crossing dermatomal confinement is the anchor for zoster; recurrence at the same limited site without full dermatomal distribution is the anchor for recurrent herpes simplex virus infection.

Summary and Key Concepts

Herpes simplex virus establishes lifelong latency and produces grouped, herpetiform vesicles that tend to recur at the same anatomic site, distinguishing it from the strictly dermatomal, non-recurring pattern of herpes zoster.

Herpes zoster reflects reactivation of latent varicella-zoster virus within a single sensory ganglion, and ophthalmic zoster with a positive Hutchinson sign warrants urgent ophthalmologic evaluation given the risk of sight-threatening complications.

Human papillomavirus-associated verrucae frequently resolve spontaneously as cell-mediated immunity develops, supporting observation as a reasonable option alongside destructive or immunotherapy-based treatment for patients desiring active management.

Molluscum contagiosum's characteristic central umbilication distinguishes it from other dome-shaped papular eruptions, though an atypically extensive presentation in an immunocompromised patient warrants biopsy to exclude an opportunistic infection mimic.

Immunocompromised patients and neonates are at risk for more severe, atypical, and diagnostically subtle presentations of every viral infection discussed in this chapter and warrant a correspondingly lower threshold for antiviral therapy and specialist involvement.

CHAPTER 10: FUNGAL INFECTIONS AND CUTANEOUS INFESTATIONS

Learning Objectives

1. Classify the dermatophyte genera and correlate their keratin-restricted growth pattern with the annular, scaling morphology seen in tinea infections at each body site.
2. Differentiate tinea capitis, tinea corporis, tinea cruris, tinea pedis, and onychomycosis by distribution, scale pattern, and predisposing factors, and distinguish each from its principal clinical mimics.
3. Select and interpret potassium hydroxide preparation, fungal culture, and dermoscopy findings appropriate to a suspected dermatophyte, candidal, or Malassezia infection.
4. Construct an evidence-based topical and systemic antifungal regimen, accounting for site, extent, nail involvement, and hepatic monitoring requirements.
5. Recognize the burrow, mite, and egg findings that confirm scabies and differentiate classic from crusted (Norwegian) scabies in immunocompromised patients.
6. Manage pediculosis capitis, corporis, and pubis, including resistance patterns and household contact treatment, within a framework of patient education and prevention.

Superficial fungal infections and cutaneous infestations occupy a disproportionate share of primary care dermatologic visits because they are common, contagious, and frequently confused with inflammatory or eczematous disease that carries an entirely different treatment. A tinea infection treated with a topical corticosteroid rather than an antifungal agent does not merely fail to improve; the anti-inflammatory effect of the steroid suppresses the host response that produces the characteristic scaling border, so the eruption spreads and blurs into a poorly marginated patch that few clinicians recognize as fungal in origin, a pattern common enough that it has been given its own name, tinea incognito. This chapter builds the recognition skills that prevent that misstep, moving from the dermatophytes through candidal and Malassezia disease to the arthropod infestations, with diagnostic confirmation and antimicrobial stewardship woven through every section.

Dermatophyte Infections: Classification and Pathophysiology

Dermatophytes are a group of keratinophilic fungi belonging to three anamorphic genera, Trichophyton, Microsporum, and Epidermophyton, each of which secretes keratinases that digest the keratin of stratum corneum, hair shaft, and nail plate. Because these organisms cannot penetrate living tissue, infection remains confined to keratinized structures, and the inflammatory changes visible clinically, erythema, scaling, and vesiculation, arise from the host immune response to fungal antigens and metabolic byproducts rather than from tissue invasion itself. This distinction explains why host immune status shapes the clinical picture more than organism virulence: a robust cell-mediated response produces the brisk, inflamed, centrifugally expanding annular lesion recognized as classic tinea, whereas an attenuated response, as in long-standing zoophilic infection or in an immunosuppressed host, produces a subtler, less inflamed, more extensive eruption that is correspondingly easier to overlook.

Anthropophilic, Zoophilic, and Geophilic Transmission

Dermatophytes are further classified by ecological reservoir, and this classification predicts both the intensity of the host response and the epidemiologic exposure that should prompt suspicion. Anthropophilic species, transmitted human to human, tend to produce a chronic, low-grade inflammatory pattern because they have coevolved with the human immune system to minimize the response that would limit transmission; Trichophyton rubrum, the most common cause of tinea pedis, tinea cruris, and onychomycosis worldwide, exemplifies this pattern. Zoophilic species, acquired from animal contact, provoke a markedly more inflammatory response in the human host, often with vesiculation, pustulation, and even kerion formation, because the organism is poorly adapted to human skin; Microsporum canis from cats and kittens and Trichophyton verrucosum from cattle are the classic examples, and a history of a new kitten or calf exposure in a patient with an inflamed, boggy scalp lesion should immediately raise suspicion for zoophilic tinea capitis. Geophilic species, acquired from soil, are less common causes of human disease but can produce inflammatory reactions similar to zoophilic organisms following direct soil contact, typically on exposed extremities.

KEY POINT: The intensity of inflammation in a tinea infection is an inverse marker of host-organism coevolution, not of organism danger: the most inflamed, dramatic-appearing tinea lesions are typically caused by zoophilic or geophilic organisms poorly adapted to humans, while the most chronic, treatment-resistant infections are typically anthropophilic organisms that have adapted to evade a brisk host response.

Tinea Corporis, Cruris, and Pedis: Clinical Presentation

Tinea corporis presents as one or more annular or arcuate plaques with an active, scaling, slightly raised border and a tendency toward central clearing as the leading edge advances centrifugally while the fungal burden at the center diminishes. The border characteristically shows the greatest scale and erythema, a pattern that distinguishes tinea from nummular eczema, in which scale and erythema are more uniform across the plaque, and from granuloma annulare, in which the border is raised and firm but non-scaling. Pruritus is variable and does not reliably distinguish tinea from its mimics. Majocchi granuloma, a follicular and often nodular variant, arises when dermatophyte organisms are driven into the follicle and dermis, most often following shaving of an affected area or application of a topical corticosteroid to unrecognized tinea, and requires systemic rather than topical antifungal therapy because the organism has escaped the reach of topical agents.

Tinea Cruris and the Groin Differential

Tinea cruris affects the groin and medial thigh with characteristic sparing of the scrotum, a feature that reliably distinguishes it from candidal intertrigo, which characteristically does involve the scrotum and produces satellite pustules beyond the main plaque margin. The active border with peripheral scale remains the diagnostic hallmark; a well-demarcated, uniformly erythematous plaque without a scaling leading edge should prompt reconsideration of inverse psoriasis or erythrasma, the latter distinguished by coral-red fluorescence under Wood lamp examination due to porphyrin production by Corynebacterium minutissimum. Chronic moisture, obesity, and occlusive clothing are the principal predisposing factors, and recurrence is common without attention to these modifiable contributors.

Tinea Pedis: Interdigital, Moccasin, and Vesiculobullous Patterns

Tinea pedis presents in three recognizable patterns that carry different treatment implications. The interdigital pattern, the most common, produces maceration, scaling, and fissuring between the toes, most often the fourth interdigital space, and serves as a frequent portal of entry for bacterial cellulitis of the lower extremity, making its treatment a component of cellulitis prevention in susceptible patients. The moccasin pattern produces diffuse, fine scaling across the sole and lateral foot in a distribution resembling the sole of a moccasin shoe, typically caused by Trichophyton rubrum, and tends toward chronicity because the thick plantar stratum corneum harbors organisms that are difficult to eradicate with topical therapy alone. The vesiculobullous pattern produces tense vesicles or bullae, usually on the instep or plantar arch, and represents the most inflammatory presentation, occasionally accompanied by an id reaction, a distant vesicular eruption on the hands representing a hypersensitivity response to fungal antigens rather than direct infection, that resolves as the primary foot infection is treated.

Pattern	Morphology	Common Mimic	Distinguishing Feature
Interdigital tinea pedis	Maceration, scaling, fissuring between toes	Erythrasma, candidal intertrigo	Wood lamp coral-red fluorescence favors erythrasma
Moccasin tinea pedis	Diffuse fine scaling of sole and lateral foot	Palmoplantar psoriasis, contact dermatitis	Psoriasis often bilateral with sharply demarcated plaques and nail pitting
Vesiculobullous tinea pedis	Tense vesicles on instep or arch	Dyshidrotic eczema, bullous impetigo	KOH preparation positive for hyphae in tinea; culture confirms in impetigo
Tinea cruris	Groin plaque with active scaling border, scrotal sparing	Candidal intertrigo, inverse psoriasis	Scrotal involvement and satellite pustules favor candidiasis

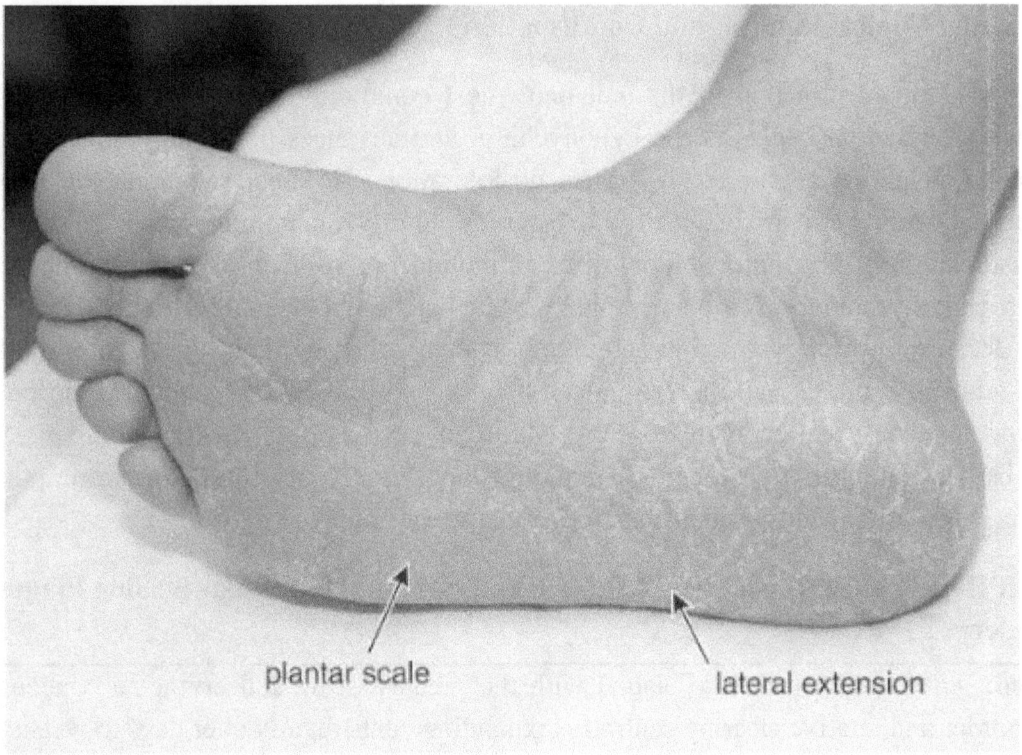

Figure 10.1 Case of moccasin-pattern tinea pedis on patient's foot.

Tinea Capitis and Onychomycosis

Tinea capitis is predominantly a disease of prepubertal children, reflecting the protective effect of postpubertal sebum composition, and presents along a spectrum from fine scaling with subtle hair loss to broken hairs at the scalp surface producing a black-dot pattern, to frank kerion formation, a boggy, exquisitely tender, pustular plaque representing an intense inflammatory response, most often to a zoophilic organism, that can scar and cause permanent alopecia if not treated promptly with systemic antifungal therapy and often a short course of oral corticosteroid to limit scarring. Posterior cervical or occipital lymphadenopathy accompanying scalp scaling and hair loss in a child is a strong clinical clue favoring tinea capitis over seborrheic dermatitis or psoriasis, neither of which typically produces regional lymphadenopathy. Topical antifungal therapy does not achieve adequate follicular penetration to treat tinea capitis, and systemic therapy, most commonly griseofulvin or terbinafine dosed by weight with a duration of six to twelve weeks, is required in every case.

CAUTION: A kerion is frequently mistaken for a bacterial abscess and incised or cultured for bacteria alone, delaying antifungal therapy. Any boggy, inflamed, pustular scalp plaque in a child, particularly with regional lymphadenopathy, warrants a KOH preparation and fungal culture before assuming a purely bacterial process, and empiric systemic antifungal therapy should not be withheld pending culture confirmation given the risk of scarring alopecia.

Onychomycosis: Clinical Patterns and Confirmation

Onychomycosis, fungal infection of the nail unit, most commonly follows a distal lateral subungual pattern in which infection begins at the hyponychium and advances proximally, producing subungual hyperkeratosis, onycholysis, and yellow-brown discoloration. Proximal subungual onychomycosis, in which infection begins at the proximal nail fold, is far less common in immunocompetent hosts and should prompt consideration of HIV infection or another immunocompromising condition when encountered. White superficial onychomycosis produces chalky white patches on the nail plate surface itself rather than beneath it. Because onychomycosis is treated with systemic therapy requiring hepatic monitoring, and because its mimics, psoriatic nail disease, lichen planus, and traumatic onycholysis, do not respond to antifungal therapy, confirmation by microscopy, culture, or periodic acid-Schiff staining of a nail clipping is required before committing a patient to a prolonged systemic course; treating presumptively without confirmation is a common and avoidable source of treatment failure.

THE MORPHOLOGY-TO-MANAGEMENT SYSTEM — The Annular Scaling Plaque With an Active Border

The Pattern: An annular or arcuate plaque with the greatest scale and erythema concentrated at the advancing border and relative clearing centrally, expanding centrifugally over days to weeks.

Presentation Variance: The border may be subtle and poorly scaling in anthropophilic infection, or markedly vesiculopustular in zoophilic infection; prior topical corticosteroid use flattens the border and blurs the annular outline, producing tinea incognito.

Trap Logic: Nummular eczema produces more uniform scale across the plaque without border accentuation; granuloma annulare produces a firm, non-scaling raised border; erythema annulare centrifugum produces a trailing scale just inside the border rather than at the leading edge. A KOH preparation resolves genuine diagnostic uncertainty in any of these comparisons.

Management Pivot: Confirm with KOH microscopy before treating; limited tinea corporis responds to a topical azole or allylamine for two to four weeks, while extensive disease, tinea capitis, onychomycosis, or Majocchi granuloma requires systemic antifungal therapy.

Pattern Anchor: Border-predominant scale plus centrifugal expansion equals tinea until KOH proves otherwise; do not treat an undiagnosed annular plaque with a topical corticosteroid alone.

Diagnostic Workup for Fungal Infections

Potassium hydroxide preparation remains the fastest and most cost-effective confirmatory test for suspected dermatophyte, candidal, or Malassezia infection. Scale is collected from the active, scaling border of the lesion, since this is where fungal density is highest, placed on a slide with ten to twenty percent potassium hydroxide solution to dissolve keratinocyte cell walls, gently heated, and examined under low then high power for septate, branching hyphae in dermatophyte infection, pseudohyphae with budding yeast in candidiasis, or the short hyphae and clustered spores producing a "spaghetti and meatballs" pattern characteristic of Malassezia in tinea versicolor. Fungal culture on Sabouraud dextrose agar provides species identification when KOH is equivocal or when treatment failure raises concern for a resistant or unusual organism, though results take one to three weeks. For nail disease, a clipping submitted for periodic acid-Schiff staining offers higher sensitivity than culture alone and is the preferred confirmatory test when systemic therapy is being considered.

1. Select the active, scaling border of the lesion for sampling, avoiding the center where fungal density is lowest.
2. Scrape scale gently with a blunt scalpel blade or the edge of a glass slide onto a collection slide.
3. Apply ten to twenty percent potassium hydroxide solution and a coverslip; gently heat to accelerate keratinocyte lysis without boiling the preparation.
4. Examine under low power to identify a region of interest, then high power to confirm septate branching hyphae, pseudohyphae with yeast forms, or short hyphae with clustered spores.
5. If KOH is negative but clinical suspicion remains high, or if species identification will change management, submit a culture on Sabouraud dextrose agar or a nail clipping for periodic acid-Schiff staining.

Antifungal Management and Treatment

Topical antifungal therapy is first-line for limited tinea corporis, tinea cruris, and interdigital or moccasin-pattern tinea pedis confined to a small surface area. Azole antifungals, such as clotrimazole and ketoconazole, and allylamines, such as terbinafine, are both effective; allylamines are fungicidal against dermatophytes and typically achieve clinical clearance in a shorter course, while azoles offer broader activity that additionally covers Candida and Malassezia, a consideration when the diagnosis is uncertain between dermatophyte and yeast infection. Topical therapy should extend one to two weeks beyond clinical clearance to reduce the risk of recurrence, since residual subclinical fungal burden at the treated border is common.

Systemic Therapy: Indications and Monitoring

Systemic antifungal therapy is required for tinea capitis in every case, for onychomycosis when treatment is pursued, for Majocchi granuloma, for extensive or treatment-refractory tinea corporis or cruris, and for tinea pedis that has failed an adequate topical trial. Terbinafine is generally preferred for dermatophyte infections given its fungicidal activity and shorter treatment duration, typically six weeks for fingernail and twelve weeks for toenail onychomycosis, though baseline and periodic liver function testing is recommended given rare hepatotoxicity, and terbinafine should be used cautiously or avoided in patients with pre-existing liver disease. Griseofulvin remains a first-line option for tinea capitis in children, particularly when caused by Microsporum species against which terbinafine is less reliably active, dosed by weight for six to twelve weeks with fatty food to enhance absorption. Itraconazole offers an alternative for onychomycosis, often given as pulse dosing, with attention to its numerous drug interactions mediated through cytochrome P450 3A4 inhibition. Fluconazole is less commonly first-line for dermatophyte disease but remains useful for candidal infections.

EVIDENCE: Comparative trials and meta-analyses of oral antifungal regimens for onychomycosis have consistently favored terbinafine over itraconazole for dermatophyte-confirmed toenail disease, with higher mycologic cure rates and lower relapse rates at long-term follow-up, supporting terbinafine as the preferred first-line systemic agent when the causative organism is a dermatophyte and hepatic status permits its use.

Emerging Terbinafine-Resistant Dermatophyte Infection

Clinicians should be aware of an emerging pattern of severe, widespread, and treatment-refractory tinea corporis and cruris caused by Trichophyton indotineae, a species that has spread beyond its initial description in South Asia to cases identified across North America and Europe, and that frequently carries mutations conferring reduced susceptibility to terbinafine and, in some isolates, to azole antifungals as well. This organism should be suspected when a patient presents with extensive, deeply pigmented, often confluent plaques covering large body surface areas that have failed an adequate trial of topical or oral terbinafine, particularly in a patient with recent travel to or contact with individuals from an endemic region, or when over-the-counter combination antifungal-corticosteroid creams have been used for a prolonged period, a practice that both masks the inflammatory response and selects for resistant organisms. When resistance is suspected, fungal culture with susceptibility testing should be pursued where available, and empiric escalation to itraconazole, often at higher or longer-duration dosing than used for typical dermatophyte infection, is a reasonable initial approach pending susceptibility data, recognizing that some isolates show reduced susceptibility across both major antifungal classes and may require specialist referral.

CAUTION: Combination antifungal-corticosteroid creams, widely available without prescription in some regions and increasingly encountered in patients who have self-treated or obtained them informally, are a recognized driver of extensive, resistant, and diagnostically confusing tinea presentations. The corticosteroid component suppresses the inflammatory border that would otherwise prompt earlier diagnosis, while providing insufficient antifungal potency to clear the infection, allowing the organism to proliferate under a clinically deceptive appearance of partial improvement.

Candidiasis and Malassezia-Associated Disease

Cutaneous candidiasis, most often caused by Candida albicans, thrives in warm, moist, occluded skin folds and presents as beefy-red, well-demarcated plaques with characteristic satellite papules and pustules extending beyond the main margin, a feature that reliably distinguishes it from tinea and from inverse psoriasis. Common sites include the inframammary and abdominal folds, the groin with scrotal involvement in men, and the interdigital web spaces of individuals with chronically wet hands, sometimes termed erosio interdigitalis blastomycetica. Predisposing factors include diabetes mellitus, obesity, systemic or topical corticosteroid use, recent antibiotic therapy that disrupts competing bacterial flora, and immunosuppression, and any patient presenting with extensive or recurrent candidal intertrigo warrants screening for undiagnosed diabetes. Treatment combines a topical azole antifungal with measures to reduce moisture and friction, such as barrier pastes and moisture-wicking fabric, and severe or refractory disease may require a short course of oral fluconazole.

Pityriasis Versicolor and Malassezia Folliculitis

Pityriasis versicolor results from conversion of the commensal yeast Malassezia furfur from its yeast to its mycelial form, producing hypopigmented, hyperpigmented, or erythematous finely scaling macules and patches predominantly on the trunk and proximal upper extremities, with pigmentary change explained by azelaic acid production that inhibits melanocyte tyrosinase in affected areas; the hypopigmentation may persist for weeks after fungal clearance since it reflects a lingering pigmentary effect rather than ongoing infection, a point worth explicit patient counseling to prevent premature abandonment of otherwise effective therapy. Wood lamp examination may show a yellow-green fluorescence in some cases, though its absence does not exclude the diagnosis. Malassezia folliculitis, a distinct entity presenting as monomorphic follicular papules and pustules on the trunk and upper back, is frequently mistaken for acne vulgaris but does not respond to standard acne therapy and instead requires topical or oral antifungal treatment; the absence of comedones in a monomorphic truncal papulopustular eruption should prompt consideration of this diagnosis. First-line treatment for both conditions is topical selenium sulfide, ketoconazole, or another azole applied to affected areas, with oral itraconazole reserved for extensive or recurrent disease given superior lipophilic penetration into sebaceous follicles compared to fluconazole.

KEY POINT: Diabetes screening should be considered in any adult presenting with extensive, recurrent, or treatment-refractory candidal intertrigo, since hyperglycemia both promotes Candida proliferation directly and impairs the cutaneous barrier and immune surveillance that would otherwise limit colonization, making recurrent candidiasis a useful clinical clue to an underlying metabolic derangement that might otherwise go unrecognized.

Scabies: Pathophysiology and Clinical Presentation

Scabies results from infestation by the mite Sarcoptes scabiei var. hominis, which burrows into the stratum corneum where the female mite lays eggs, and the intense pruritus that characterizes the disease, classically worse at night, reflects a delayed-type hypersensitivity response to mite antigens, feces, and eggs that develops over three to six weeks after initial exposure but recurs within one to two days upon reinfestation in a previously sensitized host. The burrow, a thin, serpiginous, grayish line a few millimeters long, is the pathognomonic finding but is often obscured by excoriation and secondary eczematization, and clinicians should search preferentially in the finger web spaces, flexor wrists, axillae, periumbilical skin, and genitalia, sites the mite favors for its lower skin temperature and thinner stratum corneum. In infants, the palms, soles, face, and scalp are additionally involved, sites that are typically spared in adults.

Crusted (Norwegian) Scabies

Crusted scabies, also called Norwegian scabies, occurs in immunocompromised, cognitively impaired, or institutionalized patients whose diminished immune response fails to limit mite proliferation, resulting in thick, hyperkeratotic, often fissured plaques teeming with thousands to millions of mites rather than the ten to fifteen typically present in classic scabies. This form is markedly more contagious than classic scabies despite sometimes producing less pruritus, since the itch response depends on an intact hypersensitivity reaction that is blunted in the immunocompromised host, and outbreaks in long-term care facilities are frequently traced to an unrecognized case of crusted scabies. Recognition is critical because standard contact precautions are insufficient; affected patients require combined topical and oral therapy, often with multiple treatment cycles, and environmental decontamination of the surrounding facility.

THE MORPHOLOGY-TO-MANAGEMENT SYSTEM — The Nocturnal Pruritus With Web-Space Burrows

---

The Pattern: Intense pruritus worse at night with thin, serpiginous burrows and excoriated papules concentrated in finger web spaces, flexor wrists, axillae, and genital skin.

Presentation Variance: Infants show palm, sole, face, and scalp involvement atypical for adults; immunocompromised or institutionalized patients may develop crusted scabies with thick hyperkeratotic plaques and minimal pruritus despite an enormous mite burden.

Trap Logic: Atopic dermatitis and other eczematous processes also itch and excoriate but favor flexural creases without web-space burrows and typically show a longer, non-contagious history; a new household contact with similar itching strongly favors scabies over primary eczema.

Management Pivot: Confirm by dermoscopy or skin scraping when feasible, but treat empirically when the clinical pattern is classic; treat the patient and all household and close contacts simultaneously regardless of symptoms in contacts, and launder or bag bedding and clothing.

Pattern Anchor: Nocturnal itch plus web-space burrows in more than one household member is scabies until proven otherwise, and treatment must include every close contact at the same time or reinfestation is guaranteed.

Pediculosis and Other Cutaneous Infestations

Pediculosis capitis, infestation by the head louse Pediculus humanus capitis, is most prevalent among school-age children and presents with scalp pruritus, visible nits firmly cemented to the hair shaft close to the scalp, distinguishing them from easily movable hair casts or debris, and occasionally posterior cervical lymphadenopathy from secondary excoriation and superinfection. First-line treatment is topical permethrin, though resistance is increasingly widespread, making a second application seven to nine days after the first essential regardless of the agent chosen, timed to kill newly hatched nymphs before they reach reproductive maturity. Alternative agents including malathion, spinosad, and oral ivermectin are reserved for treatment failure. Pediculosis corporis, body lice infestation, is distinct in that the organism lives and lays eggs in clothing seams rather than on the body itself, making laundering and environmental measures the primary treatment rather than topical pediculicides, and its presence in a patient should prompt attention to social circumstances such as homelessness or inadequate access to clean clothing given its strong association with crowded, unhygienic living conditions. Pediculosis pubis, pubic lice infestation typically sexually transmitted, warrants screening for other sexually transmitted infections when diagnosed.

Cutaneous Larva Migrans and Bed Bug Reactions

Cutaneous larva migrans results from percutaneous penetration by hookworm larvae, most often Ancylostoma braziliense from dog or cat feces contaminating soil or sand, producing an intensely pruritic, serpiginous, thread-like erythematous track that advances at a rate of a few millimeters to a centimeter per day as the larva migrates through the epidermis, unable to complete its life cycle in the human host. The travel history, often a recent beach vacation in a tropical or subtropical location with barefoot sand contact, combined with the classic serpiginous track, is usually sufficient for diagnosis, and treatment is oral ivermectin or albendazole. Bed bug bites from Cimex lectularius produce grouped or linear erythematous papules, often on exposed skin, classically described as occurring in a "breakfast, lunch, and dinner" pattern of three lesions in a row, though this pattern is neither universal nor specific; diagnosis relies more on history of nocturnal biting and inspection of bedding for the insects themselves than on lesion morphology alone, and treatment is symptomatic with topical corticosteroid and antihistamine while environmental pest control addresses the underlying infestation.

Agent	Indication	Typical Regimen	Key Consideration
Permethrin 5% cream	Scabies, first-line	Applied neck to soles, left 8-14 hours, repeated in 7 days	Preferred agent in pregnancy and young children
Oral ivermectin	Scabies, especially crusted or treatment-refractory disease	Weight-based single dose, repeated in 7-14 days	Avoided in pregnancy and in children below approximately 15 kg
Permethrin 1% lotion or shampoo	Pediculosis capitis, first-line	Applied to scalp and hair, repeated in 7-9 days	Rising resistance rates; second application essential
Malathion 0.5% lotion	Pediculosis capitis, treatment failure	Applied to dry hair, left 8-12 hours	Flammable formulation; avoid open flame or hair dryers during application
Oral ivermectin	Pediculosis capitis, treatment failure	Two doses one week apart	Alternative when topical resistance suspected

Laundering and environmental measures	Pediculosis corporis, first-line	Hot-water wash and hot-air drying of clothing and bedding	Topical pediculicide generally unnecessary since organism resides in clothing

Complications, Special Populations, and Prevention

Untreated or inadequately treated superficial fungal infections can seed bacterial superinfection through fissured, macerated skin, particularly at the interdigital web spaces in tinea pedis, where breaks in the epidermal barrier serve as a portal for streptococcal or staphylococcal cellulitis of the lower extremity; patients with recurrent lower extremity cellulitis should be examined for unrecognized interdigital tinea pedis as a modifiable risk factor. Chronic dermatophyte infection can also trigger an id reaction, a distant vesicular or eczematous eruption representing hypersensitivity to fungal antigens rather than direct spread, that resolves once the primary infection is treated and should not be mistaken for a new site of active infection requiring separate antifungal therapy. In diabetic patients, onychomycosis and interdigital tinea pedis carry additional weight given the risk of foot ulceration and secondary infection in the setting of neuropathy and vascular compromise, and treatment thresholds are correspondingly lower.

Pregnant patients with scabies or pediculosis should be treated with permethrin, which carries the most favorable safety profile among pediculicides and scabicides in pregnancy, while lindane is contraindicated due to neurotoxicity risk and oral ivermectin is generally avoided given limited safety data in pregnancy. Immunocompromised patients, including those with HIV infection, organ transplantation, or receiving systemic immunosuppression, are at elevated risk for atypical, extensive, or treatment-refractory presentations of every condition discussed in this chapter and warrant a lower threshold for confirmatory testing, systemic rather than topical therapy, and closer follow-up to confirm clearance rather than presumed cure based on symptom improvement alone.

PATIENT EDUCATION: Patients treated for tinea pedis or onychomycosis should be counseled that recurrence is common without attention to modifiable factors: keeping feet dry, wearing moisture-wicking socks, alternating shoes to allow full drying between wears, and treating shoes with antifungal powder can meaningfully reduce reinfection risk. Patients treated for scabies or pediculosis should be counseled that residual itching for two to four weeks after successful treatment is expected and does not indicate treatment failure or the need for repeat therapy, since it reflects the slow resolution of an established hypersensitivity reaction rather than persistent infestation.

Clinical Case: The Athlete With Recurrent Groin and Foot Eruptions

A 24-year-old competitive wrestler presented with a several-month history of an intensely itchy, scaling rash in the groin that recurred despite two courses of an over-the-counter hydrocortisone cream, along with chronic scaling and maceration between the toes of both feet. Examination of the groin revealed bilateral, well-demarcated plaques with an active, scaling, slightly raised border and clear sparing of the scrotum; the feet showed diffuse fine white scaling across both soles extending onto the lateral borders in a moccasin distribution, with maceration and mild fissuring in the fourth interdigital spaces bilaterally. A potassium hydroxide preparation from the groin's leading edge revealed abundant septate, branching hyphae, confirming tinea rather than a corticosteroid-responsive inflammatory dermatosis, and the patient was counseled that the hydrocortisone cream had likely suppressed inflammation without eradicating the organism, permitting the fungus to spread while symptoms transiently improved, an explanation that resonated with his description of the rash "getting bigger every time I stopped the cream."

Given the combined groin and foot involvement, both fed by the same reservoir of Trichophyton rubrum colonizing his feet and transferred to the groin during dressing, he was started on oral terbinafine for two weeks given the extent of disease across two body sites, alongside counseling on moisture control, daily sock changes, and antifungal shoe powder to reduce the plantar fungal reservoir that predisposes to recurrent groin involvement. He was also counseled to treat his athletic shoes and wrestling mats were flagged as a possible source of ongoing anthropophilic exposure within his training environment, prompting a broader conversation with his team's athletic trainer about mat cleaning protocols, since tinea corporis, sometimes called "tinea gladiatorum" in this context, spreads readily among wrestlers through direct skin contact and shared equipment.

Clinical Case: The Toddler With Scalp Scaling and a Boggy Plaque

A 3-year-old girl was brought in for a two-week history of scalp scaling that her mother had been treating as dandruff with an over-the-counter anti-dandruff shampoo, now with a new tender, boggy swelling on the crown that had developed over the preceding four days. The family had acquired a kitten approximately three weeks earlier. Examination revealed a two-centimeter boggy, fluctuant, exquisitely tender plaque studded with pustules on the vertex, surrounded by an area of diffuse fine scaling with several patches of broken hair shafts close to the scalp surface, and palpation revealed tender posterior cervical and occipital lymphadenopathy. The combination of an inflammatory boggy scalp plaque, broken hairs, regional lymphadenopathy, and a recent kitten exposure was recognized as a kerion, most likely caused by the zoophilic organism Microsporum canis, and a KOH preparation of extracted hair confirmed ectothrix spore invasion.

The child's pediatrician had initially considered incision and drainage for a presumed bacterial abscess, but the diagnostic pivot to fungal culture and confirmatory microscopy avoided an unnecessary procedure and correctly redirected therapy toward systemic antifungal treatment. She was started on weight-based oral griseofulvin for eight weeks given the zoophilic organism and young age, along with a short tapering course of oral prednisolone to blunt the inflammatory response and reduce the risk of scarring alopecia, a recognized adjunct in kerion management when inflammation is severe. Her mother was counseled that the family kitten, though an unlikely source of ongoing transmission once treated, should be evaluated by a veterinarian for dermatophyte infection, and that other household members should be examined for early scalp or skin lesions given the contagious nature of zoophilic tinea capitis within a household.

THE MORPHOLOGY-TO-MANAGEMENT SYSTEM — Scaling Plaques and Nocturnal Itch

Pattern Introduced This Chapter: The border-predominant annular scaling plaque of tinea, discriminated from the web-space burrows and nocturnal pruritus of scabies.

Cross-Cutting Anchor: Centrifugal expansion with border-concentrated scale anchors tinea; nocturnal itch with finger web-space and flexural burrows anchors scabies; a potassium hydroxide preparation or dermoscopy resolves genuine uncertainty between either pattern and its inflammatory mimics.

Summary and Key Concepts

Dermatophyte infections are classified by ecological reservoir (anthropophilic, zoophilic, geophilic), and the intensity of inflammation reflects host-organism adaptation rather than organism danger.

Tinea corporis, cruris, and pedis share a border-predominant scaling pattern; tinea cruris characteristically spares the scrotum, distinguishing it from candidal intertrigo.

Tinea capitis requires systemic therapy in every case; a kerion is an inflammatory complication requiring prompt treatment to prevent scarring alopecia and is often mistaken for bacterial abscess.

Onychomycosis should be confirmed by microscopy, culture, or periodic acid-Schiff staining before committing a patient to systemic therapy with hepatic monitoring, and emerging terbinafine-resistant Trichophyton indotineae warrants suspicion in extensive, treatment-refractory disease.

Candidal intertrigo is distinguished from tinea by satellite pustules and scrotal involvement; pityriasis versicolor and Malassezia folliculitis are distinct commensal-yeast-driven conditions requiring antifungal rather than antibacterial therapy.

Scabies produces nocturnal pruritus with web-space and flexural burrows; crusted scabies in immunocompromised hosts is highly contagious despite blunted pruritus and requires combined systemic and topical therapy.

Pediculosis capitis, corporis, and pubis each have distinct transmission patterns and management approaches, and household or close contacts require simultaneous treatment to prevent reinfestation.

CHAPTER 11: IMMUNOBULLOUS DISEASES

Learning Objectives

1. Distinguish the intraepidermal blistering of pemphigus from the subepidermal blistering of bullous pemphigoid on clinical, histologic, and immunofluorescence grounds.
2. Elicit and interpret the Nikolsky and Asboe-Hansen signs and correlate their presence with the plane of blister formation.
3. Select and interpret direct immunofluorescence, indirect immunofluorescence, and enzyme-linked immunosorbent assay testing appropriate to a suspected immunobullous disease.
4. Recognize dermatitis herpetiformis as a cutaneous manifestation of gluten-sensitive enteropathy and construct its confirmatory workup.
5. Construct a staged, evidence-based systemic treatment approach for pemphigus and bullous pemphigoid, including steroid-sparing and biologic options.
6. Recognize mucous membrane pemphigoid and epidermolysis bullosa acquisita and identify the complications that distinguish their management from other immunobullous diseases.

The immunobullous diseases are a family of conditions in which autoantibodies target structural proteins that hold the epidermis together or anchor it to the underlying dermis, and the level within the skin at which this adhesion fails determines nearly every clinically useful feature of the disease: the fragility of the blister roof, the presence or absence of the Nikolsky sign, the likelihood of mucosal involvement, and even the age at which the disease typically presents. Learning to read a blistering eruption for its plane of cleavage, before any biopsy is performed, is the single most valuable skill this chapter teaches, because it converts a frightening and unfamiliar presentation into a short, tractable differential that a confirmatory biopsy and immunofluorescence study can then resolve with precision.

Pemphigus Vulgaris and the Intraepidermal Blistering Diseases

Pemphigus vulgaris results from IgG autoantibodies directed against desmoglein 3, and in many patients desmoglein 1 as well, transmembrane glycoproteins that form desmosomal junctions binding adjacent keratinocytes together. Antibody binding disrupts desmosomal adhesion, a process termed acantholysis, causing keratinocytes to separate from one another within the epidermis and producing a blister whose roof is only the thin, fragile upper epidermis, explaining why pemphigus blisters rupture almost immediately after forming and why intact bullae are rarely seen clinically; most patients present instead with painful erosions, denuded skin, and a rim of collarette scale where a blister roof has sloughed away. Because desmoglein 3 is the dominant target and desmoglein 3 is more highly expressed in mucosal epithelium relative to desmoglein 1, the majority of patients with pemphigus vulgaris present first, and sometimes exclusively, with painful oral erosions that may precede cutaneous involvement by weeks to months, and unexplained oral erosions unresponsive to standard aphthous ulcer treatment should prompt consideration of this diagnosis.

Epidemiology and Genetic Predisposition

Pemphigus vulgaris is rare in the general population but shows marked variation in incidence across ethnic and geographic groups, with notably higher rates among individuals of Ashkenazi Jewish and Mediterranean descent, a pattern strongly linked to specific human leukocyte antigen class II alleles, particularly HLA-DR4 and HLA-DR6 subtypes, that confer increased susceptibility to the autoimmune response against desmoglein proteins. Onset typically occurs in the fourth to sixth decades of life, with a roughly equal distribution between sexes, though some series suggest a modest female predominance. Bullous pemphigoid, in contrast, shows a steadily rising incidence with advancing age, becoming most common after the seventh decade, a pattern that has led to increasing disease burden in aging populations globally and that correlates with age-related changes in basement membrane zone antigen expression and immune regulation, alongside a well-documented association with neurologic disease, including stroke, dementia, and Parkinson disease, that has prompted investigation into shared or cross-reactive antigenic targets between cutaneous basement membrane proteins and neuronal tissue.

The Nikolsky and Asboe-Hansen Signs

The Nikolsky sign, elicited by applying lateral shearing pressure to clinically normal-appearing skin adjacent to a lesion and observing for epidermal separation, reflects the profound loss of intraepidermal cohesion in pemphigus and is characteristically positive, whereas it is characteristically negative in bullous pemphigoid, where the blister roof is the full thickness of the epidermis and adhesion of the epidermis to itself remains intact even though its attachment to the dermis has failed. The Asboe-Hansen sign, elicited by applying direct pressure to an intact bulla and observing lateral extension of the blister into adjacent skin, similarly reflects the plane of cleavage and is positive in pemphigus. Both signs, while classically taught and clinically useful at the bedside, lack the sensitivity and specificity to replace biopsy confirmation and should be understood as supportive rather than definitive findings.

KEY POINT: A positive Nikolsky sign in a patient with widespread erosions and flaccid, easily ruptured blisters points toward pemphigus and an intraepidermal plane of cleavage; a negative Nikolsky sign with tense, intact bullae on urticarial or eczematous plaques points toward bullous pemphigoid and a subepidermal plane of cleavage. This bedside distinction should guide, but never replace, biopsy and immunofluorescence confirmation.

Drug-Induced Pemphigus and the IgA Pemphigus Variant

A subset of pemphigus cases is drug-induced, most classically associated with thiol-containing medications such as penicillamine and captopril, which are believed to interfere directly with desmosomal protein structure or function through a biochemical mechanism distinct from the idiopathic autoimmune process, and less commonly with non-thiol agents including certain other antihypertensives and nonsteroidal anti-inflammatory drugs. Drug-induced pemphigus more often resembles the more superficial pemphigus foliaceus variant clinically and on immunofluorescence testing, and, importantly, often remits after withdrawal of the offending agent, a feature that distinguishes its management and prognosis from idiopathic pemphigus and makes a thorough medication history an essential component of the initial evaluation of any newly diagnosed patient. IgA pemphigus is a separate, generally milder variant driven by IgA rather than IgG autoantibodies against desmosomal proteins, presenting with flaccid pustules and vesicles in an annular or herpetiform arrangement rather than the erosive picture of classic pemphigus vulgaris, and is generally more responsive to dapsone than to the corticosteroid and rituximab-based regimens used for IgG-mediated pemphigus.

Bullous Pemphigoid and the Subepidermal Blistering Diseases

Bullous pemphigoid, the most common autoimmune blistering disease overall and predominantly a disease of older adults, results from IgG autoantibodies targeting BP180 and BP230, components of the hemidesmosomal complex that anchors basal keratinocytes to the underlying basement membrane. Because the plane of separation is subepidermal, full-thickness epidermis forms the blister roof, producing tense, intact bullae that resist rupture on palpation and that arise on a background of urticarial, edematous plaques rather than on otherwise normal-appearing skin; this urticarial prodromal phase, which may precede frank blister formation by weeks, is a common source of diagnostic delay, since it is easily mistaken for chronic urticaria, an arthropod reaction, or a drug eruption until tense bullae eventually appear. Mucosal involvement occurs in a minority of patients with bullous pemphigoid and, when present, is typically milder and less erosive than the mucosal disease seen in pemphigus vulgaris.

Feature	Pemphigus Vulgaris	Bullous Pemphigoid
Typical age	Middle-aged adults	Older adults, typically over 60
Blister plane	Intraepidermal (suprabasal)	Subepidermal
Blister character	Flaccid, rupture easily; erosions predominate	Tense, intact bullae
Nikolsky sign	Positive	Negative
Mucosal involvement	Common, often the presenting feature	Uncommon, typically milder
Target antigen	Desmoglein 3 (and often desmoglein 1)	BP180 and BP230

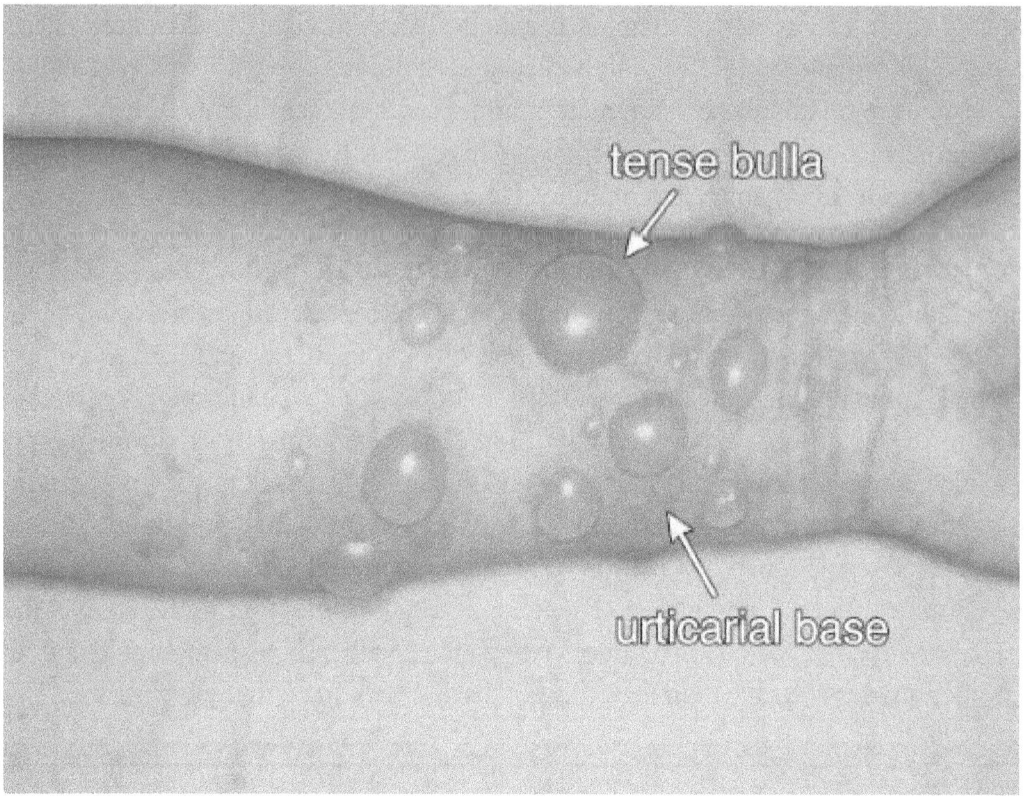

THE MORPHOLOGY-TO-MANAGEMENT SYSTEM — The Flaccid Erosion Versus the Tense Bulla

The Pattern: Widespread painful erosions with a positive Nikolsky sign favor an intraepidermal blistering process; tense, intact bullae on an urticarial base with a negative Nikolsky sign favor a subepidermal process.

Presentation Variance: Pemphigus may present as oral erosions alone for weeks to months before skin involvement; bullous pemphigoid may present as a pruritic urticarial eruption for weeks before frank bullae appear, and in older adults may be misattributed to a drug reaction.

Trap Logic: Bullous drug eruptions and bullous impetigo can mimic either pattern; a linear array of bullae along a dermatome should prompt consideration of localized herpes zoster rather than an immunobullous disease. Direct immunofluorescence of perilesional skin is the discriminating test in genuine uncertainty.

Management Pivot: Biopsy both a lesional specimen for routine histology and a perilesional specimen for direct immunofluorescence before initiating systemic immunosuppression; the immunofluorescence pattern (intercellular versus linear basement membrane zone deposition) confirms the diagnosis and guides which disease-specific treatment pathway to follow.

Pattern Anchor: Positive Nikolsky plus mucosal erosions equals pemphigus until proven otherwise; negative Nikolsky plus tense bullae on urticarial skin in an older adult equals bullous pemphigoid until proven otherwise.

Paraneoplastic Pemphigus

Paraneoplastic pemphigus is a distinct and more severe immunobullous disease arising in association with an underlying lymphoproliferative or other malignancy, most commonly non-Hodgkin lymphoma, chronic lymphocytic leukemia, or Castleman disease, and driven by a broader autoantibody response directed against multiple members of the plakin family of desmosomal and hemidesmosomal proteins in addition to desmogleins, producing a combined intraepidermal and subepidermal injury pattern that explains its distinctive and often diagnostically confusing clinical picture. Painful, severe, treatment-resistant mucosal erosions, typically more extensive and more refractory than in pemphigus vulgaris, are essentially universal and frequently involve the conjunctiva, and cutaneous lesions display a striking polymorphism, ranging from flaccid bullae resembling pemphigus vulgaris to lichenoid, violaceous papules resembling lichen planus to targetoid lesions resembling erythema multiforme, sometimes all present simultaneously in the same patient, a combination that should immediately raise suspicion for this diagnosis rather than any single immunobullous disease alone.

Diagnosis and Prognosis

Direct immunofluorescence in paraneoplastic pemphigus typically shows both intercellular and linear basement membrane zone deposition, reflecting the combined desmosomal and hemidesmosomal target profile, and indirect immunofluorescence performed on rat bladder epithelium, a substrate rich in plakin proteins but lacking desmogleins, is a distinguishing confirmatory test that is characteristically positive in paraneoplastic pemphigus and negative in pemphigus vulgaris. The disease carries a substantially worse prognosis than pemphigus vulgaris or bullous pemphigoid, both because of the severity of mucosal and cutaneous disease itself and because a subset of patients develop bronchiolitis obliterans, a progressive and often fatal pulmonary fibrosing process believed to reflect autoantibody cross-reactivity with plakin proteins expressed in bronchial epithelium; any patient with paraneoplastic pemphigus who develops dyspnea warrants urgent pulmonary evaluation. Identification and treatment of the underlying malignancy is central to management alongside immunosuppressive therapy directed at the skin and mucosal disease, and rituximab has shown benefit in this population as well, though overall outcomes remain guarded compared to the more classic immunobullous diseases.

CAUTION: A patient presenting with severe, treatment-refractory mucosal erosions accompanied by a polymorphic cutaneous eruption combining bullous, lichenoid, and targetoid features should prompt an evaluation for occult malignancy, most importantly a lymphoproliferative disorder, given the association between this clinical pattern and paraneoplastic pemphigus. Pulmonary symptoms in this setting warrant urgent evaluation for bronchiolitis obliterans.

Because paraneoplastic pemphigus can occasionally precede overt diagnosis of the associated malignancy by months, a new diagnosis of this condition should prompt a systematic malignancy evaluation even when no prior oncologic history exists, including age-appropriate imaging and consideration of lymph node or bone marrow evaluation guided by clinical findings, since earlier identification and treatment of the underlying neoplasm may favorably influence the overall disease course.

Diagnostic Workup: Immunofluorescence and Serology

Direct immunofluorescence, performed on a perilesional biopsy specimen taken from clinically normal-appearing skin immediately adjacent to a lesion rather than from the lesion itself, is the single most important confirmatory test across the immunobullous diseases, since fixation and processing of a lesional specimen for routine histology often destroys the delicate immunoreactant deposition pattern needed for diagnosis. In pemphigus, direct immunofluorescence characteristically shows an intercellular, "chicken-wire" or "fishnet" pattern of IgG and complement deposition outlining the surface of keratinocytes throughout the epidermis, reflecting antibody bound directly to desmosomal antigens. In bullous pemphigoid, direct immunofluorescence characteristically shows linear deposition of IgG and complement along the basement membrane zone, reflecting antibody bound to hemidesmosomal antigens at the dermal-epidermal junction.

Indirect Immunofluorescence and Salt-Split Skin

Indirect immunofluorescence, performed on the patient's serum rather than a biopsy specimen, detects circulating autoantibodies and is useful both for initial diagnosis and for monitoring disease activity over time, since antibody titers often correlate with clinical severity. When linear basement membrane zone deposition is identified but the specific diagnosis remains uncertain, indirect immunofluorescence performed on salt-split skin, a substrate artificially separated at the lamina lucida by incubation in sodium chloride solution, localizes antibody binding to either the epidermal (roof) or dermal (floor) side of the split, a distinction that separates bullous pemphigoid, which binds the epidermal side, from epidermolysis bullosa acquisita and most cases of mucous membrane pemphigoid, which bind the dermal side.

Histopathologic Correlation on Routine Biopsy

Routine histology from a lesional biopsy, while less specific than immunofluorescence, provides essential supportive information and should be obtained alongside the perilesional specimen at the same visit. Pemphigus vulgaris characteristically shows suprabasal acantholysis, with basal keratinocytes remaining attached to the underlying basement membrane in a pattern often described as a "row of tombstones," reflecting preserved hemidesmosomal attachment despite loss of desmosomal cohesion between basal and suprabasal cells. Pemphigus foliaceus, a more superficial variant targeting predominantly desmoglein 1, shows acantholysis at the level of the granular layer, producing superficial, crusted, scaly erosions rather than the deeper erosions of pemphigus vulgaris, and correspondingly sparing mucosal surfaces given the lower expression of desmoglein 1 in mucosal epithelium. Bullous pemphigoid shows a subepidermal blister with a characteristically eosinophil-rich infiltrate, a feature that assists in distinguishing it from other subepidermal blistering diseases with less pronounced eosinophilia, and dermatitis herpetiformis shows subepidermal blistering with neutrophilic microabscesses concentrated at the dermal papillary tips, correlating directly with the granular IgA deposition seen on immunofluorescence at the same location.

Enzyme-Linked Immunosorbent Assay Testing

Commercially available enzyme-linked immunosorbent assays quantify circulating antibody titers against desmoglein 1, desmoglein 3, and BP180, offering a less invasive alternative or adjunct to immunofluorescence testing that is particularly useful for longitudinal monitoring of disease activity and treatment response, since a falling antibody titer generally parallels clinical improvement and a rising titer often precedes clinical relapse, allowing treatment adjustment before an overt flare develops.

Dermatitis Herpetiformis

Dermatitis herpetiformis is the cutaneous manifestation of gluten-sensitive enteropathy, driven by IgA autoantibodies against tissue transglutaminase that cross-react with epidermal transglutaminase, depositing in a granular pattern at the tips of dermal papillae and triggering neutrophilic microabscess formation that produces subepidermal blistering. Clinically, the disease presents with intensely pruritic, grouped papulovesicles in a symmetric distribution favoring the elbows, knees, buttocks, and scalp, a distribution and grouping pattern that gives the condition its name, herpetiformis, referring to the herpes-like clustering rather than any relationship to herpesvirus infection. Because the intense pruritus typically leads to rapid excoriation, intact vesicles are often difficult to find on examination, and the disease frequently presents instead as grouped excoriations and crusted papules in the classic distribution, a pattern that should prompt biopsy of a fresh, unexcoriated lesion when one can be identified.

KEY POINT: Direct immunofluorescence in dermatitis herpetiformis characteristically shows granular, rather than linear, IgA deposition concentrated at the tips of dermal papillae, distinguishing it from linear IgA bullous dermatosis, in which IgA deposits in a continuous linear band along the basement membrane zone. This distinction is essential because the two conditions, despite the similarity of their names, differ in systemic association and long-term management.

Nearly all patients with dermatitis herpetiformis have some degree of gluten-sensitive enteropathy on small bowel biopsy, though gastrointestinal symptoms are frequently absent or subtle, and serologic testing for IgA anti-tissue transglutaminase and anti-endomysial antibodies supports the diagnosis and can be used to monitor dietary adherence over time. A strict, lifelong gluten-free diet is the definitive treatment, addressing both the cutaneous and intestinal manifestations of the underlying disease, though the cutaneous response to dietary change is slow, often requiring many months to a year or more, so oral dapsone is typically used for rapid symptomatic control while dietary gluten elimination takes effect, with attention to screening for glucose-6-phosphate dehydrogenase deficiency before initiation given the risk of severe hemolytic anemia in deficient patients.

Systemic Treatment of Pemphigus and Bullous Pemphigoid

Systemic corticosteroids remain the cornerstone of initial disease control in both pemphigus vulgaris and bullous pemphigoid, though the two diseases now diverge meaningfully in the steroid-sparing agents that follow. In pemphigus, rituximab, a monoclonal antibody targeting CD20-positive B lymphocytes, has shifted from a second-line to a first-line therapy in combination with corticosteroids for moderate to severe disease, reflecting trial evidence of superior rates of complete remission and lower cumulative corticosteroid exposure compared to corticosteroid therapy alone, an important consideration given the substantial long-term morbidity associated with prolonged high-dose corticosteroid use in this typically middle-aged population. Traditional steroid-sparing agents including azathioprine and mycophenolate mofetil remain used, particularly when rituximab is unavailable or contraindicated, though intravenous immunoglobulin and plasmapheresis are reserved for refractory disease given cost and logistic complexity.

Bullous Pemphigoid: Topical and Systemic Approaches

In bullous pemphigoid, which predominantly affects an older population in whom systemic corticosteroid toxicity carries particular weight given comorbid osteoporosis, diabetes, and cardiovascular disease, high-potency topical corticosteroids applied to the entire body surface have demonstrated efficacy comparable to systemic corticosteroid therapy for localized to moderate disease, with a substantially more favorable systemic side-effect profile, and represent a reasonable first-line approach in appropriately selected patients able to manage the practical demands of whole-body topical application. Doxycycline, with or without niacinamide, offers a lower-toxicity alternative for milder disease. For more extensive or refractory disease, systemic corticosteroids combined with a steroid-sparing agent, most commonly mycophenolate mofetil, azathioprine, or dapsone, remain standard, with omalizumab and dupilumab emerging as options for refractory cases given evidence linking eosinophilic and IgE-mediated inflammation to disease pathogenesis in a meaningful subset of patients.

EVIDENCE: Randomized trial evidence has established rituximab combined with a short corticosteroid taper as superior to corticosteroid therapy alone for achieving sustained complete remission in moderate to severe pemphigus vulgaris, with significantly reduced cumulative corticosteroid exposure over the treatment course, supporting a shift in practice toward earlier rituximab use rather than reserving it for corticosteroid-refractory disease.

Mucous Membrane Pemphigoid and Epidermolysis Bullosa Acquisita

Mucous membrane pemphigoid, also called cicatricial pemphigoid, is a subepidermal immunobullous disease predominantly affecting mucosal surfaces, most commonly the oral cavity and conjunctiva, with skin involvement occurring in only a minority of patients. Its clinical significance lies disproportionately in its capacity to scar, a feature far more prominent than in bullous pemphigoid and one that makes early diagnosis and treatment critical to preventing irreversible complications: ocular involvement can progress through conjunctival scarring, symblepharon formation, and ultimately blindness if untreated, while laryngeal and esophageal involvement can produce strictures with airway or swallowing compromise. Any patient with chronic, erosive, scarring conjunctivitis or oral mucosal erosions unresponsive to standard treatment warrants ophthalmologic and dermatologic evaluation with biopsy, since the window for preventing scarring complications narrows as disease duration increases.

Epidermolysis Bullosa Acquisita

Epidermolysis bullosa acquisita results from IgG autoantibodies against type VII collagen, the principal component of anchoring fibrils that secure the basement membrane to the underlying papillary dermis, and presents in two recognizable patterns: a mechanobullous variant producing tense bullae, erosions, milia, and scarring at sites of trauma such as the hands, elbows, and knees, resembling a hereditary form of epidermolysis bullosa but acquired in adulthood, and an inflammatory variant that more closely resembles bullous pemphigoid clinically, making biopsy and immunofluorescence essential to distinguish the two, since epidermolysis bullosa acquisita is generally more treatment-resistant and prone to scarring than bullous pemphigoid, altering both prognosis and counseling.

Pemphigoid Gestationis

Pemphigoid gestationis is a rare, pregnancy-associated subepidermal immunobullous disease historically termed herpes gestationis, a misnomer retained only for historical reasons since the disease bears no relationship to herpesvirus infection, driven by IgG autoantibodies against BP180 that are believed to arise from an aberrant immune response to placental tissue expressing cross-reactive basement membrane zone antigens. It classically presents in the second or third trimester, though it can occur postpartum as well, with intensely pruritic urticarial papules and plaques beginning periumbilically, a distribution distinctive enough to be a key diagnostic clue, before spreading to the trunk and extremities and evolving into tense bullae resembling bullous pemphigoid; direct immunofluorescence shows the same linear basement membrane zone C3, and often IgG, deposition pattern seen in bullous pemphigoid, reflecting the shared target antigen.

The disease typically flares at delivery and resolves over weeks to months postpartum, though it recurs in a majority of subsequent pregnancies, often with earlier onset and greater severity, and has been reported to flare with subsequent use of hormonal contraception or with menstruation, consistent with a hormonally influenced immune mechanism. A small proportion of neonates born to affected mothers develop transient cutaneous lesions from transplacental antibody transfer, which resolve spontaneously as maternal antibody clears from the neonatal circulation over the first weeks of life without long-term sequelae. Some evidence links pemphigoid gestationis with a modestly increased risk of small-for-gestational-age infants and preterm delivery, supporting closer obstetric monitoring, though the disease itself is not associated with fetal loss when appropriately monitored. Treatment emphasizes topical corticosteroids and antihistamines for mild disease, with systemic corticosteroids reserved for more extensive or refractory involvement, favoring the lowest effective dose given pregnancy; rare case reports describe a similar picture arising in association with hydatidiform mole or choriocarcinoma outside of a viable pregnancy, reflecting placental or trophoblastic tissue as the presumed antigenic trigger rather than pregnancy itself.

KEY POINT: Periumbilical onset of an intensely pruritic urticarial and bullous eruption in the second or third trimester should prompt consideration of pemphigoid gestationis rather than the far more common and benign pruritic urticarial papules and plaques of pregnancy, a distinct, non-bullous, non-immune-mediated condition typically confined to abdominal striae with periumbilical sparing; direct immunofluorescence reliably distinguishes the two when the clinical picture is ambiguous.

Coordinated care between dermatology and obstetrics is essential once pemphigoid gestationis is confirmed, both to guide the maternal treatment plan around pregnancy-safe medication choices and to ensure the obstetric team monitors fetal growth appropriately given the modest association with growth restriction, with a shared delivery plan that anticipates a likely postpartum disease flare so that treatment can be escalated promptly rather than reactively once it occurs.

Complications, Special Populations, and Patient Education

Extensive erosive disease in pemphigus vulgaris carries risks analogous to a large surface area burn, including fluid and electrolyte derangement, protein loss, and susceptibility to secondary bacterial and fungal superinfection through the disrupted epidermal barrier, and patients with widespread involvement benefit from wound care principles borrowed from burn management alongside disease-specific immunosuppressive therapy. Long-term corticosteroid and steroid-sparing immunosuppressive therapy across all the immunobullous diseases carries cumulative risk of infection, osteoporosis, hyperglycemia, and malignancy, and patients on prolonged treatment require monitoring commensurate with these risks, including bone density assessment, glucose monitoring, and age-appropriate cancer screening. Older adults with bullous pemphigoid, the population in whom the disease is most prevalent, are particularly vulnerable to the cumulative toxicity of systemic corticosteroids given coexisting comorbidities, reinforcing the preference for topical or lower-toxicity systemic approaches where disease severity permits.

PATIENT EDUCATION: Patients newly diagnosed with pemphigus vulgaris or bullous pemphigoid should be counseled that these are chronic autoimmune conditions typically requiring months to years of treatment rather than a short defined course, that gradual improvement rather than immediate resolution is the expected pattern of response, and that abrupt discontinuation of systemic corticosteroid or immunosuppressive therapy without medical guidance risks both disease flare and adrenal insufficiency. Patients with dermatitis herpetiformis should be counseled that dietary gluten elimination is a lifelong commitment addressing an underlying systemic condition, not merely a measure to control the skin eruption.

Patients on rituximab therapy require pre-treatment screening for hepatitis B given the risk of viral reactivation with B-cell depletion, along with baseline immunoglobulin levels given the risk of hypogammaglobulinemia with repeated dosing cycles, and should be counseled about a modestly increased infection risk during the months following each infusion cycle. All patients on prolonged systemic immunosuppression, regardless of the specific agent, benefit from age-appropriate vaccination review before treatment initiation where feasible, since live vaccines are generally contraindicated once significant immunosuppression is underway, and from a low threshold for evaluation of fever or new localized symptoms during treatment given both the underlying disease and its therapy predispose to infection.

Clinical Case: Oral Erosions Preceding a Cutaneous Diagnosis

A 52-year-old woman presented with a three-month history of painful oral erosions that had been treated sequentially as recurrent aphthous stomatitis and oral candidiasis without improvement, having recently developed several flaccid blisters and erosions on her upper back and scalp over the preceding two weeks. Examination revealed extensive erosions of the buccal mucosa and hard palate with denuded areas lacking intact vesicles, and on the back, several flaccid, easily ruptured bullae alongside crusted erosions with a positive Nikolsky sign elicited on adjacent clinically normal skin. A biopsy of a fresh cutaneous lesion showed suprabasal acantholysis on routine histology, and a perilesional biopsy sent for direct immunofluorescence confirmed intercellular IgG and C3 deposition in a chicken-wire pattern throughout the epidermis, establishing a diagnosis of pemphigus vulgaris; serum indirect immunofluorescence and enzyme-linked immunosorbent assay testing confirmed elevated anti-desmoglein 3 antibody titers.

Given the extent of mucocutaneous involvement, she was started on rituximab in combination with a moderate-dose oral corticosteroid taper, following the modified rituximab protocol now supported as first-line therapy for moderate to severe disease, with close dental and dermatologic follow-up to monitor oral healing and titrate the corticosteroid taper against clinical response and antibody titers. She was counseled extensively about oral hygiene modifications during the erosive phase, the expected gradual rather than immediate improvement, and the signs of infection or corticosteroid-related complications that would warrant urgent evaluation, and at three-month follow-up her oral erosions had substantially healed with only a low-dose corticosteroid taper remaining, illustrating the more rapid and durable remission achievable with early rituximab-corticosteroid combination therapy compared to historical corticosteroid monotherapy approaches.

Clinical Case: An Older Adult With a Pruritic Eruption Preceding Bullae

A 74-year-old man presented with a six-week history of an intensely pruritic eruption on his trunk and extremities that had been treated as an allergic drug reaction after a recent antibiotic course, without improvement despite discontinuation of the suspected medication and a course of oral antihistamines. Over the preceding week, several tense, fluid-filled blisters had developed on the erythematous, urticarial-appearing plaques, remaining intact rather than rupturing with minor trauma, and the Nikolsky sign was negative on adjacent skin. A lesional biopsy showed a subepidermal blister with a predominantly eosinophilic infiltrate, and perilesional direct immunofluorescence showed linear IgG and C3 deposition along the basement membrane zone, confirming bullous pemphigoid; a BP180 enzyme-linked immunosorbent assay returned a markedly elevated titer consistent with active disease.

Given his age, osteoporosis, and well-controlled type 2 diabetes, the diagnostic and treatment discussion emphasized minimizing systemic corticosteroid exposure, and he was started on twice-daily whole-body application of a high-potency topical corticosteroid, following an evidence-based regimen shown to achieve disease control comparable to systemic therapy in patients with moderate bullous pemphigoid, alongside oral doxycycline as an adjunct with a more favorable long-term safety profile than sustained systemic corticosteroid use. He and his caregiver were instructed in the technique and extent of topical application, including involvement of clinically uninvolved skin given the risk of new lesions arising outside currently affected areas, and at follow-up one month later his pruritus had substantially resolved and no new bullae had developed, allowing a gradual taper of topical corticosteroid frequency while continuing doxycycline.

Clinical Case: Refractory Mucosal Erosions With an Underlying Malignancy

A 61-year-old man with a known diagnosis of chronic lymphocytic leukemia, previously stable on observation alone, presented with a two-month history of severe, painful oral and conjunctival erosions that had failed sequential trials for presumed pemphigus vulgaris and ocular cicatricial pemphigoid, alongside a widespread cutaneous eruption that his outside dermatologist had struggled to classify, describing it as "part bullous, part lichenoid, part targetoid." Examination confirmed extensive erosive stomatitis, bilateral conjunctival injection with early symblepharon formation, and a truncal eruption combining flaccid bullae, violaceous flat-topped papules, and several targetoid lesions with dusky centers, a combination of morphologies that prompted reconsideration of the working diagnosis.

Given the combination of refractory polymorphic mucocutaneous disease and known underlying lymphoproliferative malignancy, paraneoplastic pemphigus was suspected, and biopsy showed a combined pattern of suprabasal acantholysis and interface changes, with direct immunofluorescence demonstrating both intercellular and linear basement membrane zone deposition. Indirect immunofluorescence on rat bladder epithelium returned positive, confirming the diagnosis. Given the recognized risk of bronchiolitis obliterans, pulmonary function testing was obtained promptly and showed early obstructive changes, prompting urgent pulmonology involvement alongside oncology reassessment of his leukemia and initiation of rituximab combined with systemic corticosteroids. He was counseled candidly that paraneoplastic pemphigus carries a substantially more guarded prognosis than typical pemphigus vulgaris, particularly given early pulmonary involvement, and that his ongoing management would require close coordination between dermatology, oncology, pulmonology, and ophthalmology given the multisystem nature of the disease.

Linear IgA bullous dermatosis deserves brief mention as a related subepidermal blistering disease, distinguished from dermatitis herpetiformis by its linear rather than granular IgA deposition pattern on direct immunofluorescence, and recognized clinically by its characteristic annular or polycyclic grouping of vesicles and bullae at the periphery of round plaques, sometimes described as a "cluster of jewels" or "string of pearls" pattern; it can arise idiopathically or be drug-induced, most classically by vancomycin, and dapsone remains first-line therapy for both idiopathic and drug-induced forms once the offending medication, if any, has been discontinued.

THE MORPHOLOGY-TO-MANAGEMENT SYSTEM — Reading the Plane of Cleavage

Pattern Introduced This Chapter: The Nikolsky-positive flaccid erosion of intraepidermal disease versus the Nikolsky-negative tense bulla of subepidermal disease, and the granular papillary-tip IgA pattern of dermatitis herpetiformis versus the linear basement membrane zone pattern shared by pemphigoid, linear IgA disease, and epidermolysis bullosa acquisita.

Cross-Cutting Anchor: Perilesional direct immunofluorescence, not lesional histology alone, is the anchor test across every immunobullous disease in this chapter; the deposition pattern (intercellular versus linear versus granular) and its precise localization on salt-split skin resolve the differential definitively.

Summary and Key Concepts

Pemphigus vulgaris produces intraepidermal blistering from anti-desmoglein antibody-mediated acantholysis, with a positive Nikolsky sign, flaccid erosions, and frequent early oral involvement.

Bullous pemphigoid produces subepidermal blistering from anti-BP180/BP230 antibodies, with a negative Nikolsky sign, tense bullae on an urticarial base, and a predominantly older adult population.

Perilesional direct immunofluorescence is the essential confirmatory test across the immunobullous diseases, distinguishing intercellular (pemphigus), linear basement membrane zone (pemphigoid group), and granular papillary-tip (dermatitis herpetiformis) deposition patterns.

Dermatitis herpetiformis is the cutaneous manifestation of gluten-sensitive enteropathy, treated definitively with a lifelong gluten-free diet and symptomatically with dapsone.

Rituximab combined with corticosteroids is now first-line therapy for moderate to severe pemphigus vulgaris, while whole-body topical corticosteroids offer an effective lower-toxicity alternative to systemic therapy in appropriately selected bullous pemphigoid patients.

Mucous membrane pemphigoid and epidermolysis bullosa acquisita carry a disproportionate risk of scarring complications, including blindness in ocular mucous membrane pemphigoid, making early recognition and treatment critical.

CHAPTER 12: CUTANEOUS VASCULITIS AND REACTIVE ERYTHEMAS

Learning Objectives

1. Recognize palpable purpura as the clinical hallmark of small vessel leukocytoclastic vasculitis and construct an appropriate diagnostic evaluation for its underlying cause.
2. Distinguish IgA vasculitis (Henoch-Schonlein purpura) from other causes of palpable purpura and identify its characteristic systemic involvement.
3. Differentiate urticarial vasculitis from ordinary chronic urticaria on clinical and histologic grounds.
4. Recognize erythema nodosum as a septal panniculitis and construct a systematic evaluation of its associated conditions.
5. Distinguish erythema multiforme from its target-lesion mimics and identify its principal infectious and drug-related triggers.
6. Recognize the neutrophilic dermatoses, Sweet syndrome and pyoderma gangrenosum, and identify their characteristic systemic associations and the pathergy phenomenon.

Cutaneous vasculitis and the reactive erythemas share a common conceptual thread: each represents the skin's response to an immune process occurring elsewhere, whether a circulating immune complex depositing in dermal vessels, a delayed hypersensitivity reaction to an infection or medication, or a neutrophilic infiltrate reflecting an underlying systemic inflammatory or hematologic disorder. Because these conditions are so often the cutaneous signal of a process that also involves the kidneys, joints, gastrointestinal tract, or a hidden malignancy, recognizing the specific morphologic pattern and pairing it with a targeted internal workup is often more clinically consequential than any treatment directed at the skin alone.

Leukocytoclastic Vasculitis: Pathophysiology and Recognition

Leukocytoclastic vasculitis describes a histopathologic pattern of small vessel inflammation, most often affecting postcapillary venules in the superficial dermis, characterized by neutrophilic infiltration of the vessel wall, fibrinoid necrosis, and nuclear dust from fragmenting neutrophils, termed leukocytoclasis, from which the pattern derives its name. This pattern most commonly reflects immune complex deposition within vessel walls, triggering complement activation and neutrophil recruitment, and can be triggered by a wide range of underlying processes including infection, most commonly upper respiratory streptococcal or viral illness; medications, particularly antibiotics and nonsteroidal anti-inflammatory drugs; connective tissue disease; and malignancy, most often hematologic. Clinically, the process produces palpable purpura, non-blanching purpuric papules that are raised rather than flat, reflecting the inflammatory infiltrate and edema surrounding the affected vessels rather than simple extravasation of blood alone, and this palpability is the single most important bedside finding distinguishing vasculitic purpura from the flat, non-inflammatory purpura of a primary coagulopathy or platelet disorder.

Epidemiology and Age-Related Considerations

Cutaneous small vessel vasculitis can occur at any age, but the distribution of underlying triggers shifts meaningfully across the lifespan: in children, infection, most often streptococcal, is the dominant trigger, and IgA vasculitis accounts for the large majority of cases; in adults, medications, chronic infections such as hepatitis C, and connective tissue disease become proportionally more important, and the likelihood of an underlying malignancy, while still a minority of cases overall, rises meaningfully with advancing age, particularly beyond the sixth decade, warranting a somewhat lower threshold for malignancy screening in older adults presenting with new-onset vasculitis lacking an otherwise obvious trigger. This age-stratified approach to the differential diagnosis should inform both the intensity and direction of the initial evaluation rather than applying an identical standardized workup regardless of patient age.

Distribution and Lesion Evolution

Lesions of leukocytoclastic vasculitis characteristically favor gravity-dependent areas, most often the lower extremities, reflecting the influence of hydrostatic pressure on immune complex deposition and vessel wall injury in dependent vasculature, and lesions often appear in successive crops, with new purpuric papules developing over days as older lesions fade to a brownish, hemosiderin-stained hue. Individual lesions may coalesce into larger purpuric plaques in severe cases, and hemorrhagic vesicles, bullae, or shallow ulceration can develop when the inflammatory injury is severe enough to compromise epidermal viability overlying the affected vessels. Because the process is confined to small vessels of the superficial dermis in classic leukocytoclastic vasculitis, deeper structures are spared, distinguishing it from medium vessel vasculitides that produce nodules, livedo racemosa, and ulceration reflecting deeper dermal and subcutaneous vessel involvement.

KEY POINT: Palpability is the critical bedside distinction in purpura: palpable purpura reflects an inflammatory infiltrate around affected vessels and points toward vasculitis, while flat, non-palpable purpura reflects simple blood extravasation without vessel wall inflammation and points toward a coagulopathy, thrombocytopenia, or fragile-vessel process such as senile purpura or amyloid purpura.

IgA Vasculitis (Henoch-Schonlein Purpura)

IgA vasculitis, historically termed Henoch-Schonlein purpura, is the most common vasculitis of childhood, typically arising in the wake of an upper respiratory infection and driven by IgA-dominant immune complex deposition in small vessels of the skin, joints, gastrointestinal tract, and kidneys, producing its classic tetrad: palpable purpura, typically concentrated on the lower extremities and buttocks; arthralgia or arthritis, most often affecting the knees and ankles; abdominal pain, sometimes severe enough to mimic an acute abdomen and occasionally complicated by intussusception; and renal involvement, ranging from asymptomatic microscopic hematuria to a proliferative glomerulonephritis that determines long-term prognosis more than any other feature of the disease. While most common in children between three and ten years of age, IgA vasculitis can occur in adults, in whom renal involvement tends to be more severe and persistent, warranting closer nephrology follow-up than the generally self-limited course typical in pediatric disease.

Figure 12.1 — Clinical Photography: Palpable Purpura in IgA Vasculitis

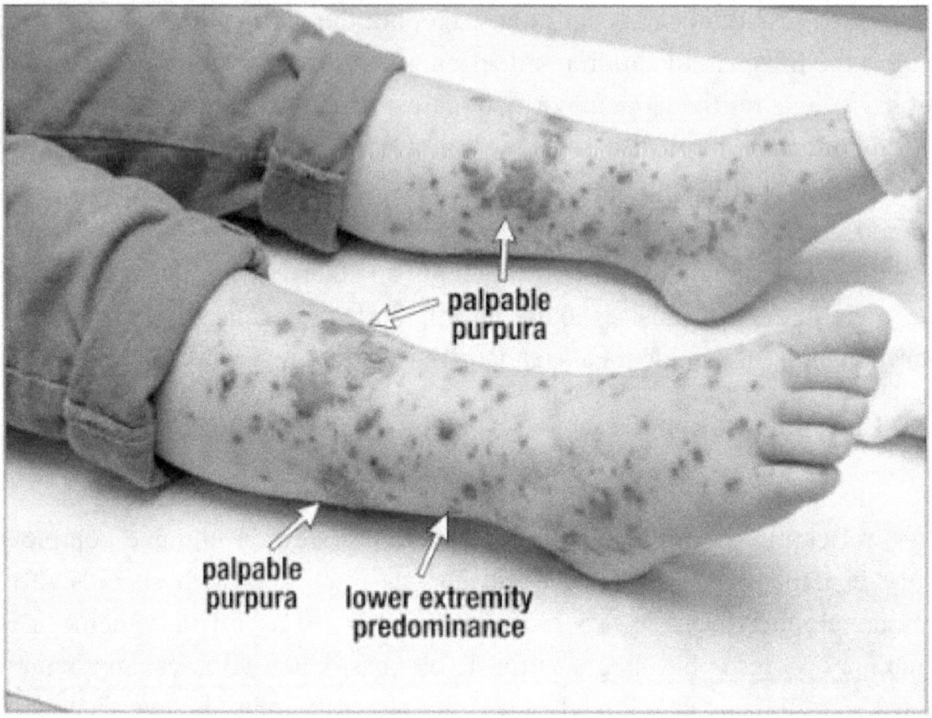

Renal Monitoring and Prognosis

Because renal involvement is the principal determinant of long-term morbidity in IgA vasculitis, urinalysis for hematuria and proteinuria should be obtained at diagnosis and repeated periodically for at least six months after resolution of cutaneous disease, since nephritis can develop or progress after the skin findings have cleared. Most cases resolve spontaneously within four to six weeks with supportive care alone, including rest, hydration, and analgesia for joint symptoms, while systemic corticosteroids are reserved for significant abdominal pain, severe joint involvement, or evidence of progressive nephritis, though corticosteroid therapy has not been shown to prevent renal involvement when used prophylactically and is not indicated for cutaneous disease alone. Referral to nephrology is warranted for any patient who develops significant proteinuria, a rising creatinine, or hypertension during follow-up, since a small proportion of patients, particularly adults, progress to chronic kidney disease requiring long-term management, and early nephrology involvement in this subset has been associated with better preservation of renal function over time.

THE MORPHOLOGY-TO-MANAGEMENT SYSTEM — Palpable Purpura on the Lower Extremities

The Pattern: Raised, non-blanching purpuric papules concentrated on gravity-dependent skin, often in successive crops of varying age and color.

Presentation Variance: In children, accompanying arthralgia, abdominal pain, and hematuria point toward IgA vasculitis; in adults, a similar pattern more often reflects a drug reaction, infection, or underlying connective tissue disease or malignancy, and renal involvement tends to be more severe and persistent.

Trap Logic: Flat, non-palpable purpura should redirect the differential toward thrombocytopenia, coagulopathy, or fragile-vessel purpura rather than vasculitis; urticarial lesions that persist beyond twenty-four hours and leave residual purpura or bruising should raise suspicion for urticarial vasculitis rather than ordinary urticaria.

Management Pivot: Obtain urinalysis, complete blood count, and a basic metabolic panel in every patient; biopsy a lesion less than forty-eight hours old for routine histology and consider direct immunofluorescence for IgA deposition when Henoch-Schonlein purpura is suspected; pursue additional workup for infection, drug exposure, connective tissue disease, or malignancy based on age and associated findings.

Pattern Anchor: Palpable purpura plus hematuria or proteinuria means renal follow-up is mandatory regardless of how quickly the skin clears, since nephritis can outlast and outweigh the cutaneous disease in long-term significance.

Urticarial Vasculitis and Medium Vessel Disease

Urticarial vasculitis presents with wheal-like lesions that closely resemble ordinary urticaria at first glance but are distinguished by their persistence beyond twenty-four hours, a burning or painful quality rather than the pruritus typical of ordinary hives, and resolution with residual purpura, bruising, or hyperpigmentation rather than complete clearing without a trace, reflecting the underlying vessel wall injury rather than the purely mast-cell-mediated process of ordinary urticaria. Biopsy shows a leukocytoclastic vasculitis pattern rather than the simple dermal edema without vessel wall injury seen in ordinary urticaria, and hypocomplementemic urticarial vasculitis, a more severe variant associated with low complement levels, carries a stronger association with systemic lupus erythematosus and systemic involvement including glomerulonephritis, obstructive pulmonary disease, and ocular inflammation, warranting a more extensive systemic evaluation than normocomplementemic disease.

Polyarteritis Nodosa: Cutaneous Manifestations

Polyarteritis nodosa, a medium vessel vasculitis, can present in a cutaneous-limited form confined to skin, subcutaneous tissue, muscle, and peripheral nerve without the visceral organ involvement of systemic polyarteritis nodosa, producing tender subcutaneous nodules along the course of affected vessels, livedo racemosa, a broken, netlike, irregular purplish pattern distinguished from the finer, regular, complete-ring pattern of livedo reticularis, and occasionally shallow, painful ulceration overlying areas of vessel occlusion. Because the vasculitic process in polyarteritis nodosa affects deeper, muscular arteries rather than the superficial dermal venules involved in leukocytoclastic vasculitis, biopsy must extend into the deep dermis or subcutaneous fat to capture an affected vessel, and a superficial punch biopsy is often non-diagnostic; a deep incisional or excisional biopsy centered on a palpable nodule is generally required for confirmation.

Feature	Livedo Reticularis	Livedo Racemosa
Pattern	Regular, complete, unbroken rings	Irregular, broken, incomplete rings
Distribution	Often symmetric, can be physiologic (cutis marmorata)	Often asymmetric, involves trunk and proximal extremities
Reversibility	Often reversible with warming	Typically fixed, does not resolve with warming
Association	Often benign or seen with cold exposure	Suggests an underlying vasculopathy or vasculitis such as polyarteritis nodosa or antiphospholipid syndrome

ANCA-Associated and Cryoglobulinemic Vasculitis

The antineutrophil cytoplasmic antibody-associated vasculitides, granulomatosis with polyangiitis, microscopic polyangiitis, and eosinophilic granulomatosis with polyangiitis, are small vessel vasculitides with prominent systemic organ involvement in which cutaneous findings, while not the dominant clinical feature, provide an accessible diagnostic clue and a convenient biopsy site when internal organ biopsy carries greater risk. Cutaneous manifestations across this group commonly include palpable purpura indistinguishable from other causes of leukocytoclastic vasculitis, tender subcutaneous nodules, and, less commonly, ulceration or digital ischemia reflecting more severe vessel involvement; granulomatosis with polyangiitis can additionally produce oral ulceration and a characteristic strawberry-like gingival hyperplasia, while eosinophilic granulomatosis with polyangiitis, formerly termed Churg-Strauss syndrome, occurs in patients with a preceding history of asthma and eosinophilia and can produce palpable purpura alongside subcutaneous nodules concentrated on the scalp and extremities.

Serologic Correlation and Organ Screening

Antineutrophil cytoplasmic antibody testing, distinguishing a cytoplasmic pattern targeting proteinase 3, more characteristic of granulomatosis with polyangiitis, from a perinuclear pattern targeting myeloperoxidase, more characteristic of microscopic polyangiitis and eosinophilic granulomatosis with polyangiitis, supports the diagnosis when cutaneous vasculitis is accompanied by systemic features such as sinusitis, pulmonary nodules or hemorrhage, or renal impairment, though a meaningful minority of patients, particularly with limited cutaneous disease, test ANCA-negative, so a negative result does not exclude the diagnosis when clinical suspicion remains high. Any patient with biopsy-confirmed vasculitis and unexplained sinus, pulmonary, or renal findings warrants prompt rheumatologic evaluation, since these conditions carry substantial morbidity and mortality if systemic involvement is not recognized and treated promptly with immunosuppressive therapy, typically combining glucocorticoids with rituximab or cyclophosphamide depending on severity.

Cryoglobulinemic vasculitis results from circulating immunoglobulins that precipitate reversibly at reduced temperature, most often in the setting of chronic hepatitis C infection for the mixed cryoglobulinemia subtype, and produces palpable purpura with a distinctly acral, cold-sensitive distribution favoring the lower extremities and worsening in cold weather, sometimes accompanied by livedo reticularis, digital ulceration, and peripheral neuropathy. Screening for hepatitis C, along with hepatitis B and, in the appropriate context, an underlying lymphoproliferative disorder or connective tissue disease, is an essential component of the evaluation once cryoglobulinemic vasculitis is suspected or confirmed by a properly collected and transported cryoglobulin assay, since the specimen must be maintained at body temperature during collection and transport to avoid a false-negative result from premature precipitation and loss of the cryoprecipitate before laboratory analysis.

KEY POINT: Cryoglobulin testing requires special handling: blood must be collected in a pre-warmed tube and transported to the laboratory at body temperature, since cryoglobulins that precipitate prematurely during a cold transport process will be lost from the serum fraction before analysis, producing a falsely negative result despite genuinely active cryoglobulinemic disease.

Diagnostic Workup for Cutaneous Vasculitis

A punch biopsy of a lesion less than forty-eight hours old, timed to capture the acute inflammatory infiltrate before it resolves or becomes nonspecific, is the essential first diagnostic step for any suspected cutaneous vasculitis, with a second specimen sent for direct immunofluorescence when IgA vasculitis or another immune complex-mediated process is suspected, since IgA-dominant vessel wall deposition supports that diagnosis specifically. Laboratory evaluation should be tailored to the clinical picture but generally includes a complete blood count, comprehensive metabolic panel with renal function, urinalysis to screen for renal involvement, erythrocyte sedimentation rate and C-reactive protein to assess systemic inflammatory activity, and complement levels, particularly when urticarial vasculitis is suspected. Additional testing, including antineutrophil cytoplasmic antibody testing, antinuclear antibody testing, hepatitis B and C serologies, cryoglobulins, and age-appropriate malignancy screening, should be guided by the specific clinical context, associated systemic findings, and patient age rather than ordered indiscriminately in every case.

A thorough medication history deserves particular emphasis in the vasculitis workup, since a substantial proportion of adult-onset cutaneous vasculitis is drug-induced, with antibiotics, particularly beta-lactams and sulfonamides, nonsteroidal anti-inflammatory drugs, thiazide diuretics, and, as detailed below, certain recreational drug adulterants among the most frequently implicated agents; identifying and discontinuing a culprit medication is often the single most important management step in drug-induced vasculitis and can obviate the need for systemic immunosuppressive therapy altogether when recognized promptly and the offending agent withdrawn before significant systemic organ involvement develops.

1. Identify a lesion less than forty-eight hours old for biopsy, since older lesions may show only nonspecific changes.
2. Obtain a punch biopsy for routine histology to confirm the leukocytoclastic vasculitis pattern and assess vessel size and depth of involvement.
3. Obtain a second perilesional or lesional specimen for direct immunofluorescence when IgA vasculitis or another immune complex-mediated process is suspected.
4. Screen for renal and systemic involvement with urinalysis, complete blood count, metabolic panel, and inflammatory markers in every patient.
5. Tailor further serologic, infectious, and malignancy evaluation to the patient's age, associated systemic findings, and clinical context rather than pursuing an exhaustive standardized panel in every case.

Erythema Nodosum: A Septal Panniculitis

Erythema nodosum is the most common form of panniculitis, an inflammatory process centered in the subcutaneous fat, and reflects a delayed-type hypersensitivity reaction occurring in the septa between fat lobules rather than a primary vasculitis, though the two conditions are frequently discussed together given their overlapping list of triggers and shared status as reactive cutaneous processes. It presents as tender, erythematous to violaceous subcutaneous nodules, most characteristically on the bilateral anterior shins, that never ulcerate, a feature that reliably distinguishes erythema nodosum from other panniculitides such as pancreatic panniculitis or nodular vasculitis, which do ulcerate. Individual lesions evolve through a color progression resembling a resolving bruise, from red to violaceous to a yellow-green hue, a phenomenon termed erythema contusiforme, over one to two weeks, even as new lesions may continue to appear over several weeks.

Systematic Evaluation of Erythema Nodosum

Because erythema nodosum is a reactive process rather than a primary disease, its clinical significance lies chiefly in identifying the underlying trigger, and a systematic evaluation should include screening for streptococcal infection, the most common trigger overall, particularly in children; inflammatory bowel disease, in which erythema nodosum can precede gastrointestinal symptoms and serves as a useful marker of disease activity; sarcoidosis, in which erythema nodosum combined with bilateral hilar lymphadenopathy, fever, and arthralgia constitutes Lofgren syndrome, a presentation with a favorable prognosis for spontaneous remission; medications, particularly oral contraceptives and sulfonamide antibiotics; and, less commonly, deep fungal infection or pregnancy. A chest radiograph is a reasonable component of the initial evaluation given the diagnostic and prognostic significance of identifying Lofgren syndrome, alongside a throat culture or streptococcal serology, complete blood count, and inflammatory markers, with additional testing directed by the review of systems and physical examination.

EVIDENCE: Lofgren syndrome, the combination of erythema nodosum, bilateral hilar lymphadenopathy, fever, and polyarthralgia as an acute presentation of sarcoidosis, carries a favorable prognosis, with spontaneous remission occurring in the substantial majority of patients within several months, distinguishing it from the more chronic, progressive course that can characterize sarcoidosis presenting through other manifestations, and generally obviating the need for biopsy confirmation when the clinical constellation is classic.

Erythema Multiforme

Erythema multiforme is an acute, self-limited hypersensitivity reaction characterized by the target or iris lesion, a papule or plaque with three concentric zones, a dusky or blistered center, a surrounding pale ring of edema, and an outer erythematous ring, distributed classically in an acral, symmetric pattern favoring the extensor surfaces of the extremities, palms, and soles. The overwhelming majority of cases are triggered by infection rather than medication, with herpes simplex virus responsible for the large majority of recurrent erythema multiforme, and Mycoplasma pneumoniae a well-recognized trigger, particularly in children and adolescents, sometimes producing a distinct pattern with more prominent mucosal involvement termed Mycoplasma-induced rash and mucositis. Erythema multiforme is subdivided into a minor form, with absent or limited mucosal involvement at only one site and no systemic symptoms, and a major form, with involvement of at least two mucosal surfaces and systemic symptoms including fever and malaise, though even major erythema multiforme is distinguished from Stevens-Johnson syndrome by the presence of true target lesions rather than the atypical, flat, purpuric targets and widespread epidermal detachment characteristic of that more severe, distinct condition.

CAUTION: Erythema multiforme and Stevens-Johnson syndrome are frequently confused but are distinct entities with different triggers, morphology, and management: erythema multiforme is overwhelmingly infection-triggered with true, well-formed target lesions in an acral distribution, while Stevens-Johnson syndrome is overwhelmingly medication-triggered with atypical, flat, purpuric targets and progressive epidermal detachment predominantly on the trunk. Correctly distinguishing the two shapes the entire management approach, since discontinuing a culprit medication is central to Stevens-Johnson syndrome but often irrelevant to infection-triggered erythema multiforme.

Recurrent Erythema Multiforme and Suppressive Therapy

Recurrent herpes-associated erythema multiforme, defined as multiple episodes occurring over months to years, is managed with continuous suppressive antiviral therapy, typically oral acyclovir or valacyclovir, even when an individual herpes labialis outbreak preceding the erythema multiforme episode was clinically inapparent or forgotten by the patient, since the immunologic trigger, deposition of herpes simplex viral antigen in keratinocytes with a subsequent T-cell-mediated response, can occur even after subclinical viral reactivation. Suppressive therapy is typically continued for six months to a year before a trial discontinuation, with resumption if recurrences reappear, and this approach is markedly more effective at preventing recurrence than episodic treatment of the herpes outbreak itself, since the erythema multiforme reaction is triggered by an immunologic cascade that begins before clinically apparent lesions develop. Patients whose recurrent disease persists despite adequate antiviral suppression, or in whom no herpes trigger can be identified despite thorough evaluation, warrant reconsideration of the diagnosis and evaluation for other recurrent triggers, including contact allergens and, rarely, an underlying autoinflammatory predisposition.

Neutrophilic Dermatoses: Sweet Syndrome and Pyoderma Gangrenosum

Sweet syndrome, also termed acute febrile neutrophilic dermatosis, presents with the abrupt onset of tender, edematous, erythematous to violaceous plaques and nodules, often with a pseudovesicular or "juicy" surface quality reflecting dense dermal edema, accompanied by fever, peripheral neutrophilia, and elevated inflammatory markers. The classic form is idiopathic or follows an upper respiratory or gastrointestinal infection, while a malignancy-associated form, most often linked to acute myeloid leukemia or myelodysplastic syndrome, and a drug-induced form, classically triggered by granulocyte colony-stimulating factor, are important variants to recognize given their distinct evaluation and management implications; new-onset Sweet syndrome in an older adult, or Sweet syndrome accompanying unexplained cytopenias, should prompt hematologic evaluation. Histology shows a dense dermal neutrophilic infiltrate without evidence of true vasculitis, a feature that helps distinguish Sweet syndrome from vasculitic processes despite some clinical overlap in appearance, and treatment with systemic corticosteroids produces a rapid, often dramatic response that itself carries some diagnostic value.

Pyoderma Gangrenosum and the Pathergy Phenomenon

Pyoderma gangrenosum begins as a tender papulopustule or nodule that rapidly ulcerates, producing a characteristic deeply undermined, violaceous, overhanging border surrounding a purulent, necrotic ulcer base, most often on the lower extremities, and is strongly associated with inflammatory bowel disease, rheumatoid arthritis, and hematologic disorders including myelodysplastic syndrome and monoclonal gammopathy, though a substantial proportion of cases remain idiopathic. Pyoderma gangrenosum is a diagnosis of exclusion, since its clinical appearance can be mimicked by infection, vasculitis, vasculopathy, and malignancy, each of which must be reasonably excluded before committing a patient to immunosuppressive therapy, and biopsy, while nonspecific, is valuable primarily to rule out these mimics rather than to confirm pyoderma gangrenosum itself. The pathergy phenomenon, in which minor trauma such as a biopsy, surgical debridement, or injection triggers new lesions or dramatic enlargement of an existing ulcer at the site of injury, is a hallmark feature that has direct clinical implications: surgical debridement of a pyoderma gangrenosum ulcer, a reasonable intervention for many other chronic wounds, can substantially worsen the condition and should be avoided until the diagnosis is confirmed and systemic immunosuppressive therapy has been initiated.

CAUTION: Aggressive surgical debridement of a presumed infected or non-healing ulcer that is actually pyoderma gangrenosum can dramatically worsen the wound through the pathergy phenomenon. Any atypical, rapidly progressive ulcer with a violaceous, undermined border, particularly in a patient with inflammatory bowel disease, rheumatoid arthritis, or a hematologic disorder, should prompt dermatologic consultation before surgical intervention is pursued.

Treatment Approaches for Pyoderma Gangrenosum

Treatment intensity for pyoderma gangrenosum is generally matched to lesion severity and extent: localized, early lesions may respond to high-potency topical or intralesional corticosteroid or topical calcineurin inhibitor therapy combined with gentle wound care, while more extensive or rapidly progressive disease requires systemic therapy, most often systemic corticosteroids as initial treatment given their rapid onset of action, with cyclosporine as an alternative first-line systemic option particularly effective for rapid disease control. Biologic therapy, most notably tumor necrosis factor-alpha inhibitors such as infliximab and adalimumab, has become an important component of the treatment armamentarium, particularly for patients with associated inflammatory bowel disease in whom the biologic addresses both the cutaneous and gastrointestinal disease simultaneously, and offers a corticosteroid-sparing option for long-term maintenance once acute control is achieved. Wound care for pyoderma gangrenosum emphasizes moisture balance and gentle, non-adherent dressings, explicitly avoiding sharp debridement given the pathergy risk discussed above, and pain control deserves particular attention given the often severe pain disproportionate to wound size that characterizes this condition.

Complications, Special Populations, and Patient Education

Levamisole-Induced Vasculopathy

A distinctive drug-induced vasculopathy has emerged among users of cocaine adulterated with levamisole, an antihelminthic agent widely used as a cutting agent, producing painful, retiform purpura, meaning purpura with an angulated, branching, stellate configuration reflecting vascular occlusion rather than simple inflammatory leakage, with a striking predilection for the ears, cheeks, and nose in addition to the extremities, a distribution distinctly unusual for other forms of cutaneous vasculitis and a valuable diagnostic clue when present. Serologic testing often reveals a distinctive combination of both perinuclear and cytoplasmic ANCA positivity simultaneously, an unusual dual pattern rarely seen in idiopathic ANCA-associated vasculitis, alongside neutropenia in a meaningful proportion of affected patients, reflecting a direct toxic effect of levamisole on the bone marrow. Recognition of this entity depends heavily on a candid substance use history, which patients may be reluctant to volunteer, and management centers on cessation of the offending exposure alongside supportive wound care, since the vasculopathy typically improves once levamisole-adulterated cocaine use stops, though recognition can be delayed when the history is not proactively elicited.

The most consequential long-term complication across the cutaneous vasculitides is renal involvement, and any patient with vasculitic purpura warrants at least a single screening urinalysis regardless of the presumed trigger, with more extended monitoring in children with IgA vasculitis and in any patient with an ANCA-associated or other systemic vasculitis. Pregnant patients with erythema nodosum should be evaluated for pregnancy itself as a potential trigger alongside the standard evaluation, since erythema nodosum can arise as a physiologic reactive process in pregnancy without another identifiable cause, generally resolving after delivery. Patients on immunosuppressive therapy for pyoderma gangrenosum or Sweet syndrome require the same infection and vaccination precautions discussed elsewhere in this text for other immunosuppressive regimens, and children with recurrent erythema multiforme benefit from pediatric infectious disease or dermatology co-management to optimize suppressive antiviral dosing and monitor for breakthrough recurrence.

PATIENT EDUCATION: Patients diagnosed with a reactive erythema or vasculitis should be counseled explicitly that the skin finding is often a signal of a process occurring elsewhere in the body, and that the evaluation is directed at identifying that underlying cause rather than simply treating the visible rash; this framing helps patients understand why extensive laboratory testing, imaging, or referral to other specialists may be recommended even when the skin lesions themselves are not severe or particularly bothersome.

Compression therapy and leg elevation offer useful adjunctive symptomatic relief for the lower extremity edema and discomfort that frequently accompany leukocytoclastic vasculitis and erythema nodosum alike, given the gravity-dependent nature of both conditions, and patients should be counseled that new crops of lesions appearing over the days following diagnosis do not necessarily indicate treatment failure but rather reflect the expected evolution of an already-triggered inflammatory process working its way through resolution. Rest and limb elevation additionally reduce hydrostatic pressure on affected dependent vasculature, and prolonged standing or ambulation during an active flare can visibly worsen purpura, a mechanistic point worth explaining to patients who might otherwise attribute new lesions solely to disease progression rather than partly to activity level.

Clinical Case: A Child With Purpura, Joint Pain, and Abdominal Discomfort

A 6-year-old boy presented with a five-day history of a rash on his lower legs and buttocks, accompanied by pain and swelling in both ankles and intermittent, crampy abdominal pain, two weeks after an upper respiratory illness treated supportively at home. Examination revealed numerous palpable, purpuric papules and small plaques concentrated on the lower legs, ankles, and buttocks, with mild swelling and tenderness of both ankle joints but full range of motion, and a soft abdomen without rebound or guarding despite his reported discomfort. Urinalysis revealed microscopic hematuria without significant proteinuria, and a punch biopsy of a purpuric papule showed leukocytoclastic vasculitis with direct immunofluorescence demonstrating prominent IgA deposition within vessel walls, confirming a diagnosis of IgA vasculitis.

Given the presence of hematuria, he was started on a monitoring plan with repeat urinalysis every one to two weeks for the following two months to watch for progression to proteinuria or declining renal function, alongside supportive care for his joint pain with acetaminophen, since his arthralgia was not severe enough to warrant systemic corticosteroid therapy. His parents were counseled that the cutaneous and joint symptoms would likely resolve within four to six weeks without specific treatment, but that renal monitoring was the most important ongoing component of his care regardless of how quickly the visible rash improved, and that any development of visibly bloody or notably reduced urine output should prompt immediate re-evaluation. At two-month follow-up, his skin and joint symptoms had fully resolved and repeat urinalysis remained free of proteinuria, allowing him to be transitioned to a lower-frequency monitoring schedule, with a final urinalysis planned at the six-month mark from symptom onset before formal discharge from renal surveillance, consistent with guideline-recommended monitoring duration for this condition.

Clinical Case: A Rapidly Enlarging Leg Ulcer After a Biopsy

A 44-year-old woman with a history of ulcerative colitis presented with a two-week history of a painful, rapidly enlarging ulcer on her shin that had been initially treated by an outside clinician as a presumed infected wound with oral antibiotics and a surgical debridement, after which the ulcer had roughly doubled in size over the following week. Examination revealed a four-centimeter ulcer with a deeply undermined, violaceous, boggy border and a purulent, necrotic base, with no surrounding cellulitis or lymphangitic streaking to suggest an ongoing untreated bacterial process, and wound cultures from the prior visit had grown only mixed skin flora without a clear pathogen.

The combination of a rapidly enlarging ulcer with a violaceous undermined border, a history of inflammatory bowel disease, and clear worsening following surgical debridement was recognized as classic for pyoderma gangrenosum with pathergy, and further surgical intervention was explicitly avoided. After reasonable exclusion of infection, vasculitis, and vascular insufficiency through wound culture, biopsy showing a dense neutrophilic infiltrate without vasculitis, and arterial and venous duplex studies, she was started on systemic corticosteroid therapy with a plan to transition to a corticosteroid-sparing agent given her underlying inflammatory bowel disease, which was also reassessed by gastroenterology given the recognized link between pyoderma gangrenosum activity and underlying bowel disease activity. She and her wound care team were explicitly counseled that debridement should be avoided going forward given the pathergy phenomenon, and gentle, non-traumatic local wound care alongside systemic immunosuppressive therapy was emphasized as the appropriate combined approach, with her ulcer showing early margin flattening and reduced purulence within two weeks of starting treatment.

THE MORPHOLOGY-TO-MANAGEMENT SYSTEM — Reading the Reactive Skin as a Systemic Signal

Pattern Introduced This Chapter: Palpable purpura as the marker of small vessel vasculitis, non-ulcerating pretibial nodules as the marker of erythema nodosum, and target lesions as the marker of infection-triggered erythema multiforme, each requiring a distinct systemic evaluation.

Cross-Cutting Anchor: Every condition in this chapter is a cutaneous signal of a process elsewhere in the body; biopsy timing (a lesion under forty-eight hours old), lesion palpability, and ulceration versus non-ulceration are the anchors that separate the vasculitides and reactive erythemas from one another and guide the direction of systemic workup.

Summary and Key Concepts

Palpable purpura is the clinical hallmark of small vessel leukocytoclastic vasculitis and should be distinguished from flat, non-inflammatory purpura, which points toward a coagulopathy or platelet disorder instead.

IgA vasculitis (Henoch-Schonlein purpura) presents with the tetrad of palpable purpura, arthralgia, abdominal pain, and renal involvement, and requires extended urinary monitoring given the prognostic weight of nephritis.

Urticarial vasculitis is distinguished from ordinary urticaria by wheals persisting beyond twenty-four hours, a burning quality, and residual purpura or hyperpigmentation on resolution.

Erythema nodosum is a septal panniculitis presenting as non-ulcerating pretibial nodules, and its evaluation should focus on identifying an underlying trigger such as streptococcal infection, inflammatory bowel disease, or sarcoidosis.

Erythema multiforme is overwhelmingly infection-triggered, most often by herpes simplex virus, and is distinguished from Stevens-Johnson syndrome by its true target lesions, acral distribution, and generally milder course.

Sweet syndrome and pyoderma gangrenosum are neutrophilic dermatoses associated with hematologic malignancy and inflammatory bowel disease respectively, and the pathergy phenomenon in pyoderma gangrenosum means surgical debridement should be avoided until the diagnosis is confirmed.

CHAPTER 13: CONNECTIVE TISSUE DISEASE AND THE SKIN

Learning Objectives

1. Classify the cutaneous manifestations of lupus erythematosus into acute, subacute, and chronic forms and correlate each with its characteristic morphology, photosensitivity, and likelihood of systemic disease.
2. Recognize the pathognomonic and characteristic cutaneous findings of dermatomyositis and understand their association with underlying malignancy and systemic muscle disease.
3. Distinguish localized morphea from systemic sclerosis and correlate each with its expected pattern of internal organ involvement.
4. Select and interpret antinuclear antibody testing and its associated specific autoantibody panels appropriate to a suspected connective tissue disease.
5. Construct an evidence-based approach to photoprotection and systemic therapy across the cutaneous connective tissue diseases.
6. Recognize nailfold capillary changes and calcinosis cutis as clinically useful examination findings across this disease group.

The connective tissue diseases discussed in this chapter, lupus erythematosus, dermatomyositis, and scleroderma, each announce themselves on the skin before, alongside, or sometimes entirely without overt systemic involvement, making the dermatologist and the primary care clinician frequently the first physician to recognize a disease that will ultimately be managed by rheumatology, yet whose cutaneous findings remain a lifelong marker of disease activity requiring ongoing dermatologic attention. Because photosensitivity, nailfold capillary changes, and the specific morphology of an eruption carry diagnostic weight that a general description of "a rash" cannot capture, this chapter emphasizes the examination technique and pattern recognition that transform a nonspecific-appearing eruption into a named, actionable diagnosis.

Cutaneous Lupus Erythematosus: Classification

Cutaneous lupus erythematosus is classified into three principal forms based on lesion morphology, duration, and scarring potential, a classification that carries direct prognostic weight regarding the likelihood of systemic lupus erythematosus. Acute cutaneous lupus erythematosus presents classically as the malar, or butterfly, rash, an erythematous to edematous eruption across the cheeks and nasal bridge that characteristically spares the nasolabial folds, a sparing pattern that helps distinguish it from rosacea and seborrheic dermatitis, both of which tend to involve the nasolabial folds more prominently. Acute cutaneous lupus erythematosus is strongly associated with concurrent systemic disease activity, often flaring alongside other systemic manifestations such as arthritis, serositis, or nephritis, and resolves without scarring as the systemic flare is controlled.

Subacute Cutaneous Lupus Erythematosus

Subacute cutaneous lupus erythematosus presents as annular, polycyclic, or papulosquamous plaques with a predilection for sun-exposed skin, the upper trunk, extensor arms, and neck, sparing the face somewhat more than acute cutaneous lupus, and is strongly associated with anti-Ro/SSA and, less consistently, anti-La/SSB antibodies. A meaningful proportion of subacute cutaneous lupus is drug-induced, most classically by hydrochlorothiazide, terbinafine, proton pump inhibitors, and calcium channel blockers, and identifying and discontinuing a culprit medication is an essential step in management, since the eruption typically improves, sometimes dramatically, following withdrawal of the offending agent. Systemic disease activity in subacute cutaneous lupus tends to be milder than in acute cutaneous lupus, often limited to musculoskeletal symptoms, though renal and central nervous system disease can still occur and should be screened for at diagnosis.

Chronic Cutaneous (Discoid) Lupus Erythematosus

Chronic cutaneous lupus erythematosus, most commonly presenting as discoid lupus erythematosus, produces well-demarcated, erythematous plaques with adherent scale, follicular plugging visible as small keratotic plugs within dilated follicular openings, and, critically, a tendency toward scarring, atrophy, and dyspigmentation as lesions resolve, a feature that distinguishes it from the non-scarring acute and subacute forms and that carries substantial cosmetic and psychosocial consequence, particularly when lesions involve the scalp, where discoid lupus is a well-recognized cause of scarring alopecia, or the conchal bowl of the ear, a characteristic and easily overlooked site. Discoid lupus erythematosus is the most common cutaneous lupus subtype to occur in the absence of systemic lupus erythematosus, with only a minority of patients presenting with discoid lesions alone eventually developing systemic disease, though this risk rises with more widespread or disseminated discoid involvement.

Subtype	Morphology	Scarring	Systemic Disease Association
Acute cutaneous lupus	Malar erythema sparing nasolabial folds; can be generalized	None	Strong; parallels systemic disease activity
Subacute cutaneous lupus	Annular or papulosquamous plaques, photodistributed	None	Moderate; strongly anti-Ro/SSA associated; consider drug cause
Chronic (discoid) cutaneous lupus	Scaly plaques with follicular plugging	Yes, with atrophy and dyspigmentation	Lower when discoid lesions are the sole manifestation

Figure 13.1 — Clinical Photography: Discoid Lupus Erythematosus of the Conchal Bowl

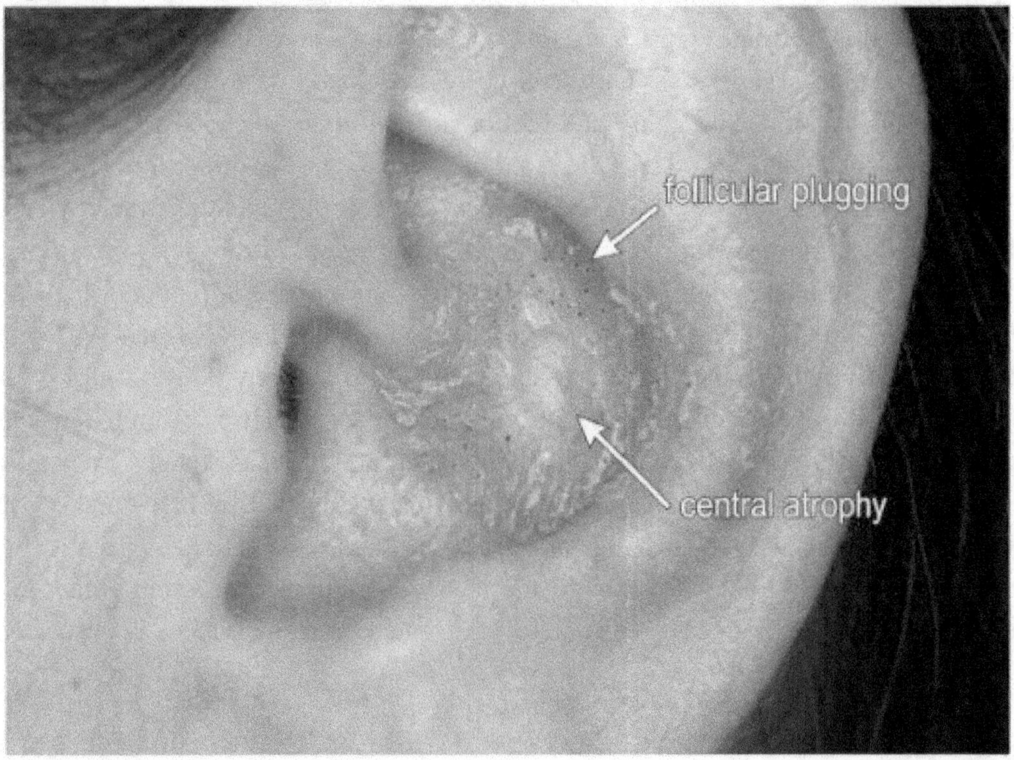

THE MORPHOLOGY-TO-MANAGEMENT SYSTEM — Photodistributed Erythema That Does or Does Not Scar

The Pattern: A photodistributed eruption, ranging from malar erythema to annular plaques to discoid scaly plaques, with scarring potential the single most important morphologic distinction to establish.

Presentation Variance: Acute cutaneous lupus spares the nasolabial folds and parallels systemic flares; subacute cutaneous lupus favors the upper trunk and is frequently drug-induced; discoid lupus favors the face, ears, and scalp and produces follicular plugging with eventual scarring.

Trap Logic: Rosacea and seborrheic dermatitis both involve the nasolabial folds, unlike acute cutaneous lupus; tinea faciei and polymorphous light eruption can mimic subacute cutaneous lupus but lack its serologic associations; scarring alopecia from other causes can mimic scalp discoid lupus, making biopsy essential when hair loss with scarring is present.

Management Pivot: Biopsy for routine histology and direct immunofluorescence (the lupus band test) when the diagnosis is uncertain; obtain antinuclear antibody testing and an extended autoantibody panel including anti-Ro/SSA in every newly diagnosed patient; review medications for a subacute cutaneous lupus-inducing drug; initiate rigorous photoprotection in every subtype regardless of systemic status.

Pattern Anchor: Scarring plus follicular plugging equals discoid lupus and demands early, aggressive treatment to prevent permanent disfigurement; non-scarring photodistributed erythema, whether malar or annular, should prompt a search for the specific systemic associations of acute versus subacute disease.

Diagnostic Workup for Cutaneous Lupus Erythematosus

Biopsy of an active lesion for routine histology, showing interface dermatitis with vacuolar change at the dermal-epidermal junction, a superficial and deep perivascular and periadnexal lymphocytic infiltrate, and, in discoid lesions, follicular plugging and basement membrane thickening, supports the diagnosis across all cutaneous lupus subtypes, while a second specimen sent for direct immunofluorescence, the lupus band test, showing granular deposition of IgG, IgM, and complement along the basement membrane zone, provides additional confirmatory support, particularly valuable in discoid lupus where a positive band in lesional, sun-protected, uninvolved skin correlates with a higher likelihood of systemic disease. Serologic evaluation should include antinuclear antibody testing as an initial screen, with reflex testing to anti-double-stranded DNA and anti-Smith antibodies, both relatively specific for systemic lupus erythematosus, and anti-Ro/SSA and anti-La/SSB antibodies, particularly relevant to subacute cutaneous lupus and to screening for the risk of neonatal lupus in women of childbearing age. A negative antinuclear antibody test does not exclude cutaneous lupus erythematosus confined to the skin, since a meaningful proportion of patients, particularly those with isolated discoid disease, never develop a positive antinuclear antibody test despite unambiguous biopsy-confirmed cutaneous lupus, reinforcing that the skin biopsy, not the serology, remains the primary diagnostic anchor when cutaneous lupus is suspected on clinical grounds.

1. Obtain a lesional biopsy for routine histology to confirm an interface dermatitis pattern consistent with cutaneous lupus erythematosus.
2. Obtain a second specimen, ideally including some non-lesional but sun-exposed skin, for direct immunofluorescence (lupus band test) when systemic disease risk assessment is needed.
3. Screen with antinuclear antibody testing, reflexing to anti-double-stranded DNA, anti-Smith, anti-Ro/SSA, and anti-La/SSB antibodies as clinically indicated.
4. Screen for systemic disease with a complete blood count, complement levels, and urinalysis in every newly diagnosed patient regardless of cutaneous subtype.
5. Review the medication list for agents associated with drug-induced subacute cutaneous lupus, particularly hydrochlorothiazide, terbinafine, and proton pump inhibitors.

Treatment of Cutaneous Lupus Erythematosus

Rigorous photoprotection, including broad-spectrum sunscreen with both ultraviolet A and B coverage, protective clothing, and behavioral sun avoidance, is foundational across every cutaneous lupus subtype, since ultraviolet exposure is a well-established trigger for both new lesion development and disease flare, and patients should be counseled that photoprotection is a treatment in its own right rather than a supplementary lifestyle recommendation. High-potency topical corticosteroids and topical calcineurin inhibitors form the first line of localized treatment, with intralesional corticosteroid injection useful for thick, resistant discoid plaques. Antimalarial therapy, most commonly hydroxychloroquine, is the systemic treatment of choice across all cutaneous lupus subtypes when topical therapy alone is insufficient, offering the additional benefit of reducing systemic disease flares and providing a cardiovascular risk-modifying effect in patients with systemic lupus erythematosus, though periodic ophthalmologic screening for hydroxychloroquine retinopathy is required given cumulative dose-related risk with long-term use.

CAUTION: Smoking has been shown to reduce the efficacy of antimalarial therapy for cutaneous lupus erythematosus, and patients who continue to smoke while on hydroxychloroquine show a demonstrably poorer treatment response than nonsmokers; smoking cessation counseling should be incorporated as a component of cutaneous lupus management rather than treated as an unrelated general health recommendation.

Dermatomyositis: Cutaneous Findings

Dermatomyositis is an idiopathic inflammatory myopathy with characteristic and often pathognomonic cutaneous findings that frequently precede or accompany proximal muscle weakness, making cutaneous recognition central to timely diagnosis. Gottron papules, violaceous to erythematous flat-topped papules and plaques overlying the extensor surfaces of the metacarpophalangeal and interphalangeal joints, are considered pathognomonic when present, distinguishing them from the more diffuse Gottron sign, a similar violaceous erythema without discrete papules overlying the same extensor surfaces as well as the elbows and knees. The heliotrope rash, a violaceous discoloration of the upper eyelids, often accompanied by periorbital edema, is similarly a highly characteristic finding, though it can be subtle, particularly in richly pigmented skin, where the violaceous hue may be more easily appreciated under natural light or by comparison to the patient's baseline coloring than under typical examination room lighting.

Additional Cutaneous Signs

The shawl sign, a photodistributed erythema across the posterior neck, shoulders, and upper back in a distribution resembling a shawl, and the V-sign, a similar photodistributed erythema across the anterior chest and neck, reflect the pronounced photosensitivity characteristic of dermatomyositis. Periungual and cuticular changes, including dilated, tortuous nailfold capillaries visible on careful examination or dermoscopy, ragged cuticles, and cuticular hemorrhage, are common and clinically useful findings, while mechanic's hands, a symmetric hyperkeratotic, fissured, and roughened change along the radial and palmar aspects of the fingers, resembling the calluses of manual laborers, is associated with the antisynthetase syndrome subset of dermatomyositis, characterized by the additional combination of interstitial lung disease and inflammatory arthritis alongside myositis and a specific set of anti-synthetase autoantibodies, most commonly anti-Jo-1.

KEY POINT: Gottron papules occur over the joints themselves, while the clinically similar-appearing violaceous erythema of psoriasis or lichen planus more typically involves the periarticular skin without the same joint-centered distribution; careful attention to whether violaceous change is centered precisely over the joint or more diffusely distributed around it assists in distinguishing dermatomyositis from its inflammatory dermatosis mimics.

Dermatomyositis: Malignancy Association and Subtypes

Adult-onset dermatomyositis carries a well-established association with underlying malignancy, particularly ovarian, lung, pancreatic, gastric, and colorectal cancers and non-Hodgkin lymphoma, with risk highest in the year surrounding diagnosis and declining, though not disappearing, over subsequent years; this association warrants age- and sex-appropriate malignancy screening at diagnosis, with some experts recommending more extensive screening, including computed tomography of the chest, abdomen, and pelvis, particularly in patients with specific clinical features associated with higher malignancy risk, such as rapid disease onset, cutaneous necrosis, or certain myositis-specific autoantibodies including anti-transcriptional intermediary factor 1-gamma. Clinically amyopathic dermatomyositis, in which characteristic cutaneous findings occur without clinically detectable muscle weakness for at least six months despite adequate evaluation, still carries the same malignancy association and interstitial lung disease risk as classic dermatomyositis and should be evaluated and monitored with equivalent rigor despite the absence of overt myopathy.

CAUTION: Clinically amyopathic dermatomyositis should never be regarded as a milder or lower-risk variant simply because muscle weakness is absent; the malignancy association and the risk of rapidly progressive interstitial lung disease, particularly linked to anti-MDA5 antibody positivity, can be equally or even more severe than in classic dermatomyositis with overt myopathy, and anti-MDA5-associated disease in particular warrants urgent pulmonary evaluation given its potential for fulminant, life-threatening lung involvement.

Localized Morphea Versus Systemic Sclerosis

Morphea, also termed localized scleroderma, produces sclerotic, indurated plaques with an inflammatory violaceous border during active disease, termed the lilac ring, and a smooth, ivory-colored, hairless center as the plaque matures, confined to skin and subcutaneous tissue without the internal organ involvement, digital ischemia, or Raynaud phenomenon characteristic of systemic sclerosis; this distinction is the single most important branch point in this section, since morphea, despite its alarming sclerotic appearance, carries a fundamentally different prognosis and management approach than systemic sclerosis. Morphea subtypes include plaque morphea, the most common and generally most limited form; linear morphea, which follows a linear band along an extremity or, when affecting the frontoparietal scalp and forehead, produces the characteristic en coup de sabre pattern resembling a sword strike, occasionally accompanied by underlying facial hemiatrophy (Parry-Romberg syndrome) when deeper tissue is involved; and generalized morphea, involving multiple body sites with confluent plaques, which can produce functional limitation from cutaneous and subcutaneous sclerosis across joints even without the systemic organ involvement of true systemic sclerosis.

Systemic Sclerosis: Cutaneous and Vascular Findings

Systemic sclerosis is subdivided into limited and diffuse cutaneous forms based on the extent of skin sclerosis, a distinction that carries substantial prognostic and monitoring implications: limited cutaneous systemic sclerosis confines sclerosis to the skin distal to the elbows and knees, plus the face, historically recognized through the CREST acronym, calcinosis cutis, Raynaud phenomenon, esophageal dysmotility, sclerodactyly, and telangiectasia, and carries a slower disease course with pulmonary arterial hypertension as its most concerning late complication, while diffuse cutaneous systemic sclerosis involves proximal skin including the trunk, progresses more rapidly, and carries higher risk of early, severe interstitial lung disease and scleroderma renal crisis, a hypertensive emergency with acute kidney injury requiring prompt recognition and angiotensin-converting enzyme inhibitor therapy. Raynaud phenomenon, a triphasic color change of the digits, pallor from vasospasm, cyanosis from deoxygenation, and rubor from reperfusion, typically precedes other manifestations of systemic sclerosis by months to years and, when accompanied by abnormal nailfold capillaroscopy findings, digital ulceration, or a positive specific autoantibody, substantially raises the likelihood of an evolving connective tissue disease rather than primary Raynaud phenomenon alone.

Feature	Morphea	Systemic Sclerosis
Distribution	Localized plaques or bands, asymmetric	Distal (limited) or diffuse including trunk (diffuse)
Raynaud phenomenon	Absent	Present, often an early feature
Nailfold capillary changes	Absent	Dilated loops with dropout, visible on capillaroscopy
Internal organ involvement	Absent (except rare deep morphea variants)	Common: lung, esophagus, kidney, heart
Autoantibody associations	Less consistent; some ANA positivity	Anti-centromere (limited), anti-Scl-70/topoisomerase (diffuse), anti-RNA polymerase III (diffuse, renal crisis risk)

KEY POINT: Nailfold capillaroscopy, examining the periungual skin under magnification, ideally with a drop of oil to improve optical clarity, for dilated capillary loops, capillary dropout, and hemorrhage, is a simple, in-office technique that distinguishes primary Raynaud phenomenon, which shows a normal capillary pattern, from secondary Raynaud phenomenon associated with an evolving connective tissue disease, which shows these characteristic abnormalities often before other diagnostic features become apparent.

Treatment of Morphea and Systemic Sclerosis

Treatment of morphea is guided by disease activity and depth rather than applied uniformly to every plaque, since the lilac ring border indicating active inflammation is the signal that treatment can still meaningfully alter the disease course, whereas long-standing, burned-out, ivory-colored plaques without an active border reflect established fibrosis that treatment is unlikely to reverse. Superficial, limited plaque morphea often responds to high-potency topical corticosteroids or topical calcineurin inhibitors combined with phototherapy, most commonly ultraviolet A1 phototherapy, which penetrates deeply enough to reach the dermis where the sclerotic process is centered, while linear or generalized morphea, particularly when crossing a joint or affecting a growing child at risk of limb length discrepancy or facial asymmetry, warrants systemic therapy, typically methotrexate with or without a corticosteroid bridge, given the more significant functional and cosmetic stakes involved in these subtypes.

Systemic Sclerosis: Organ-Directed Management

Management of systemic sclerosis is organized around its distinct organ-specific complications rather than a single unified treatment protocol, reflecting the multisystem nature of the disease. Raynaud phenomenon is managed with cold avoidance and, when needed, calcium channel blockers as first-line pharmacologic therapy, with phosphodiesterase-5 inhibitors or endothelin receptor antagonists reserved for more severe disease or digital ulceration. Interstitial lung disease, now recognized as a leading cause of mortality in systemic sclerosis, is treated with immunosuppressive therapy, most commonly mycophenolate mofetil, and antifibrotic agents originally developed for idiopathic pulmonary fibrosis have shown benefit in slowing progression of scleroderma-associated interstitial lung disease specifically. Scleroderma renal crisis, a hypertensive emergency more common in diffuse cutaneous disease and early in the disease course, is treated urgently with angiotensin-converting enzyme inhibitor therapy regardless of baseline renal function, a critical point since these agents are otherwise used cautiously in acute kidney injury but are specifically indicated here given the renin-mediated pathophysiology of this particular crisis. Esophageal dysmotility and reflux, nearly universal in systemic sclerosis, are managed with proton pump inhibitor therapy and positional and dietary modification, given the risk of aspiration and esophageal stricture with inadequately controlled reflux over time.

CAUTION: Unlike most causes of acute kidney injury, in which angiotensin-converting enzyme inhibitors are typically avoided or used cautiously, scleroderma renal crisis is a specific exception where these agents are the cornerstone of urgent treatment regardless of renal function at presentation, reflecting the renin-angiotensin-mediated pathophysiology unique to this complication; delaying angiotensin-converting enzyme inhibitor therapy while awaiting nephrology consultation in a patient with suspected scleroderma renal crisis can meaningfully worsen outcomes.

Sjogren Syndrome and Mixed Connective Tissue Disease

Sjogren syndrome, an autoimmune exocrinopathy targeting the salivary and lacrimal glands and producing the characteristic sicca symptoms of dry mouth and dry eyes, carries several cutaneous manifestations relevant to this chapter's framework, most notably an annular erythema that can closely resemble subacute cutaneous lupus erythematosus, reflecting the shared anti-Ro/SSA and anti-La/SSB antibody profile between the two conditions, and cutaneous vasculitis, most often presenting as palpable purpura on the lower extremities and carrying particular significance in Sjogren syndrome given its association with cryoglobulinemia and a modestly increased long-term risk of lymphoma, particularly mucosa-associated lymphoid tissue lymphoma arising within chronically inflamed salivary gland tissue. Xerosis and generalized cutaneous dryness are near-universal in Sjogren syndrome, reflecting the broader exocrine gland dysfunction that defines the condition, and can be sufficiently severe to warrant dedicated emollient therapy alongside management of the sicca symptoms themselves.

Mixed Connective Tissue Disease

Mixed connective tissue disease describes an overlap syndrome combining clinical features of systemic lupus erythematosus, systemic sclerosis, and dermatomyositis or polymyositis within a single patient, unified serologically by a high-titer anti-U1 ribonucleoprotein antibody that is considered essentially required for the diagnosis. Cutaneously, patients often display a combination of findings drawn from each contributing disease, puffy, edematous fingers progressing toward sclerodactyly, Raynaud phenomenon, and photosensitive or lupus-like skin changes, and the puffy hands finding in particular, diffuse non-pitting edema of the fingers giving them a sausage-like appearance, is often an early and distinctive clue that should prompt consideration of this overlap diagnosis when combined with Raynaud phenomenon and a positive antinuclear antibody test. The clinical course of mixed connective tissue disease is variable and can evolve over time to more closely resemble one of its constituent diseases, particularly systemic sclerosis, making longitudinal follow-up and periodic reassessment of organ involvement, especially pulmonary and cardiac, an essential component of long-term management regardless of how the disease presented initially.

KEY POINT: Puffy, sausage-like swelling of the fingers without clear pitting edema, particularly when accompanied by Raynaud phenomenon and a positive antinuclear antibody test, should prompt anti-U1 ribonucleoprotein antibody testing to evaluate for mixed connective tissue disease, since this finding often precedes the more classic sclerodactyly or myositis features that would otherwise suggest the diagnosis.

Myositis-Specific Autoantibody Testing in Dermatomyositis

Myositis-specific autoantibody testing has become an increasingly important component of the dermatomyositis workup, since specific antibodies correlate with distinct clinical phenotypes, complication risks, and, in some cases, prognosis, allowing a more individualized approach to evaluation and monitoring than was possible when dermatomyositis was treated as a single homogeneous entity. Anti-Mi-2 antibodies are associated with a more classic dermatomyositis phenotype with a relatively lower malignancy risk and generally favorable treatment response; anti-transcriptional intermediary factor 1-gamma antibodies carry the strongest association with underlying malignancy among the myositis-specific antibodies and warrant particularly thorough age-appropriate cancer screening when identified; anti-nuclear matrix protein 2 antibodies are associated with a higher risk of calcinosis cutis, particularly in juvenile dermatomyositis, and with more severe cutaneous ulceration; and anti-MDA5 antibodies, discussed above in the context of clinically amyopathic disease, carry the strongest association with rapidly progressive, potentially fatal interstitial lung disease and a distinctive cutaneous phenotype including painful palmar papules, cutaneous ulceration, and oral pain.

Myositis-Specific Antibody	Key Clinical Association
Anti-Mi-2	Classic dermatomyositis phenotype; relatively lower malignancy risk
Anti-TIF1-gamma	Strongest malignancy association; warrants thorough cancer screening
Anti-NXP2	Calcinosis cutis, especially in juvenile dermatomyositis; severe cutaneous ulceration
Anti-MDA5	Rapidly progressive interstitial lung disease; painful palmar papules and oral pain; can occur with minimal or absent myopathy
Anti-Jo-1 and other antisynthetase antibodies	Antisynthetase syndrome: myositis, interstitial lung disease, arthritis, mechanic's hands

Calcinosis Cutis and Additional Shared Findings

Calcinosis cutis, the deposition of insoluble calcium salts within the skin and subcutaneous tissue, occurs across several of the conditions in this chapter, most notably limited cutaneous systemic sclerosis and juvenile dermatomyositis, presenting as firm, sometimes tender nodules that can extrude a chalky white material through overlying ulceration and that are frequently complicated by secondary infection and significant functional impairment when they occur over pressure points or near joints. Radiographic imaging confirms the diagnosis and delineates the extent of deposits, and management remains challenging, with surgical excision reserved for symptomatic, well-localized, accessible lesions and medical therapies, including diltiazem, bisphosphonates, and sodium thiosulfate, showing variable and generally modest efficacy, reflecting the overall limited evidence base for calcinosis cutis treatment across the connective tissue diseases. Telangiectasias, small dilated superficial blood vessels most prominent on the face, lips, and hands, are another shared finding across limited cutaneous systemic sclerosis and, to a lesser degree, dermatomyositis, and while they carry no direct medical risk in isolation, they can be a source of significant cosmetic concern and are amenable to vascular laser treatment once the underlying disease is otherwise stable.

Panniculitis and Additional Overlap Findings

Lupus panniculitis, also termed lupus profundus, produces firm, tender subcutaneous nodules and plaques that heal with characteristic depressed, lipoatrophic scarring, most often affecting the face, upper arms, and buttocks, and can occur in isolation, in association with discoid lupus lesions overlying the same area, or as part of systemic lupus erythematosus; recognizing this variant matters both because the residual lipoatrophy can be cosmetically significant and permanent and because the differential diagnosis for tender subcutaneous nodules includes several other panniculitides, such as erythema nodosum discussed in the preceding chapter, that carry entirely different underlying associations and management approaches. Rheumatoid nodules, though technically a manifestation of rheumatoid arthritis rather than the three conditions emphasized in this chapter, deserve brief mention as a commonly encountered subcutaneous nodule in patients with overlapping connective tissue disease features, presenting as firm, mobile, non-tender nodules over extensor surfaces and pressure points, most classically the olecranon, and correlating with seropositive, often more erosive rheumatoid arthritis when present.

Complications, Special Populations, and Patient Education

Neonatal lupus erythematosus results from transplacental passage of maternal anti-Ro/SSA and anti-La/SSB antibodies and produces annular, photodistributed cutaneous lesions resembling subacute cutaneous lupus in the affected infant, typically resolving spontaneously over months as maternal antibody clears, but carries a more serious risk of congenital heart block, a permanent and potentially life-threatening cardiac conduction abnormality that, unlike the cutaneous findings, does not resolve and may require permanent pacemaker placement; women with anti-Ro/SSA or anti-La/SSB antibodies who are pregnant or planning pregnancy warrant fetal cardiac monitoring during pregnancy given this risk. Children with juvenile dermatomyositis show a distinct pattern compared to adult disease, with a substantially lower malignancy association but a higher prevalence of calcinosis cutis and vasculopathic complications including gastrointestinal vasculitis, underscoring those as the areas of particular monitoring concern in the pediatric population. Pregnancy in women with systemic sclerosis warrants particular attention to blood pressure monitoring given the overlapping risk profile between scleroderma renal crisis and preeclampsia, both of which can present with new hypertension and require prompt, accurate differentiation since their management diverges substantially despite superficially similar presentations.

PATIENT EDUCATION: Patients across every condition in this chapter benefit from explicit counseling that rigorous, consistent sun protection is a core component of disease management, not merely a general health recommendation, given the well-documented role of ultraviolet exposure in triggering both new lesions and disease flares in lupus erythematosus and dermatomyositis alike, and that Raynaud phenomenon management through cold avoidance, layered clothing, and prompt rewarming techniques can meaningfully reduce the frequency and severity of digital ischemic episodes.

Patients with any connective tissue disease discussed in this chapter benefit from a coordinated, multidisciplinary care model rather than a purely dermatology-centered approach, given the frequency and severity of internal organ involvement across this disease group; establishing early relationships with rheumatology, and pulmonology or nephrology when indicated, before a complication develops rather than only after one is recognized, supports more timely intervention and better long-term outcomes.

Clinical Case: Photodistributed Plaques With a Surprising Trigger

A 58-year-old woman presented with a three-month history of annular, scaly, erythematous plaques across her upper back, shoulders, and the extensor surfaces of both arms, sparing her face almost entirely, that had progressively worsened despite treatment with a topical antifungal for a presumed diagnosis of tinea corporis. Her medication list, reviewed carefully given the photodistributed and annular morphology, revealed that she had started hydrochlorothiazide for hypertension approximately five months earlier. Examination confirmed multiple annular, polycyclic, erythematous plaques with fine scale in a strictly photodistributed pattern, without evidence of induration, follicular plugging, or scarring, and a biopsy showed an interface dermatitis pattern consistent with subacute cutaneous lupus erythematosus; serologic testing returned strongly positive for anti-Ro/SSA antibodies with a negative anti-double-stranded DNA and normal complement levels, arguing against significant systemic disease activity.

Her hydrochlorothiazide was discontinued in coordination with her primary care physician, who transitioned her antihypertensive regimen to an alternative agent, and she was started on a high-potency topical corticosteroid alongside rigorous photoprotection counseling. Over the following two months, her eruption showed substantial improvement even before initiating hydroxychloroquine, which was nonetheless started given the extent of her initial presentation and the desire to prevent recurrence, and she was scheduled for baseline and annual ophthalmologic screening given the plan for long-term antimalarial therapy. She was counseled that while her presentation had been drug-induced, the presence of anti-Ro/SSA antibodies meant she would benefit from periodic monitoring for lupus-related symptoms even after her eruption resolved, since these antibodies can persist and carry implications for any future pregnancy given the associated risk of neonatal lupus and congenital heart block. She was also advised that any future pregnancy should be flagged to her obstetric team given her antibody status, so that fetal cardiac monitoring could be arranged proactively rather than only after a concerning finding prompted the referral.

Clinical Case: Hand Changes Preceding a Systemic Diagnosis

A 47-year-old man presented for evaluation of progressively thickening, tight skin on both hands over eight months, accompanied by new Raynaud phenomenon and difficulty fully extending his fingers, alongside a six-month history of a dry cough that his primary care physician had attributed to seasonal allergies. Examination revealed sclerodactyly with taut, shiny skin over the fingers, several small pitted scars at the fingertips consistent with digital ulceration, and dilated, tortuous nailfold capillaries with areas of capillary dropout visible on capillaroscopy examination. Given the combination of sclerodactyly, Raynaud phenomenon, digital ulceration, and an unexplained chronic cough, systemic sclerosis was suspected and pulmonary function testing was obtained promptly, revealing a restrictive pattern with reduced diffusing capacity consistent with early interstitial lung disease; serologic testing returned positive for anti-Scl-70 (anti-topoisomerase) antibodies, supporting a diagnosis of diffuse cutaneous systemic sclerosis given the extent of proximal skin involvement subsequently identified on more complete examination of his forearms and chest.

He was promptly referred to rheumatology and pulmonology for coordinated management, given the recognized importance of early interstitial lung disease treatment in altering long-term outcomes in this specific antibody subset, and was counseled extensively about scleroderma renal crisis, including the importance of home blood pressure monitoring and urgent evaluation for any new headache, visual change, or significantly elevated blood pressure reading, given his diffuse cutaneous subtype and the life-threatening but treatable nature of this complication when recognized early and treated with angiotensin-converting enzyme inhibitor therapy. He was also referred to occupational therapy for hand function preservation and counseled on rigorous cold avoidance and layered clothing strategies to reduce the frequency of Raynaud episodes, with a coordinated follow-up plan established across dermatology, rheumatology, and pulmonology given the multisystem nature of his diagnosis. At his three-month follow-up visit, mycophenolate mofetil had been initiated for his interstitial lung disease with early stabilization of his pulmonary function testing, and he reported no further digital ulceration since beginning a calcium channel blocker for Raynaud phenomenon, illustrating the value of the coordinated, organ-directed treatment approach established at diagnosis.

THE MORPHOLOGY-TO-MANAGEMENT SYSTEM — Reading Photosensitivity and Sclerosis for Systemic Risk

Pattern Introduced This Chapter: Scarring versus non-scarring photodistributed erythema across the lupus subtypes, pathognomonic Gottron papules and heliotrope rash in dermatomyositis, and the localized sclerotic plaque of morphea versus the Raynaud-associated, capillary-abnormal sclerodactyly of systemic sclerosis.

Cross-Cutting Anchor: Nailfold capillary examination and a targeted autoantibody panel are the anchors that separate a purely cutaneous process from one carrying internal organ risk across every condition in this chapter; abnormal capillaries or a specific disease-associated autoantibody should always prompt systemic evaluation regardless of how limited the cutaneous findings appear.

Summary and Key Concepts

Cutaneous lupus erythematosus is classified into acute, subacute, and chronic (discoid) forms, distinguished by morphology, scarring potential, and systemic disease association; only discoid lupus scars.

Subacute cutaneous lupus erythematosus is frequently drug-induced, most classically by hydrochlorothiazide, and identifying and discontinuing the culprit medication is central to management.

Gottron papules and the heliotrope rash are characteristic cutaneous findings of dermatomyositis, which carries a significant malignancy association in adults, present even in clinically amyopathic disease.

Localized morphea is confined to skin and subcutaneous tissue without Raynaud phenomenon or internal organ involvement, distinguishing it fundamentally from systemic sclerosis.

Limited and diffuse cutaneous systemic sclerosis differ in the extent of skin involvement and in the timing and severity of pulmonary, renal, and cardiac complications, with anti-centromere, anti-Scl-70, and anti-RNA polymerase III antibodies carrying distinct prognostic associations.

Nailfold capillaroscopy is a simple in-office technique that distinguishes primary from secondary Raynaud phenomenon and should prompt systemic evaluation when abnormal.

CHAPTER 14: DISORDERS OF PIGMENTATION

Learning Objectives

1. Explain the autoimmune melanocyte destruction underlying vitiligo and distinguish its clinical patterns and management options from other causes of hypopigmentation.
2. Recognize melasma and construct a management approach addressing both pigment reduction and its high relapse tendency.
3. Differentiate post-inflammatory hyperpigmentation and hypopigmentation from primary pigmentary disorders and counsel patients on their expected time course.
4. Recognize the major congenital and acquired causes of hyperpigmentation, including cafe-au-lait macules and their syndromic associations.
5. Identify medications and systemic conditions that produce drug-induced and endocrine-associated pigmentary change.
6. Construct an evidence-based photoprotection and topical treatment regimen appropriate to each major pigmentary disorder.

Disorders of pigmentation occupy a distinctive place in dermatology: they rarely threaten physical health, yet they carry a disproportionate psychosocial burden, particularly in patients with richly pigmented skin where contrast against surrounding normal skin is often more visually striking and where the condition may be misread by others as contagious or as a marker of poor hygiene. Effective management in this chapter therefore depends as much on setting realistic expectations, particularly regarding the slow time course of repigmentation and the high relapse tendency of several of these conditions, as it does on selecting the correct topical or procedural therapy, and clinicians who fail to prepare patients for this reality risk a discouraged patient who abandons an otherwise appropriate treatment plan too early to see benefit.

Vitiligo: Pathophysiology and Classification

Vitiligo results from autoimmune-mediated destruction of melanocytes, driven by cytotoxic CD8-positive T lymphocytes that target melanocyte antigens, producing depigmented, not merely hypopigmented, macules and patches with a characteristic chalk-white or milk-white color and well-demarcated borders, a distinction that matters clinically because complete depigmentation reflects total melanocyte loss rather than reduced melanocyte activity, with direct implications for which treatments retain any chance of success. The Koebner phenomenon, the development of new lesions at sites of skin trauma such as friction, cuts, or sunburn, occurs in a meaningful proportion of patients and both supports the diagnosis when present and offers practical counseling value, since patients can be advised to minimize unnecessary skin trauma in areas where new lesions would be particularly noticeable or distressing.

Non-Segmental Versus Segmental Vitiligo

Non-segmental vitiligo, the more common form, produces bilateral, often symmetric patches with a predilection for periorificial skin, the hands, and areas of repeated friction or trauma, tends to progress unpredictably over years with periods of stability interspersed with flares, and carries a meaningful association with other autoimmune conditions, most notably autoimmune thyroid disease, but also alopecia areata, pernicious anemia, and type 1 diabetes mellitus, reflecting a shared underlying predisposition to autoimmunity rather than a direct causal relationship between vitiligo and these conditions. Segmental vitiligo, in contrast, presents unilaterally in a band-like or dermatomal-appearing distribution, typically develops rapidly over months before stabilizing, usually presents earlier in life, and carries little to no association with other autoimmune disease, reflecting a distinct pathophysiology believed to involve a mosaic population of melanocytes with heightened susceptibility to immune-mediated destruction rather than the more diffusely distributed autoimmune process of non-segmental disease. This distinction carries direct prognostic and treatment-planning value: segmental vitiligo, once stable, is often more amenable to surgical repigmentation techniques given its typically limited, stable extent, while non-segmental disease requires ongoing management of an unpredictable, potentially progressive course. A minority of patients present with a mixed pattern combining features of both forms, and halo nevi, melanocytic nevi surrounded by a ring of depigmentation, can be an early cutaneous clue preceding more widespread vitiligo in a susceptible individual, though halo nevi also occur as an isolated, benign finding without necessarily progressing to generalized vitiligo.

Feature	Non-Segmental Vitiligo	Segmental Vitiligo
Distribution	Bilateral, often symmetric, periorificial and acral predilection	Unilateral, band-like or dermatomal-appearing
Onset and course	Variable age of onset, unpredictable progression over years	Often earlier onset, rapid progression then stabilization
Autoimmune associations	Common (thyroid disease, alopecia areata, others)	Rare
Surgical treatment candidacy	Less predictable given ongoing activity	Often favorable once stable given limited, fixed extent

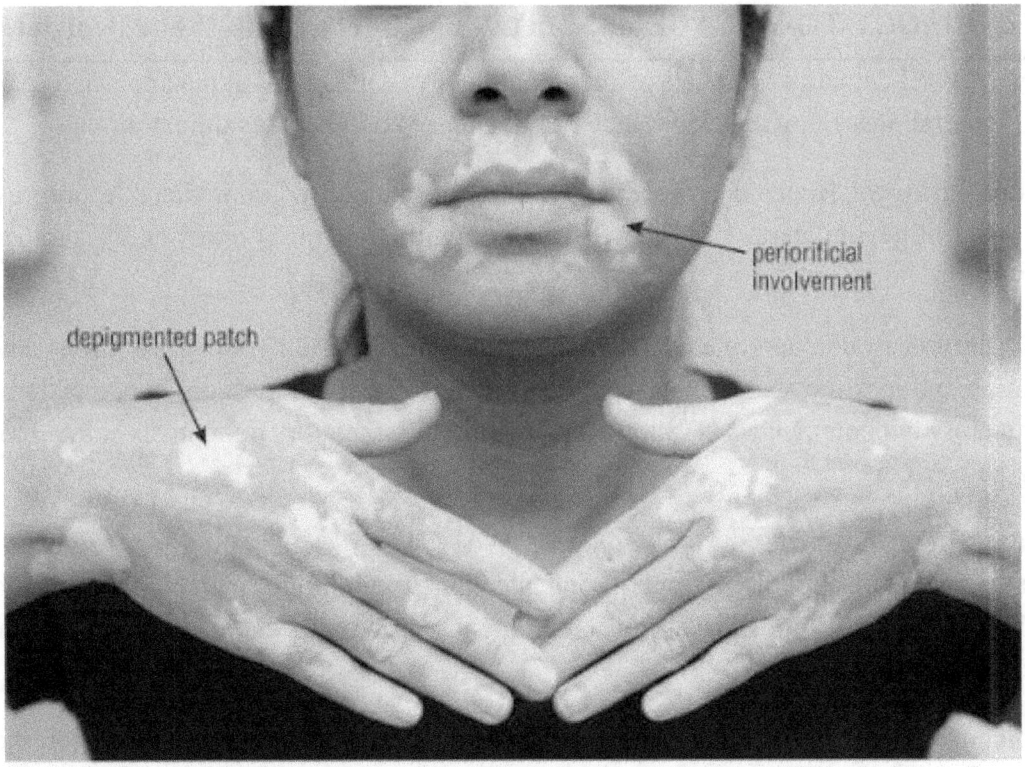

Figure 14.1 — Clinical Photography: Symmetric Depigmented Patches of Non-Segmental Vitiligo.

Vitiligo: Diagnostic Confirmation and Associated Conditions

Wood lamp examination is a valuable bedside tool for vitiligo, since depigmented lesions fluoresce a bright blue-white color that accentuates the border and extent of involvement, often revealing lesions not readily apparent under ambient room lighting, particularly in lightly pigmented patients where the contrast between depigmented and normal skin is otherwise subtle; this examination is especially useful for establishing a baseline extent of disease against which future treatment response or progression can be measured. Biopsy is rarely necessary for classic vitiligo but can be helpful in atypical or inflammatory presentations, showing a complete absence of melanocytes on special staining, distinguishing it from other hypopigmented conditions in which melanocytes remain present but are functionally suppressed or reduced in number rather than entirely absent. Baseline screening for thyroid dysfunction with thyroid-stimulating hormone testing is a reasonable component of the initial evaluation given the well-established association, with additional autoimmune screening guided by symptoms and review of systems rather than pursued indiscriminately in every patient. Standardized photography at baseline and at regular follow-up intervals, taken under consistent lighting conditions, provides an objective record of extent and treatment response that is considerably more reliable than subjective visual comparison alone, particularly over the many months typically required to judge whether a given treatment approach is working.

The Pattern: Well-demarcated, chalk-white, completely depigmented macules and patches, often periorificial or acral, that fluoresce bright blue-white under Wood lamp examination.

Presentation Variance: Bilateral, symmetric distribution with slow, unpredictable progression favors non-segmental vitiligo, unilateral, band-like distribution with rapid onset followed by stabilization favors segmental vitiligo.

Trap Logic: Pityriasis alba and tinea versicolor produce incomplete hypopigmentation rather than true depigmentation and lack the sharp, chalk-white quality and Wood lamp fluorescence pattern of vitiligo; post-inflammatory hypopigmentation follows a preceding inflammatory dermatosis at the same site rather than arising de novo.

Management Pivot: Confirm the pattern with Wood lamp examination and screen for thyroid dysfunction; initiate topical corticosteroid or topical calcineurin inhibitor therapy for limited disease, and consider phototherapy for more extensive involvement, setting expectations for a slow, months-long treatment course from the outset.

Pattern Anchor: Complete depigmentation with sharp borders and Wood lamp fluorescence equals vitiligo until proven otherwise; incomplete, ill-defined hypopigmentation should redirect the differential toward a post-inflammatory or infectious cause instead.

Vitiligo: Treatment Approaches

Topical corticosteroids and topical calcineurin inhibitors form the first line of treatment for limited vitiligo, with calcineurin inhibitors particularly favored for facial and periorificial involvement given the risk of cutaneous atrophy from prolonged corticosteroid use in these thinner-skinned areas. Topical Janus kinase inhibitors, most notably ruxolitinib cream, represent a newer addition to the topical armamentarium, targeting the interferon-gamma-driven inflammatory pathway now understood to be central to vitiligo pathogenesis, and have demonstrated meaningful repigmentation in clinical trials, particularly for facial disease, though as with all vitiligo treatments, response requires sustained therapy over months rather than weeks. Narrowband ultraviolet B phototherapy is the treatment of choice for more extensive disease, typically administered two to three times weekly over many months, and can be combined with topical therapy for enhanced effect; excimer laser, delivering a more targeted and higher-intensity form of narrowband ultraviolet B, is particularly useful for limited, localized lesions where whole-body phototherapy would be unnecessarily broad.

Surgical and Systemic Options

Surgical repigmentation techniques, including punch grafting, suction blister grafting, and melanocyte-keratinocyte cell suspension transplantation, are reserved for stable, treatment-resistant vitiligo, generally requiring at least six to twelve months of documented disease stability before consideration, since surgical intervention in actively progressing disease risks Koebnerization at both donor and recipient sites and poor graft take. For rapidly progressive or extensive disease, a short course of systemic corticosteroids or other systemic immunosuppressive therapy can help halt progression, though this approach addresses disease activity rather than achieving repigmentation itself, and depigmentation therapy, using topical monobenzone to permanently remove residual pigment in patients with extensive vitiligo covering the large majority of the body surface, is a specialized option chosen by a minority of patients who prefer a uniform depigmented appearance over the patchy contrast of partial disease, a deeply personal decision that should be discussed thoroughly, including its irreversibility, before proceeding. Systemic Janus kinase inhibitors, already established for other autoimmune skin diseases, are an area of active investigation for extensive, rapidly progressive vitiligo not adequately controlled by topical or phototherapy-based approaches, reflecting the broader shift in vitiligo treatment strategy toward directly targeting the interferon-gamma-driven immune pathway rather than relying solely on nonspecific anti-inflammatory or repigmentation-stimulating approaches.

PATIENT EDUCATION: Patients beginning any vitiligo treatment should be counseled explicitly that visible repigmentation typically requires three to six months of consistent therapy to become apparent, and often longer to achieve maximal benefit, and that perifollicular repigmentation, small dots of pigment reappearing around hair follicles within a depigmented patch, is the earliest and most encouraging sign of treatment response, appearing well before the patch fills in completely.

Additional Causes of Hypopigmentation

Idiopathic guttate hypomelanosis produces small, discrete, well-demarcated, porcelain-white macules, typically two to five millimeters in diameter, on sun-exposed extremities, most commonly the shins and forearms of older adults, reflecting a combination of cumulative photodamage and age-related decline in melanocyte density and function; while cosmetically bothersome to some patients, it is entirely benign and increasingly common with advancing age, requires no treatment beyond reassurance and ongoing photoprotection to limit further lesion development, and is distinguished from vitiligo by its small, discrete, guttate (drop-like) morphology, its confinement to chronically sun-exposed skin, and the absence of the confluent patches and Wood lamp fluorescence pattern characteristic of vitiligo. Chemical leukoderma results from occupational or consumer exposure to certain phenolic and catechol compounds found in some rubber products, adhesives, and skin-lightening agents, which are directly toxic to melanocytes, producing depigmented patches that can closely mimic vitiligo both clinically and, in some cases, histologically, making a careful occupational and product-use history essential when hypopigmentation develops in a distribution corresponding to glove use, footwear contact, or application of a specific cosmetic product.

Pityriasis Alba

Pityriasis alba, most common in children and adolescents and considered a subtle, minor manifestation of the atopic diathesis, produces ill-defined, faintly scaly, hypopigmented patches most often on the face, particularly the cheeks, that become considerably more noticeable during summer months as surrounding normal skin tans while the affected patches, with their relatively reduced melanocyte activity, do not tan to the same degree, creating an apparent seasonal worsening that actually reflects a fixed underlying process made more visible by contrast rather than a true flare of disease activity. Management is generally conservative, emphasizing emollients and photoprotection of the affected areas, with low-potency topical corticosteroids reserved for periods of more active scaling and inflammation, and parents should be reassured that pityriasis alba resolves spontaneously over months to a few years as the child ages, without permanent pigmentary consequence.

Melasma

Melasma is an acquired hyperpigmentation disorder producing symmetric, blotchy, tan to brown patches typically affecting the face in a centrofacial, malar, or mandibular distribution, driven by a combination of ultraviolet exposure, hormonal influence, most notably pregnancy and estrogen-containing oral contraceptives, and genetic predisposition, with a strong female predominance and higher prevalence in individuals with darker skin phototypes given the greater baseline melanocyte reactivity to these triggers. Wood lamp examination can help characterize the depth of pigment, with epidermal melasma showing enhanced contrast under Wood lamp illumination and dermal melasma showing minimal enhancement, reflecting deeper pigment deposition less accessible to topical therapy, though in practice many cases show a mixed pattern with both epidermal and dermal components, and this distinction, while conceptually useful, has only modest practical impact on initial treatment selection given the mixed pattern's prevalence.

Treatment and the Challenge of Relapse

Rigorous, consistent broad-spectrum photoprotection, including sunscreens that provide visible light protection through iron oxide or other tinting agents given evidence that visible light itself, not only ultraviolet radiation, can trigger melasma in susceptible individuals, is the foundation of both treatment and relapse prevention and should be emphasized as at least as important as any prescribed topical agent. First-line topical therapy typically combines hydroquinone, a tyrosinase inhibitor that reduces new melanin synthesis, with a retinoid to accelerate epidermal turnover and a mild topical corticosteroid to reduce irritation, a combination commonly formulated as a single triple-combination cream, and this regimen typically requires eight to twelve weeks of consistent use before meaningful improvement becomes apparent. Oral tranexamic acid has emerged as a valuable adjunct for more extensive or treatment-resistant melasma, believed to act by reducing plasmin-mediated stimulation of melanocyte activity, though it requires screening for contraindications including a personal or strong family history of thromboembolic disease before initiation given its antifibrinolytic mechanism. Discontinuation of an estrogen-containing oral contraceptive, when feasible and appropriate in coordination with the prescribing clinician, should also be discussed as a contributing modifiable factor in patients whose melasma appeared or clearly worsened around the time of starting hormonal contraception.

CAUTION: Melasma carries a notably high relapse tendency, and both patients and clinicians should understand from the outset that achieving improvement is often only the first phase of management, with an ongoing maintenance strategy, typically lower-potency topical therapy combined with unwavering photoprotection, required indefinitely to sustain results; aggressive procedural treatments such as high-fluence laser therapy, without a clear treatment and maintenance plan, can paradoxically worsen melasma through post-inflammatory hyperpigmentation triggered by the procedure itself, particularly in darker skin phototypes.

Procedural Adjuncts and Periorbital Hyperpigmentation

Chemical peels, most commonly formulated with glycolic acid, salicylic acid, or trichloroacetic acid, and certain laser and light-based devices can serve as useful adjuncts to topical therapy for melasma in appropriately selected patients, but carry a genuine risk of triggering post-inflammatory hyperpigmentation, particularly in darker skin phototypes, and should generally be reserved for patients who have demonstrated tolerance of and partial response to topical therapy first, introduced cautiously with conservative settings, and always undertaken with the same rigorous photoprotection expectations applied to every other aspect of melasma management. Periorbital hyperpigmentation, commonly referred to as under-eye dark circles, is a related but distinct concern frequently presenting alongside or independent of melasma, arising from a combination of factors including genuine dermal pigment deposition, visibility of underlying vasculature through thin periorbital skin, structural shadowing from tear trough hollowing, and postinflammatory change from chronic eye rubbing in atopic individuals; because the relative contribution of these mechanisms varies considerably between patients, an accurate assessment of which factor predominates is essential before selecting a treatment approach, since a purely vascular or structural component will not respond to pigment-directed therapy such as topical hydroquinone.

Post-Inflammatory Hyperpigmentation and Hypopigmentation

Post-inflammatory hyperpigmentation and hypopigmentation are secondary pigmentary changes following a preceding inflammatory or traumatic insult to the skin, such as acne, eczema, psoriasis, a burn, or a cutaneous procedure, and are distinguished from primary pigmentary disorders by their direct correspondence to the distribution of the preceding inflammatory process rather than arising independently. Post-inflammatory hyperpigmentation results from inflammation-triggered stimulation of melanocyte activity and transfer of melanin to surrounding keratinocytes and, in some cases, into the dermis via melanin incontinence, and is more common and more persistent in darker skin phototypes, reflecting the greater baseline melanocyte reactivity in these populations; epidermal post-inflammatory hyperpigmentation generally fades over months, while dermal melanin incontinence can persist for a year or longer given the much slower clearance of pigment once it has been deposited in the dermis. Post-inflammatory hypopigmentation, in contrast, reflects transient suppression of melanocyte function by the preceding inflammatory process rather than melanocyte destruction, and therefore has a favorable prognosis for spontaneous repigmentation over weeks to months as the inflammatory trigger resolves and melanocyte activity recovers, an important distinction from vitiligo, in which melanocytes are permanently destroyed rather than merely suppressed.

KEY POINT: The single most important counseling point for post-inflammatory pigmentary change is that both hyperpigmentation and hypopigmentation are generally temporary and self-resolving once the underlying inflammatory trigger is controlled, in sharp contrast to vitiligo, and setting this expectation early prevents patients from prematurely seeking aggressive or unnecessary pigment-correcting treatment for a condition that would likely have resolved on its own with time and control of the original inflammatory dermatosis.

Management of post-inflammatory hyperpigmentation begins with controlling the underlying inflammatory trigger, since ongoing active disease, most commonly acne in clinical practice, will continue generating new pigmentary change faster than existing pigment can fade; once the primary process is controlled, rigorous daily photoprotection prevents further darkening of existing pigment, since ultraviolet exposure stimulates additional melanin production in already-hyperactive melanocytes at the affected site, and topical agents including azelaic acid, topical retinoids, and, for more persistent cases, hydroquinone can accelerate fading, though patients should be counseled that even with active treatment the natural resolution timeline, typically several months for epidermal pigment and up to a year or more for dermal melanin incontinence, cannot be dramatically shortened and that consistent, patient adherence to a straightforward regimen outperforms an aggressive but poorly tolerated one.

Congenital and Acquired Hyperpigmentation

Cafe-au-lait macules, well-demarcated, uniformly tan to light brown patches present at birth or developing in early childhood, are common in the general population as isolated findings but carry syndromic significance when multiple lesions are present: six or more cafe-au-lait macules larger than five millimeters in prepubertal children, or larger than fifteen millimeters in postpubertal individuals, is one of the diagnostic criteria for neurofibromatosis type 1, and the presence of this finding should prompt a careful examination for other diagnostic features, including axillary or inguinal freckling (Crowe sign), neurofibromas, and Lisch nodules on ophthalmologic examination, alongside a family history and consideration of genetic counseling and referral. McCune-Albright syndrome should be considered when cafe-au-lait macules are larger, fewer in number, and demonstrate a characteristically irregular, jagged border often likened to the coastline of Maine, in contrast to the smoother border of neurofibromatosis-associated macules, in a patient with accompanying precocious puberty or polyostotic fibrous dysplasia.

Becker Nevus and Other Acquired Hyperpigmentation

Becker nevus is an acquired, unilateral, tan to brown patch, most commonly appearing on the shoulder or upper trunk around puberty, frequently developing overlying coarse terminal hair growth (hypertrichosis) and occasionally an underlying smooth muscle hamartoma producing subtle piloerection or a slightly elevated, cobblestoned surface texture; it is a benign finding requiring no treatment beyond reassurance, though patients bothered by its cosmetic appearance may pursue laser hair removal for the associated hypertrichosis and laser or other pigment-directed therapy for the patch itself, generally with only modest and variable results given its typically dermal component. Acanthosis nigricans, velvety, hyperpigmented, thickened plaques most commonly affecting the neck, axillae, and other flexural areas, serves as a valuable cutaneous marker of underlying insulin resistance and should prompt screening for type 2 diabetes mellitus and metabolic syndrome, particularly in children and adolescents where its presence is an important, often earlier clue to emerging insulin resistance than laboratory abnormalities alone; rapidly progressive, extensive acanthosis nigricans in an older adult, particularly with mucosal involvement or an atypical distribution, should prompt consideration of malignant acanthosis nigricans, a rare paraneoplastic phenomenon most often associated with gastric adenocarcinoma.

Physiologic and Benign Pigmentary Variants

Linea nigra, a vertical band of hyperpigmentation extending along the midline from the pubis toward the umbilicus, is a common physiologic finding in pregnancy, reflecting hormonally driven melanocyte stimulation analogous to that seen in melasma, and resolves gradually postpartum without specific treatment required. Longitudinal melanonychia, a brown to black linear band running the length of the nail plate, is common and typically benign in darker skin phototypes, where it can affect multiple nails and reflects physiologic melanocyte activity within the nail matrix, but a single band, particularly one that is new, widening, darkening, or accompanied by pigment extending onto the surrounding proximal or lateral nail fold skin, termed a positive Hutchinson sign, should prompt urgent evaluation to exclude subungual melanoma, since this presentation is otherwise indistinguishable at a glance from benign melanonychia yet carries an entirely different, potentially life-threatening significance. Dermatosis papulosa nigra, small, benign, hyperpigmented papules most commonly on the face and neck of individuals with darker skin phototypes, represents a benign proliferation related to seborrheic keratosis and requires no treatment beyond reassurance unless removal is desired for cosmetic reasons, in which case gentle techniques such as light electrodesiccation or scissor excision are preferred given the elevated risk of post-inflammatory pigmentary change from more aggressive removal methods in this skin type.

CAUTION: A single, new, or changing band of longitudinal melanonychia, especially with pigment extension onto the adjacent nail fold skin (a positive Hutchinson sign), should never be assumed to be a benign physiologic variant without further evaluation, since this presentation can represent subungual melanoma, a diagnosis where delayed recognition carries serious prognostic consequences.

Drug-Induced and Endocrine-Associated Pigmentary Change

A range of systemic medications can produce distinctive patterns of hyperpigmentation that should be recognized to avoid an unnecessary and potentially invasive workup for a primary pigmentary disorder when the true cause is pharmacologic. Minocycline, used extensively for acne and rosacea, produces at least three distinct patterns of pigmentation: a blue-gray discoloration within scars or areas of prior inflammation, a blue-gray discoloration of normal skin, particularly on the shins, and a more diffuse muddy-brown discoloration of sun-exposed skin, each reflecting a different proposed mechanism of pigment or drug-metabolite deposition, and all of which can be slow to resolve, sometimes over years, even after the medication is discontinued. Amiodarone produces a distinctive blue-gray to violaceous discoloration concentrated in sun-exposed areas, particularly the face, reflecting drug and drug-metabolite accumulation in the dermis with secondary photosensitization, and antimalarial agents, including hydroxychloroquine, can produce blue-gray pigmentation of the shins, hard palate, and nail beds through a related mechanism of drug-pigment complex deposition.

Endocrine Causes of Pigmentary Change

Primary adrenal insufficiency (Addison disease) produces diffuse hyperpigmentation, most pronounced in sun-exposed areas, skin folds, pressure points, and mucosal surfaces, resulting from markedly elevated adrenocorticotropic hormone levels that, due to shared precursor cleavage from proopiomelanocortin, also stimulate melanocyte activity through cross-reactivity with melanocortin receptors; this finding, particularly when accompanied by fatigue, weight loss, and orthostatic hypotension, should prompt endocrine evaluation given the potentially life-threatening nature of untreated adrenal insufficiency. Hyperthyroidism can produce a more subtle, diffuse hyperpigmentation in some patients, while hypothyroidism more classically produces a pale, sallow complexion with associated dry, coarse skin, illustrating how thyroid dysfunction in either direction can manifest through cutaneous pigmentary and textural change that offers a clinical clue to the underlying systemic endocrine abnormality. Nutritional deficiencies, particularly vitamin B12 deficiency, can likewise produce a diffuse hyperpigmentation, sometimes most prominent over the knuckles and skin creases, and should be considered in patients with an appropriate dietary history, malabsorptive condition, or accompanying macrocytic anemia, since the pigmentary change often improves once the underlying deficiency is corrected with appropriate supplementation.

Complications, Special Populations, and Patient Education

Vitiligo carries a well-documented psychosocial burden, including anxiety, depression, and reduced quality of life, that can rival or exceed the burden of many medically more severe dermatologic conditions, particularly in patients with darker skin phototypes where the visual contrast is more pronounced and in cultures where vitiligo carries additional social stigma; screening for psychosocial impact and offering appropriate support or referral is an important, often underemphasized component of comprehensive vitiligo care. Melasma occurring in pregnancy, sometimes termed the mask of pregnancy or chloasma, often improves substantially after delivery as hormonal levels normalize, and definitive pigment-directed treatment is generally deferred until the postpartum period both because several first-line topical agents carry pregnancy safety concerns and because a meaningful proportion of pregnancy-associated melasma improves spontaneously without treatment. Children with extensive cafe-au-lait macules or other pigmentary findings suggestive of a genetic syndrome benefit from early referral to genetics and appropriate subspecialty follow-up, since early diagnosis of conditions such as neurofibromatosis type 1 allows for proactive surveillance of associated complications rather than reactive management after a complication has already developed. All patients with a depigmenting or hypopigmenting condition, most importantly vitiligo, require heightened photoprotection counseling specific to their affected skin, since depigmented patches lack the natural ultraviolet protection provided by melanin and are therefore more susceptible to sunburn than surrounding normally pigmented skin, an important and sometimes overlooked point given that the overall discussion of photoprotection in these patients often centers on preventing pigmentary change in unaffected skin rather than on the distinct, elevated burn risk within the depigmented areas themselves.

PATIENT EDUCATION: Patients with any pigmentary disorder benefit from clear counseling that pigmentary conditions are neither contagious nor a reflection of poor hygiene, a misconception that unfortunately remains common and can compound the psychosocial burden these conditions already carry; providing patients with accurate, simple language to explain their condition to others, alongside appropriate treatment, is a meaningful and often underappreciated part of comprehensive care.

Camouflage cosmetics, including specialized concealers and self-tanning products designed to blend depigmented or hyperpigmented areas with surrounding normal skin, offer a valuable adjunctive tool for patients across nearly every condition in this chapter while definitive treatment is underway, and referral to a cosmetic counselor or patient support organization familiar with camouflage techniques for vitiligo in particular can meaningfully improve quality of life during the often lengthy treatment course; this option should be offered proactively rather than only in response to a patient specifically asking about cosmetic coverage, since many patients are unaware such resources exist.

Clinical Case: Depigmented Patches With a Family History of Thyroid Disease

A 29-year-old woman presented with a two-year history of gradually enlarging, symmetric depigmented patches around her eyes, mouth, and on the dorsal aspects of both hands, noting that her mother had a history of hypothyroidism. Examination confirmed multiple well-demarcated, chalk-white, completely depigmented patches in a periorificial and acral distribution, and Wood lamp examination revealed additional subtle patches not readily visible under ambient lighting, along with sharper delineation of the extent of her known lesions. The bilateral, symmetric distribution and slow progressive course over two years were consistent with non-segmental vitiligo, and given the strong family history of autoimmune thyroid disease, thyroid-stimulating hormone testing was obtained as part of her initial workup, returning mildly elevated and prompting referral to endocrinology, where she was subsequently diagnosed with subclinical hypothyroidism.

She was started on a topical calcineurin inhibitor for her facial and periorificial lesions, given the sensitivity of this skin to long-term corticosteroid use, and narrowband ultraviolet B phototherapy was initiated for the more extensive hand involvement, with explicit counseling that meaningful repigmentation would likely take several months of consistent treatment to become apparent and that early perifollicular pigment dots, rather than complete patch resolution, would be the first sign of a positive response. She was also counseled about the association between vitiligo and other autoimmune conditions and advised to report any new symptoms suggestive of additional autoimmune disease, given her demonstrated predisposition, and at her four-month follow-up visit, early perifollicular repigmentation was visible within several of her facial patches, providing encouraging, tangible evidence of treatment response that reinforced her motivation to continue the lengthy treatment course. She was additionally counseled about her elevated sunburn risk within the depigmented patches themselves and provided with a mineral-based, higher-protection sunscreen specifically for use over these areas, distinct from the routine daily sunscreen she already used on the rest of her face.

Clinical Case: Facial Hyperpigmentation With a Hormonal Trigger

A 34-year-old woman presented six months postpartum with persistent, symmetric, blotchy brown patches across her cheeks, upper lip, and forehead that had first appeared during her pregnancy and had not improved despite delivery several months earlier. She reported considerable distress about the appearance of the patches, which she felt made her look perpetually "dirty" or unwashed despite normal hygiene, and noted that the patches appeared to worsen with sun exposure, including through her car window during her daily commute, a detail that prompted specific counseling that ordinary window glass blocks most ultraviolet B but transmits a substantial proportion of ultraviolet A and visible light, both of which are relevant triggers for her condition. Examination revealed symmetric, centrofacial hyperpigmented patches with a mixed pattern on Wood lamp examination, consistent with melasma showing both epidermal and dermal pigment components.

She was counseled extensively that broad-spectrum sunscreen providing visible light protection, applied daily regardless of weather or planned sun exposure, was the single most important intervention both for treatment and for preventing recurrence, and was started on a triple-combination topical cream containing hydroquinone, a retinoid, and a mild corticosteroid, with explicit counseling about the expected eight-to-twelve-week timeline before meaningful improvement and about the high likelihood that some maintenance therapy would be needed indefinitely to sustain results given melasma's well-recognized relapse tendency. She was also counseled against pursuing aggressive laser treatment that she had researched online, given the risk that such treatment could paradoxically worsen her pigmentation through post-inflammatory hyperpigmentation in her skin type, and was instead offered a conservative, stepwise treatment plan with realistic expectations set from the outset; at three-month follow-up she reported meaningful improvement in the visibility of her patches and had maintained consistent sunscreen use, which she now understood as a permanent component of her skincare routine rather than a temporary measure. She was also reassured that any hormonal contraception she might consider in the future carried a risk of triggering or worsening her melasma, information she found useful for an upcoming discussion with her primary care physician about postpartum contraceptive options.

THE MORPHOLOGY-TO-MANAGEMENT SYSTEM — Complete Loss Versus Excess or Transient Change

Pattern Introduced This Chapter: The chalk-white, Wood lamp-fluorescent, complete depigmentation of vitiligo versus the symmetric centrofacial hyperpigmentation of melasma versus the transient, distribution-matched pigmentary change following a preceding inflammatory dermatosis.

Cross-Cutting Anchor: Whether melanocytes are destroyed (vitiligo, permanent), overactive (melasma and hyperpigmentation, treatable but relapse-prone), or merely transiently suppressed (post-inflammatory hypopigmentation, self-resolving) is the anchor question that determines both prognosis and how aggressively to intervene across every pigmentary disorder in this chapter.

Summary and Key Concepts

Vitiligo results from autoimmune melanocyte destruction, producing chalk-white, completely depigmented, Wood lamp-fluorescent patches, and is classified into non-segmental (bilateral, autoimmune-associated) and segmental (unilateral, typically non-associated) forms.

Vitiligo treatment, whether topical, phototherapy-based, or surgical, requires months of sustained therapy before meaningful repigmentation is apparent, and setting this expectation is essential to treatment adherence.

Melasma is a hormonally and ultraviolet-influenced hyperpigmentation disorder with a high relapse tendency, managed with rigorous photoprotection, combination topical therapy, and, for resistant cases, oral tranexamic acid.

Post-inflammatory hyperpigmentation and hypopigmentation follow a preceding inflammatory dermatosis in the same distribution and are generally self-resolving, distinguishing them from primary pigmentary disorders such as vitiligo.

Six or more cafe-au-lait macules above a size threshold should prompt evaluation for neurofibromatosis type 1, while acanthosis nigricans serves as a cutaneous marker of underlying insulin resistance warranting metabolic screening.

Minocycline, amiodarone, and antimalarial agents produce recognizable drug-induced pigmentary patterns, and diffuse hyperpigmentation with fatigue and weight loss should prompt evaluation for primary adrenal insufficiency.

CHAPTER 15: HAIR DISORDERS AND ALOPECIA

Learning Objectives

1. Distinguish non-scarring from scarring alopecia on clinical and trichoscopic grounds and explain why this distinction determines both urgency and treatment approach.
2. Recognize the patterned distribution of androgenetic alopecia and construct an evidence-based treatment approach for both male and female patients.
3. Differentiate alopecia areata from androgenetic alopecia and telogen effluvium using pull test findings, exclamation point hairs, and trichoscopic features.
4. Identify the common triggers of telogen effluvium and anagen effluvium and distinguish each from the more gradual course of androgenetic alopecia.
5. Recognize the major scarring (cicatricial) alopecias and understand why early diagnosis and treatment are critical to preventing permanent hair loss.
6. Distinguish trichotillomania from alopecia areata and construct an appropriate evaluation and referral pathway.

Hair loss carries a psychosocial weight disproportionate to its physical severity, and patients presenting with alopecia are frequently anxious, having often already searched extensively online and arrived with strong preconceptions about diagnosis and prognosis. The single most important organizing question in this chapter, one that should be answered within the first minute of examination, is whether the follicular openings are preserved or lost: preserved follicular ostia indicate a non-scarring process with potential for full recovery, while obliterated follicular openings indicate a scarring process in which lost hair is permanently gone, a distinction that reframes the entire encounter from a discussion of treatment options to one of urgency, since scarring alopecia treated early can be stabilized before further permanent loss occurs, while scarring alopecia recognized late offers only damage control.

The Non-Scarring Versus Scarring Framework

A thorough hair loss history, including onset and time course, pattern of shedding versus thinning, family history, medication and supplement use, dietary history, recent illness or major life stressors, and hairstyling practices, provides essential context that often narrows the differential substantially before the physical examination even begins. Trichoscopy, dermoscopic examination of the scalp and hair, is the essential bedside tool for making the scarring versus non-scarring distinction quickly and reliably. In non-scarring alopecia, follicular openings remain visible, often with characteristic findings specific to the underlying cause, such as miniaturized hairs of varying diameter in androgenetic alopecia or exclamation point hairs in alopecia areata, while the follicular unit itself, capable of regenerating a normal hair shaft once the underlying process resolves or is treated, remains structurally intact. In scarring alopecia, follicular openings are replaced by smooth, shiny areas of fibrosis, sometimes with perifollicular erythema or scale at the actively inflamed periphery of the process, reflecting destruction of the follicular stem cell niche located in the bulge region, an injury from which the follicle cannot recover regardless of subsequent treatment; the histologic distinction mirrors this bedside finding, with non-scarring alopecia showing preserved follicular architecture and scarring alopecia showing follicular destruction and replacement by fibrous tissue.

KEY POINT: The presence or absence of visible follicular openings on trichoscopy is the single most valuable piece of information in the entire alopecia evaluation, since it immediately separates a group of conditions with potential for full recovery from a group of conditions in which lost hair is permanently gone and treatment goals shift to halting further progression rather than restoring what has already been lost.

Androgenetic Alopecia

Androgenetic alopecia, the most common cause of hair loss in both sexes, results from progressive miniaturization of genetically susceptible hair follicles under the influence of dihydrotestosterone, a more potent androgen derived from testosterone through the action of 5-alpha-reductase, causing each successive hair cycle to produce a shorter, finer, less pigmented hair until the follicle eventually produces only a vellus-like hair or ceases to cycle altogether. In men, the process follows a characteristic patterned progression classified by the Hamilton-Norwood scale, beginning with bitemporal recession and vertex thinning that can progress to complete loss across the vertex and frontal scalp while the occipital and lateral scalp, whose follicles are relatively resistant to androgen-mediated miniaturization, remain preserved, a preservation that is precisely why hair transplantation, which relocates these androgen-resistant follicles to affected areas, is an effective long-term solution. In women, androgenetic alopecia (sometimes termed female pattern hair loss) more typically produces diffuse thinning concentrated over the crown and part line, following the Ludwig or Sinclair classification scales, with frontal hairline preservation more common than in male-pattern disease, though a subset of women do show a more male-pattern-like distribution, particularly when associated with an underlying hyperandrogenic condition.

Evaluation and the Role of Underlying Hyperandrogenism in Women

While androgenetic alopecia in men rarely requires evaluation for an underlying endocrine abnormality, women presenting with a pattern suggestive of androgenetic alopecia, particularly when accompanied by hirsutism, irregular menses, or acne, warrant screening for polycystic ovary syndrome and other causes of hyperandrogenism, including total and free testosterone, dehydroepiandrosterone sulfate, and, when clinically indicated, evaluation for a virilizing tumor if the hair loss and hyperandrogenic features have developed with unusually rapid onset or severity. A gradual, patterned onset over years without other hyperandrogenic features is reassuring and typically does not warrant extensive endocrine workup, while rapid onset combined with other signs of hyperandrogenism should prompt a more thorough evaluation given the possibility of an underlying androgen-secreting process requiring its own specific management beyond the hair loss itself.

Feature	Male Pattern (Androgenetic)	Female Pattern (Androgenetic)
Distribution	Bitemporal recession, vertex thinning, classified by Hamilton-Norwood scale	Diffuse crown/part-line thinning, frontal hairline often preserved, classified by Ludwig/Sinclair scale
Typical onset	Can begin in late teens to twenties	Often perimenopausal, though can begin earlier
Endocrine workup	Not routinely needed	Consider if accompanied by hirsutism, acne, or menstrual irregularity
First-line topical treatment	Topical minoxidil	Topical minoxidil
First-line additional systemic option	Oral finasteride or dutasteride	Spironolactone or other antiandrogen (off-label)

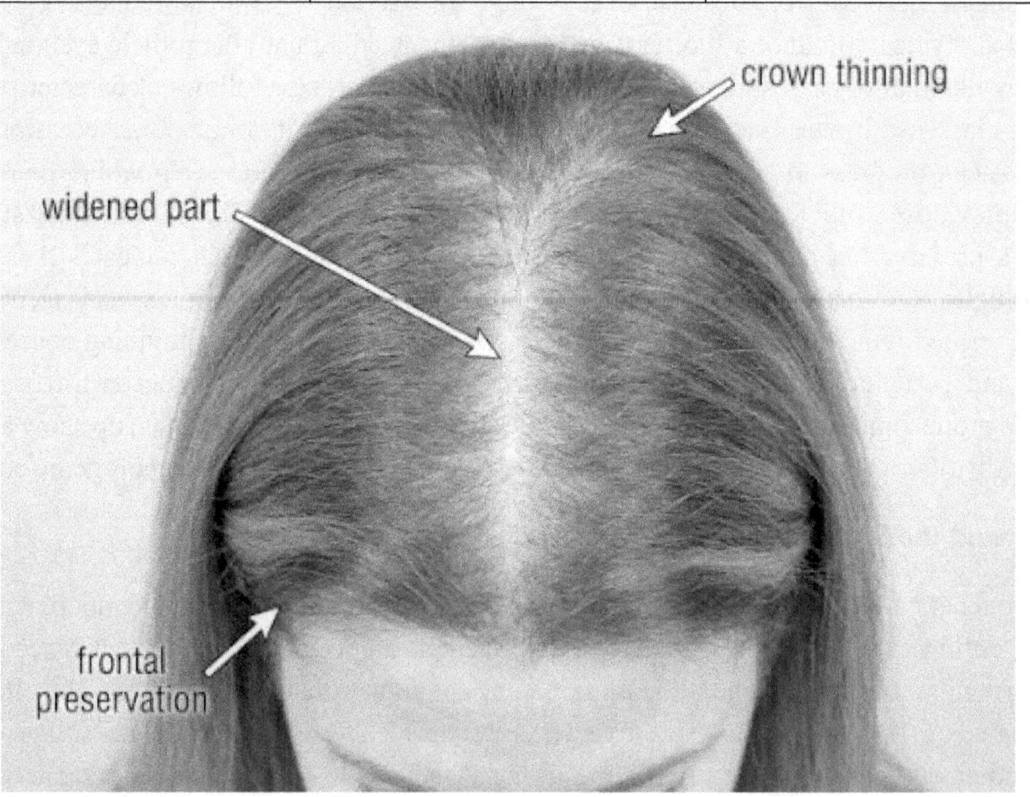

Treatment of Androgenetic Alopecia

Topical minoxidil, available over the counter in multiple strengths and formulations, is first-line therapy for both sexes, believed to act by prolonging the anagen (growth) phase and increasing follicular size, though its precise mechanism remains incompletely understood; efficacy requires consistent, indefinite use, since discontinuation results in gradual loss of any gained benefit over several months as the underlying miniaturization process resumes unopposed, a point that should be emphasized clearly at treatment initiation to set realistic long-term expectations. Low-dose oral minoxidil has emerged as a useful and generally well-tolerated alternative or adjunct for patients who find the topical formulation cosmetically inconvenient or who experience local scalp irritation, though it requires attention to potential systemic effects, including fluid retention and reflex tachycardia, particularly at higher doses or in patients with underlying cardiovascular disease. Oral finasteride, a 5-alpha-reductase type 2 inhibitor, and dutasteride, which inhibits both type 1 and type 2 isoenzymes, reduce dihydrotestosterone levels and are effective additional options for male androgenetic alopecia, with counseling required regarding rare but recognized sexual side effects and, in patients who might father children, the theoretical risk to male fetal development given the drug's mechanism, making pregnancy avoidance counseling relevant for partners. Spironolactone, an antiandrogen with aldosterone receptor antagonist activity, is commonly used off-label for female pattern hair loss, particularly in women with accompanying signs of hyperandrogenism, though it requires pregnancy avoidance given feminization risk to a male fetus and periodic potassium monitoring in patients with relevant renal or cardiac risk factors.

Procedural and Emerging Options

Low-level laser therapy devices, available as combs, helmets, and caps for home use, have modest supporting evidence as an adjunct to topical and oral therapy, though they are generally considered a secondary rather than primary treatment option given their more limited efficacy relative to minoxidil and finasteride. Platelet-rich plasma injection, in which a concentrated preparation of the patient's own platelets is injected into the affected scalp to deliver growth factors that may support follicular health, has shown benefit in some studies, though protocols vary considerably between practices and long-term comparative data against established therapies remain limited. Hair transplantation, relocating androgen-resistant follicular units from the occipital and lateral scalp to areas of pattern loss, remains the definitive procedural option for patients with sufficient donor density who desire a permanent cosmetic solution, though it does not halt ongoing miniaturization of the patient's remaining native hair, meaning that concurrent medical therapy is generally recommended to preserve surrounding native hair even after a successful transplant procedure.

THE MORPHOLOGY-TO-MANAGEMENT SYSTEM — Patterned Thinning With Preserved Follicular Openings

The Pattern: Gradual, patterned hair thinning, bitemporal and vertex in men, crown and part-line in women, with preserved follicular ostia and miniaturized hairs of varying shaft diameter on trichoscopy.

Presentation Variance: Frontal hairline recession predominates in men, while diffuse crown thinning with frontal preservation predominates in women; rapid onset with other hyperandrogenic signs in a woman should prompt endocrine evaluation rather than a purely cosmetic approach.

Trap Logic: Diffuse, non-patterned, acute-onset shedding without miniaturization favors telogen effluvium rather than androgenetic alopecia; patchy, well-circumscribed areas of complete hair loss with exclamation point hairs favor alopecia areata instead.

Management Pivot: Confirm the patterned distribution and miniaturization pattern on trichoscopy; initiate topical minoxidil in every patient as first-line therapy, adding oral finasteride or dutasteride in men and considering spironolactone in women with hyperandrogenic features, and set expectations for indefinite maintenance therapy from the outset.

Pattern Anchor: Patterned distribution plus miniaturized hairs of varying diameter equals androgenetic alopecia, and treatment benefit is maintenance-dependent: stopping therapy resumes the underlying miniaturization process that was never actually cured, only suppressed.

Alopecia Areata

Alopecia areata is an autoimmune, non-scarring hair loss condition in which a T-cell-mediated inflammatory infiltrate attacks the hair follicle during the anagen phase, collapsing immune privilege at the follicular bulb and producing well-circumscribed, round to oval patches of complete hair loss, most classically on the scalp but potentially affecting any hair-bearing site. The exclamation point hair, a short, broken hair that is narrower at its proximal end near the scalp than at its distal tip, reflects a follicle in the acute process of shutting down hair production and is a highly characteristic finding at the active periphery of an expanding patch, while a positive pull test, in which gentle traction on hairs at the margin of a patch easily removes multiple hairs, indicates active disease progression, a useful marker both for diagnosis and for monitoring treatment response over time. More extensive variants include alopecia totalis, complete loss of scalp hair, and alopecia universalis, complete loss of all body hair including eyebrows, eyelashes, and other body hair, both of which carry a more guarded prognosis for spontaneous regrowth than limited patch-stage disease.

Nail Findings and Associated Autoimmune Conditions

Nail pitting, presenting as small, regularly spaced depressions across the nail plate, is a common accompanying finding in alopecia areata and, when present alongside patchy hair loss, supports the diagnosis, while trachyonychia, a rough, sandpapered nail surface texture, occurs in more severe or longstanding disease. Alopecia areata carries an association with other autoimmune conditions, most notably autoimmune thyroid disease and vitiligo, reflecting shared underlying autoimmune predisposition, and atopic disease, particularly atopic dermatitis, is also more prevalent among patients with alopecia areata than in the general population, an association whose mechanism remains an area of active investigation given the traditionally distinct immunologic pathways (T-helper 1 versus T-helper 2 predominant) historically ascribed to each condition.

Treatment of Alopecia Areata

Intralesional corticosteroid injection is first-line therapy for limited patch-stage alopecia areata, typically repeated every four to six weeks, with regrowth often apparent within two to three months of initiating treatment, while high-potency topical corticosteroids offer an alternative for patients who prefer to avoid injections or for widespread disease not amenable to injection therapy alone, and contact irritant or sensitizing agents such as anthralin have also been used historically for more diffuse disease, though largely supplanted by newer treatment options where available. Topical immunotherapy, using a sensitizing contact allergen such as diphenylcyclopropenone applied regularly to induce a controlled, mild allergic contact dermatitis intended to divert the immune response away from the follicle, is reserved for more extensive disease resistant to first-line measures and requires careful patient counseling given the deliberately induced dermatitis central to its mechanism. Oral Janus kinase inhibitors have transformed the treatment landscape for extensive and refractory alopecia areata, including alopecia totalis and universalis, with clinical trials demonstrating meaningful regrowth in a substantial proportion of previously treatment-resistant patients by directly targeting the interferon-gamma and interleukin-15 signaling pathway now understood to be central to disease pathogenesis, representing the first systemic, mechanism-targeted therapy specifically approved for this condition.

EVIDENCE: Randomized, placebo-controlled trials of oral Janus kinase inhibitors in severe alopecia areata have demonstrated clinically meaningful scalp hair regrowth in a substantial proportion of treated patients over six months of therapy, a response rate that represents a marked advance over historical treatment options for extensive disease, though relapse after treatment discontinuation is common, supporting the current understanding of these agents as effective suppressive rather than curative therapy requiring sustained treatment to maintain benefit.

Telogen Effluvium and Anagen Effluvium

Telogen effluvium describes a diffuse, non-scarring shedding of hair resulting from a synchronized shift of an abnormally large proportion of follicles from the anagen (growth) phase into the telogen (resting) phase, typically triggered two to three months prior by a significant physiologic stressor such as major surgery, high fever, severe illness, significant weight loss, childbirth, or a major psychological stressor, with the delay between the trigger and clinically apparent shedding reflecting the normal duration of the telogen phase before the affected hairs are shed. The hair pull test in telogen effluvium yields easily extracted telogen hairs, recognizable by their small, non-pigmented, club-shaped root, distinguishing them from the anagen hairs with a pigmented, gel-like root sheath extracted in anagen effluvium, and the diffuse, non-patterned nature of the shedding, without the patterned distribution of androgenetic alopecia or the well-circumscribed patches of alopecia areata, is itself a key diagnostic clue on history and examination.

Chronic Telogen Effluvium and Anagen Effluvium

Chronic telogen effluvium, persisting beyond six months, warrants a more thorough evaluation for an ongoing underlying trigger, including iron deficiency, assessed through serum ferritin given its correlation with hair cycle disruption even in the absence of frank anemia, thyroid dysfunction, and, in some cases, medications, since certain drugs, including beta-blockers, retinoids, and anticoagulants, are recognized triggers of a telogen effluvium-like pattern, and a careful, dated timeline of medication changes relative to shedding onset can help identify a culprit agent when one exists. Anagen effluvium, in contrast, results from an acute insult severe enough to abruptly halt hair production during the active growth phase itself rather than triggering a delayed, synchronized shift into telogen, most classically from cytotoxic chemotherapy, and therefore produces much more rapid, often near-total hair loss within days to a few weeks of the causative exposure, since a much larger proportion of scalp follicles are actively cycling in anagen at any given time compared to the smaller proportion in telogen affected in ordinary telogen effluvium; hair regrowth in anagen effluvium is generally expected once the causative chemotherapy is completed, since the follicular structure itself, unlike in scarring alopecia, remains intact despite the abrupt cessation of hair production.

PATIENT EDUCATION: Patients experiencing telogen effluvium should be reassured that the underlying follicles remain structurally intact and capable of producing normal hair once the triggering stressor resolves, that the observed shedding, however alarming in volume, reflects an event that occurred two to three months earlier rather than an ongoing new problem, and that spontaneous, full recovery over six to twelve months is the expected course for most cases once the underlying trigger has resolved or been addressed.

Scarring (Cicatricial) Alopecia

Lichen planopilaris, the most common primary scarring alopecia, produces perifollicular erythema and scale at the active margin of expanding patches of hair loss, with progressive loss of follicular openings as the disease advances, and biopsy showing a lichenoid, lymphocytic infiltrate targeting the follicular epithelium analogous to the interface changes of cutaneous lichen planus discussed elsewhere in this text. Frontal fibrosing alopecia, now understood as a clinical variant of lichen planopilaris affecting predominantly postmenopausal women, produces a band-like recession of the frontotemporal hairline accompanied by loss of eyebrows in a large proportion of affected patients, a finding valuable enough diagnostically that eyebrow loss in an older woman with frontal hairline recession should prompt strong consideration of this diagnosis even before scalp biopsy is performed; the perifollicular erythema and scale at the advancing hairline, along with frequently observed loss of the fine vellus hairs normally present just anterior to the frontal hairline, are additional supportive trichoscopic findings.

Central Centrifugal Cicatricial Alopecia and Folliculitis Decalvans

Central centrifugal cicatricial alopecia produces progressive, centrifugally expanding scarring hair loss beginning at the vertex and spreading outward in a roughly symmetric pattern, occurring predominantly in women of African descent, and while its precise etiology remains incompletely understood, mechanical and thermal traction from certain hairstyling practices, including chemical relaxers, heat styling, and tight braiding or weaving, has been implicated as a contributing factor in at least a subset of cases, making a sensitive, nonjudgmental discussion of hair care practices and, where appropriate, gentle modification of high-traction styling an important component of management alongside medical therapy directed at halting inflammatory progression. Folliculitis decalvans produces painful, pustular, crusted patches of scarring alopecia, often with tufted folliculitis, multiple hairs emerging from a single dilated follicular opening, reflecting scarring and follicular unit fusion from recurrent inflammatory injury, and is understood to involve an abnormal host response to Staphylococcus aureus colonization, supporting a treatment approach that combines anti-inflammatory and antistaphylococcal antibiotic therapy rather than anti-inflammatory therapy alone.

CAUTION: Every scarring alopecia in this section shares a common urgency: hair lost to follicular destruction does not regrow regardless of subsequent treatment, so the goal of therapy is to halt active inflammation and further progression as early as possible rather than to restore already-lost hair. Any patient presenting with perifollicular erythema, scale, or pustules accompanying progressive hair loss warrants prompt biopsy and treatment initiation rather than a period of watchful waiting, given the irreversible nature of established follicular scarring.

Treatment of Scarring Alopecia

Treatment across the primary scarring alopecias is directed at suppressing the active inflammatory process rather than restoring lost hair, and typically combines high-potency topical or intralesional corticosteroids at the active margin with systemic anti-inflammatory or immunomodulatory therapy for more extensive or rapidly progressive disease; hydroxychloroquine and oral tetracycline-class antibiotics, valued here for their anti-inflammatory rather than antimicrobial properties, are commonly used first-line systemic options for lichen planopilaris and frontal fibrosing alopecia, while more refractory disease may require additional immunosuppressive agents. Folliculitis decalvans treatment centers on combination oral antibiotic therapy targeting Staphylococcus aureus, often for a prolonged course, given the condition's presumed relationship to abnormal host response to colonization, sometimes combined with topical or intralesional corticosteroid therapy to address the inflammatory component directly. Across all scarring alopecias, treatment response is measured by cessation of further progression and resolution of active inflammatory signs, perifollicular erythema, scale, and pustules, rather than by hair regrowth, and this distinction in treatment goals should be communicated clearly and repeatedly to patients who may otherwise measure success solely by whether new hair appears in already-scarred areas.

Trichotillomania and Traction Alopecia

Trichotillomania is a body-focused repetitive behavior disorder in which patients, often unconsciously or during periods of stress, boredom, or concentration, pull out their own hair, producing patches of hair loss with an irregular, geometric border and hairs broken at variable, unusually short lengths, in contrast to the more uniform, well-circumscribed patches and characteristic exclamation point hairs of alopecia areata; the eyebrows and eyelashes are commonly affected in addition to the scalp, and the pattern often follows the patient's dominant hand distribution given the mechanics of the pulling behavior itself. Trichoscopy can assist in distinguishing the two conditions, showing broken hairs of markedly variable length and, in some cases, coiled hairs reflecting hair that has been pulled and partially regrown, rather than the more uniform exclamation point hairs of alopecia areata, and biopsy, when performed, shows evidence of trauma to the follicle, including perifollicular hemorrhage and pigment casts, rather than the lymphocytic inflammatory infiltrate characteristic of alopecia areata.

Traction Alopecia

Traction alopecia results from chronic mechanical tension on the hair shaft from certain hairstyling practices, including tight ponytails, braids, weaves, and extensions, and initially presents as a reversible, non-scarring thinning most classically along the frontotemporal hairline, marked by the fringe sign, a rim of thin, fragile hairs remaining at the very margin of the hairline while hair loss has already occurred just behind it; if the traction is not modified, the process can progress to permanent, scarring hair loss over time, making early recognition and prompt counseling on protective hairstyling modification essential to preventing the transition from a reversible to an irreversible process. Both trichotillomania and traction alopecia benefit from a nonjudgmental, collaborative counseling approach: trichotillomania warrants referral for cognitive behavioral therapy, specifically habit reversal training, which has the strongest evidence base among behavioral interventions for this condition, while traction alopecia warrants a sensitive discussion of hairstyling practices that avoids shaming a patient for culturally significant or personally meaningful hair care choices while still conveying the urgency of modification before scarring becomes established.

Hirsutism and Hypertrichosis

Hirsutism describes excess terminal hair growth in women in a male-pattern distribution, the face, chest, and lower abdomen, reflecting increased androgen production, increased peripheral androgen sensitivity, or both, and is quantified clinically using the modified Ferriman-Gallwey score, which assigns a severity rating across nine androgen-sensitive body areas to provide a standardized, reproducible measure of severity useful both for initial assessment and for tracking treatment response over time. Polycystic ovary syndrome is the most common underlying cause of hirsutism, typically accompanied by irregular menses, acne, and, as discussed earlier in this chapter, androgenetic alopecia, while less common but more concerning causes, including congenital adrenal hyperplasia, androgen-secreting ovarian or adrenal tumors, and Cushing syndrome, should be considered particularly when hirsutism develops with rapid onset, is severe, or is accompanied by frank virilization, including clitoromegaly, voice deepening, or significant increase in muscle mass, findings that warrant more urgent endocrine evaluation and imaging rather than a routine outpatient workup timeline.

Management of Hirsutism

Management of hirsutism combines treatment of any identified underlying endocrine cause with direct cosmetic and pharmacologic approaches to the excess hair itself, since even successful treatment of an underlying hormonal abnormality does not reverse hair follicles that have already been converted from vellus to terminal hair by prior androgen exposure. Combined oral contraceptives, which reduce ovarian androgen production and increase sex hormone-binding globulin, thereby reducing free androgen levels, are frequently used as first-line pharmacologic therapy, often combined with an antiandrogen such as spironolactone for more significant hirsutism, with the combination requiring several months of use before meaningful reduction in hair growth becomes apparent given the long hair growth cycle involved. Direct hair removal methods, including electrolysis, which individually destroys each treated follicle and can achieve permanent results, and laser hair removal, most effective in patients with lighter skin and darker, coarser terminal hair given the pigment-based mechanism of most hair removal lasers, offer complementary approaches to the pharmacologic management of the underlying hormonal driver, and combining medical therapy with a direct hair removal method generally produces a more satisfying outcome than either approach used in isolation.

KEY POINT: Hypertrichosis, excess hair growth that is not confined to androgen-dependent areas and not driven by androgen excess, should be distinguished from hirsutism, since it can reflect an entirely different set of causes, including certain medications such as minoxidil and cyclosporine, and rare congenital hypertrichosis syndromes, and does not respond to antiandrogen therapy given its androgen-independent mechanism.

Complications, Special Populations, and Patient Education

Postpartum telogen effluvium, occurring roughly two to four months after delivery as estrogen-mediated prolongation of the anagen phase during pregnancy reverses and a large cohort of hairs synchronously enters telogen, is an extremely common and entirely physiologic occurrence that should be distinguished clearly from a pathologic process, with reassurance regarding the expected several-month recovery course forming the cornerstone of counseling for new mothers who are often especially anxious about hair loss during an already stressful postpartum period. Children presenting with patchy hair loss deserve particular attention to the possibility of tinea capitis, discussed in an earlier chapter, and trichotillomania, both of which are more common considerations in pediatric patch-stage hair loss than in adults, alongside alopecia areata itself. Iron deficiency, even without frank anemia, is an important and readily correctable contributing factor to hair shedding across multiple conditions in this chapter and deserves screening with serum ferritin in appropriate patients, particularly menstruating women and those with dietary restrictions, given the ease of correction relative to its potential contribution to ongoing symptoms. Patients considering finasteride, dutasteride, or spironolactone should also have a thorough medication reconciliation and relevant baseline laboratory testing performed before initiation, and women of childbearing potential prescribed any of these agents require clear, repeated counseling on reliable contraception given the shared risk of fetal harm across this drug class.

PATIENT EDUCATION: Patients across every condition in this chapter benefit from being shown, ideally with side-by-side trichoscopic images or photographs, exactly what feature (miniaturization, exclamation point hairs, perifollicular scale, or an irregular pulled-hair border) supports their specific diagnosis, since this visual, evidence-based explanation both improves understanding of a sometimes emotionally difficult diagnosis and reinforces confidence in the recommended treatment plan, particularly when that plan requires many months of patience before results become apparent. Referral to a mental health professional should be offered without hesitation when hair loss of any type is accompanying or contributing to significant anxiety, depression, or social withdrawal, since the psychological burden of hair loss is frequently underestimated relative to its objective physical severity.

Clinical Case: An Expanding Patch With a Deceptively Simple Explanation

A 34-year-old woman presented with a six-month history of a slowly enlarging, tender, scaling patch of hair loss on her crown, which she had initially attributed to a new shampoo and had treated with an over-the-counter anti-dandruff formulation without improvement. Examination revealed a patch of hair loss with absent follicular openings on trichoscopy, surrounded by an active, scaling, erythematous border with perifollicular hyperkeratosis, and no exclamation point hairs or other features suggestive of alopecia areata were present. A scalp biopsy taken from the active margin, rather than the center of established hair loss, showed a lichenoid lymphocytic infiltrate targeting the follicular epithelium, confirming a diagnosis of lichen planopilaris.

Given the clear evidence of active, ongoing inflammation at the margin and the risk of continued permanent hair loss, she was started on a combination of intralesional corticosteroid injections at the active border and oral hydroxychloroquine, with explicit counseling that treatment was directed at halting further progression of the scarring process rather than regrowing hair in the already-affected central area, an important distinction she had not previously understood despite months of self-treatment with cosmetic hair products. At three-month follow-up, the previously active, scaling border had quieted considerably with no evidence of further centrifugal expansion of the patch, representing a treatment success by the appropriate metric even though the existing bald patch itself remained visually unchanged, and she was scheduled for ongoing monitoring given the chronic, relapsing nature of lichen planopilaris even with adequate initial treatment response. She was additionally counseled that periodic reassessment, including repeat trichoscopic examination at follow-up visits, would guide any need for treatment adjustment, since recurrence of active inflammatory signs after a period of quiescence is common in this condition and would warrant prompt escalation of therapy rather than a wait-and-see approach.

Clinical Case: Diffuse Shedding Three Months After a Difficult Delivery

A 29-year-old woman presented at four months postpartum with several weeks of alarming, diffuse hair shedding, reporting clumps of hair coming out with routine washing and brushing to a degree she had never previously experienced, and expressing significant anxiety that she might be going bald. Her delivery had been complicated by significant postpartum hemorrhage requiring transfusion. Examination revealed diffuse thinning without a patterned distribution and without well-circumscribed patches, and a gentle pull test at multiple scalp sites easily extracted numerous hairs with a small, club-shaped, non-pigmented root consistent with telogen hairs; trichoscopy showed no evidence of miniaturization, exclamation point hairs, or loss of follicular openings.

The diffuse, non-patterned distribution, the telogen-predominant pull test findings, and the clear temporal relationship to both delivery and the additional physiologic stress of postpartum hemorrhage were recognized as classic for telogen effluvium, and serum ferritin was checked given the blood loss history, returning low-normal and prompting a recommendation for iron supplementation as a supportive measure alongside reassurance. She was counseled at length that the shedding she was experiencing reflected an event that had been set in motion months earlier by the physiologic stress of delivery and blood loss, that her follicles remained fundamentally healthy and intact, and that the expected course was gradual improvement over the following several months as the affected follicles cycled back into active growth; she was given a specific timeline of expected improvement to reference, and at six-month follow-up her shedding had resolved substantially with visibly regrowing hair along her temples and part line, an outcome she reported had considerably eased the anxiety that had accompanied her initial presentation.

THE MORPHOLOGY-TO-MANAGEMENT SYSTEM — Preserved Versus Lost Follicular Openings

Pattern Introduced This Chapter: Preserved follicular ostia with miniaturization (androgenetic alopecia), exclamation point hairs (alopecia areata), and easily extracted telogen hairs (telogen effluvium) as non-scarring patterns, versus perifollicular erythema and lost follicular openings as the scarring pattern requiring urgent treatment.

Cross-Cutting Anchor: Trichoscopic assessment of follicular ostia is the anchor examination for every hair loss presentation in this chapter; its presence or absence determines whether the treatment conversation is about restoring lost hair or about racing to prevent further permanent loss.

Summary and Key Concepts

The distinction between non-scarring and scarring alopecia, determined chiefly by whether follicular openings are preserved or lost on trichoscopy, is the single most important organizing question in the evaluation of hair loss.

Androgenetic alopecia produces patterned, progressive miniaturization treated with topical minoxidil as first-line therapy in both sexes, with oral finasteride or dutasteride added in men and spironolactone often used off-label in women.

Alopecia areata produces well-circumscribed patches of complete hair loss with exclamation point hairs and a positive pull test, and oral Janus kinase inhibitors have transformed treatment of extensive and refractory disease.

Telogen effluvium produces diffuse, non-patterned shedding roughly two to three months after a physiologic stressor and generally resolves spontaneously over six to twelve months, while anagen effluvium produces much more rapid, near-total hair loss from an acute insult such as chemotherapy.

The primary scarring alopecias, including lichen planopilaris, frontal fibrosing alopecia, central centrifugal cicatricial alopecia, and folliculitis decalvans, cause permanent hair loss, making early recognition and prompt anti-inflammatory treatment essential to prevent further irreversible progression.

Trichotillomania and traction alopecia are distinguished from alopecia areata by their irregular borders and variable hair breakage lengths, and both benefit from a nonjudgmental counseling approach paired with appropriate behavioral or hairstyling interventions.

CHAPTER 16: NAIL DISORDERS

Learning Objectives

1. Describe the functional anatomy of the nail unit and correlate specific structural components with the clinical findings they produce when disrupted.
2. Distinguish acute from chronic paronychia and construct an appropriate management approach for each.
3. Recognize the nail findings of psoriasis and correlate them with the specific nail unit structure involved.
4. Differentiate benign longitudinal melanonychia from subungual melanoma using the ABCDEF criteria and the Hutchinson sign.
5. Recognize systemic disease associations of nail findings, including clubbing, koilonychia, and Beau lines.
6. Identify the common benign nail unit tumors and select an appropriate management approach for each.

The nail unit is a small, frequently overlooked structure that nonetheless offers a remarkably efficient diagnostic window into both localized nail disease and systemic illness occurring elsewhere in the body, and a systematic nail examination, evaluating the nail plate, the surrounding folds, and the lunula in turn, takes only moments yet routinely yields findings that redirect an entire diagnostic workup. This chapter builds the structural literacy needed to read the nail unit accurately: because different diseases target different anatomic components of this small but functionally complex structure, understanding which component produces which finding transforms an isolated nail abnormality from a cosmetic curiosity into a precise diagnostic clue.

Functional Anatomy of the Nail Unit

The nail matrix, located beneath the proximal nail fold and visible in part as the lunula, the pale, crescent-shaped structure at the base of the nail, is the site of nail plate production, and disease affecting the matrix produces changes in the nail plate's surface texture, thickness, and shape, such as pitting, ridging, or thinning, since the plate is generated here and carries forward any disruption to its formation as it grows distally. Fingernails grow considerably faster than toenails, roughly three millimeters per month compared to roughly one millimeter per month, a difference with direct practical relevance for estimating the timing of a Beau line or other transient matrix insult and for counseling patients on the expected duration of onychomycosis treatment, which must span the full growth-out period of the affected nail to be considered a completed course. The nail bed, the vascular structure beneath the nail plate distal to the lunula, is responsible for the pink color visible through the healthy, translucent plate and for firmly adhering the plate to the underlying tissue; disease affecting the nail bed rather than the matrix, such as psoriasis affecting this specific structure, characteristically produces onycholysis, separation of the plate from the bed, and changes in the color visible through the plate, such as the oil drop sign, rather than changes to the plate's own surface texture. The proximal and lateral nail folds form the cuticle and lateral borders that seal the nail unit against the external environment, and disruption of this seal, whether through chronic moisture exposure, trauma, or infection, is the starting point for both acute and chronic paronychia.

KEY POINT: Determining whether a nail abnormality reflects matrix disease (affecting the surface, texture, and shape of the plate itself) or nail bed disease (affecting the plate's adherence and the color visible through it) is the single most useful structural question to ask when examining an abnormal nail, since it directs attention to the correct underlying process and its likely differential diagnosis.

The hyponychium, the small strip of skin beneath the free edge of the nail plate at its distal margin, and the eponychium, the thin band of modified cuticle tissue immediately overlying the proximal nail plate, together complete the seal that protects the nail unit from the external environment and from pathogen entry, and disruption of either structure, much like disruption of the nail folds themselves, predisposes to secondary infection and inflammatory change.

Acute and Chronic Paronychia

Acute paronychia presents as a rapidly developing, painful, erythematous, and often fluctuant swelling of the proximal or lateral nail fold, typically following a break in the protective seal of the nail fold from minor trauma such as nail biting, aggressive manicure, or a hangnail, and is most commonly caused by Staphylococcus aureus, occasionally with streptococcal co-infection; when a discrete abscess has formed, incision and drainage is required in addition to antibiotic therapy, since antibiotics alone are unlikely to adequately address a walled-off collection of purulent material. Chronic paronychia, in contrast, develops gradually over weeks to months, producing persistent, less acutely painful swelling and erythema of the proximal nail fold with loss of the cuticle, and reflects a fundamentally different process: repeated exposure to moisture and irritants, common in individuals whose hands are frequently wet, such as dishwashers, healthcare workers, and bartenders, disrupts the nail fold seal chronically, allowing secondary colonization by Candida species and various bacteria that perpetuate a low-grade inflammatory state rather than an acute infection driving the process.

Distinguishing Treatment Approaches

Because chronic paronychia is fundamentally an inflammatory response to barrier disruption from chronic moisture exposure rather than a primary infection, treatment directed solely at eradicating the secondarily colonizing organisms with antifungal or antibacterial therapy alone is frequently disappointing; the cornerstone of management instead is rigorous moisture and irritant avoidance, including glove use during wet work, combined with a topical corticosteroid to address the underlying inflammation, an approach that has been shown in comparative studies to outperform antifungal therapy alone for this condition. Patients who fail conservative measures despite adequate adherence may benefit from a minor surgical procedure, eponychial marsupialization, which removes a crescent of tissue from the proximal nail fold to improve drainage and allow the nail fold to reseal against the nail plate, reserved for genuinely refractory cases given its more invasive nature relative to the topical and behavioral measures that resolve the majority of cases.

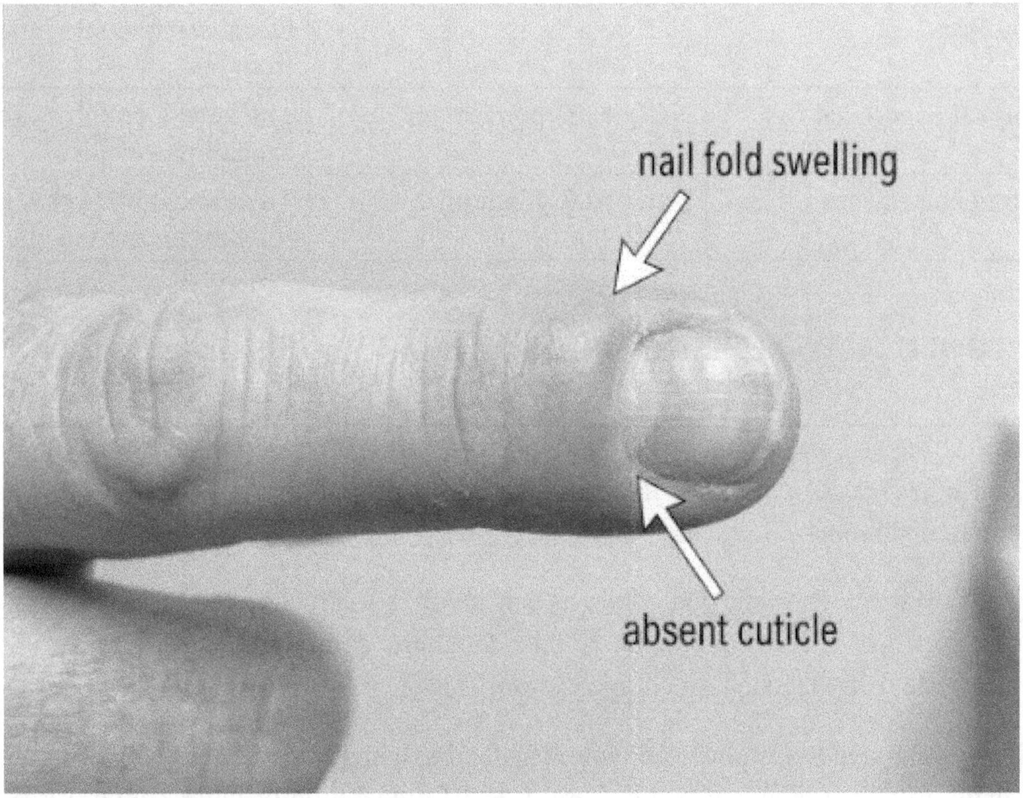

Nail Findings in Psoriasis

Psoriatic nail disease occurs in a substantial proportion of patients with cutaneous psoriasis and an even higher proportion of those with psoriatic arthritis, making nail examination a valuable component of psoriasis assessment, since certain nail findings correlate specifically with the presence of joint involvement and can prompt earlier rheumatologic evaluation. Nail pitting, small, discrete depressions scattered across the nail plate, reflects matrix involvement and results from parakeratotic foci within the proximal matrix that are subsequently shed as the nail grows, while the oil drop sign, a yellow-brown, translucent discoloration visible through the nail plate, reflects nail bed involvement from psoriatic plaques beneath the plate itself and is considered one of the more specific psoriatic nail findings. Onycholysis, distal separation of the nail plate from the bed, and subungual hyperkeratosis, thickened, crumbly debris accumulating beneath the distal nail plate, both reflect nail bed disease and can be difficult to distinguish clinically from onychomycosis, making fungal studies a valuable and frequently necessary step before attributing nail changes to psoriasis alone, particularly since the two conditions can and frequently do coexist in the same patient.

Finding	Nail Unit Structure Involved	Clinical Appearance
Pitting	Matrix	Small, discrete surface depressions
Oil drop sign	Nail bed	Yellow-brown translucent discoloration

Onycholysis	Nail bed	Distal separation of plate from bed
Subungual hyperkeratosis	Nail bed/hyponychium	Thickened, crumbly debris beneath the plate
Splinter hemorrhages	Nail bed (longitudinal vessels)	Thin, linear, red-brown streaks beneath the plate

THE MORPHOLOGY-TO-MANAGEMENT SYSTEM — Matrix Signature Versus Nail Bed Signature

The Pattern: Pitting and surface texture change point to matrix disease; onycholysis, the oil drop sign, and subungual hyperkeratosis point to nail bed disease, a distinction that applies across psoriasis and several other nail conditions.

Presentation Variance: Psoriatic nail disease can show a matrix-predominant pattern, a nail bed-predominant pattern, or, most commonly, a mixed pattern combining both, and severity does not necessarily correlate with the extent of cutaneous psoriasis present elsewhere on the body.

Trap Logic: Onychomycosis produces onycholysis and subungual hyperkeratosis that can be visually indistinguishable from psoriatic nail bed disease; a KOH preparation or nail clipping for periodic acid-Schiff staining is required to distinguish the two, and coexistence of both conditions in the same nail is common.

Management Pivot: Confirm or exclude coexisting onychomycosis before attributing nail bed changes to psoriasis alone; treat matrix-predominant disease (pitting) with intralesional or systemic therapy targeting the proximal matrix, and consider systemic psoriasis therapy for extensive nail involvement given the relatively limited efficacy of topical treatment for nail disease.

Pattern Anchor: Nail findings correlating with joint symptoms should prompt psoriatic arthritis evaluation regardless of how limited the cutaneous psoriasis appears, since nail disease is a recognized independent marker of joint involvement risk.

Diagnostic Workup and Treatment of Nail Bed Disease

A nail clipping submitted for periodic acid-Schiff staining, taken from the most proximal, least degraded portion of affected nail along with any accessible subungual debris, offers higher diagnostic yield than a simple KOH preparation for distinguishing onychomycosis from psoriatic or other nail bed disease and should be pursued whenever the distinction will change management, particularly before committing a patient to systemic antifungal therapy or, conversely, before attributing nail changes to psoriasis without adequately excluding a treatable fungal component. Treatment of nail psoriasis is notably more challenging than treatment of cutaneous psoriasis, given the relative inaccessibility of the nail matrix and bed to topical therapy penetration; intralesional corticosteroid injection into the proximal nail fold can be effective for matrix-predominant disease but is limited by the pain of the injection itself, while systemic or biologic therapy for psoriasis, when indicated for cutaneous or joint disease, generally improves nail findings as well, making nail disease severity a relevant factor in decisions about escalating to systemic therapy even when cutaneous disease alone might not otherwise meet a systemic treatment threshold.

Longitudinal Melanonychia and Subungual Melanoma

Longitudinal melanonychia, discussed briefly in the preceding chapter on pigmentation, warrants more detailed attention here given the serious consequences of a missed subungual melanoma diagnosis. The ABCDEF mnemonic provides a structured framework for assessing a pigmented nail band: Age (peak incidence in the fifth to seventh decades, and darker-skinned populations in whom subungual melanoma represents a disproportionately higher percentage of all melanoma given lower rates of cutaneous melanoma overall), Brown to black coloration with Breadth exceeding three millimeters or occupying more than two-thirds of the nail plate, irregular or blurred Borders, a single digit most commonly affected (the great toe and thumb are the most frequently involved sites), rapid Change in size, color, or growth rate, and Extension of pigment onto the surrounding periungual skin, the Hutchinson sign, along with a personal or Family history of melanoma or dysplastic nevus syndrome.

Distinguishing Benign From Concerning Melanonychia

Benign longitudinal melanonychia, common as an incidental finding affecting multiple nails in individuals with darker skin phototypes, typically presents as a narrow, evenly pigmented, parallel-sided band that remains stable in width and color over time, in contrast to the widening, irregular, and rapidly changing bands more characteristic of melanoma. Dermoscopy of the nail plate can assist in this distinction, with a regular, parallel-lined pattern of pigmentation favoring a benign process and an irregular pattern with disruption of the parallel lines, variation in color and line spacing, or triangular pigment bands favoring a concerning process, though dermoscopic findings should be interpreted alongside the full clinical picture rather than relied upon in isolation. Any band meeting concerning ABCDEF criteria, particularly a new, solitary, widening band with a positive Hutchinson sign, warrants biopsy, generally performed as a matrix biopsy by a clinician experienced with nail unit procedures given the technical considerations involved in sampling this structure without producing permanent nail plate deformity, since inadequate or improperly performed biopsy technique both risks missing the diagnosis and risks unnecessary permanent nail dystrophy.

CAUTION: Subungual melanoma is frequently diagnosed at a more advanced stage than cutaneous melanoma at other sites, in part because early lesions are often mistaken for trauma-related subungual hematoma or a benign nevus and observed rather than biopsied; any pigmented nail band that does not clearly correspond to a known, recent trauma history, or that fails to grow out and migrate distally over several months as a hematoma would, warrants prompt evaluation and a low threshold for biopsy.

Traumatic Nail Conditions

Subungual hematoma results from acute trauma to the nail bed, producing a sharply demarcated area of red, purple, or black discoloration beneath the nail plate that, unlike a pigmented lesion, grows out distally with the nail plate over subsequent weeks and eventually resolves as the affected portion of the plate is trimmed away, a distal migration pattern that serves as the single most important distinguishing feature from a true pigmented nail lesion, which remains fixed in its position relative to the matrix rather than migrating distally with plate growth. Acute, painful subungual hematomas involving a substantial proportion of the nail bed, particularly following a crush injury, may warrant trephination, creating a small hole through the nail plate to relieve pressure and drain accumulated blood, which can provide significant pain relief and reduce the risk of secondary nail plate loss from the pressure effect of the underlying hematoma; radiographic imaging should be considered when the mechanism of injury raises concern for an underlying distal phalanx fracture, since a substantial subungual hematoma is frequently associated with fracture given the shared mechanism of significant direct trauma to the digit tip.

Distinguishing Hematoma From Melanonychia in Practice

When the history of trauma is clear, temporally appropriate, and consistent with the appearance and location of the discoloration, and when the patient can be reliably followed to confirm distal migration and eventual resolution as the nail grows out over the following weeks to months, observation is reasonable; however, when the trauma history is vague, remote, unwitnessed, or inconsistent with the finding, when the discoloration fails to demonstrate the expected distal migration on interval examination, or when any Hutchinson sign or ABCDEF concerning feature is present, the presumption of benign trauma should be abandoned in favor of biopsy, since subungual melanoma is disproportionately misattributed to trauma by both patients and clinicians, a recognized and preventable contributor to diagnostic delay in this disease.

Nail Findings as Markers of Systemic Disease

Clubbing, characterized by increased curvature of the nail plate in both the longitudinal and transverse planes, loss of the normal angle between the nail plate and proximal nail fold, and a spongy or floating sensation on palpation of the proximal nail fold, reflects soft tissue proliferation at the distal digit believed to result from megakaryocyte fragments and platelet clumps bypassing the pulmonary capillary bed and releasing growth factors locally, a mechanism that explains its classic association with conditions that create a right-to-left shunt or impaired pulmonary filtration, including cyanotic congenital heart disease, lung cancer, interstitial lung disease, and chronic suppurative lung conditions such as bronchiectasis and cystic fibrosis, alongside inflammatory bowel disease and cirrhosis. Koilonychia, a spoon-shaped concavity of the nail plate capable of holding a drop of water, classically reflects iron deficiency anemia, though it can also be seen as a normal, transient finding in infants and in certain occupational settings involving repeated nail trauma, making correlation with the broader clinical picture, particularly symptoms and laboratory findings consistent with iron deficiency, important before attributing this finding definitively to a systemic cause.

Beau Lines, Splinter Hemorrhages, and Half-and-Half Nails

Beau lines, transverse depressions or grooves running across the width of the nail plate, reflect a temporary disruption of matrix activity from a significant systemic stressor, such as high fever, major illness, chemotherapy, or severe nutritional deficiency, analogous in concept to the synchronized follicular shift underlying telogen effluvium, and the distance of the line from the proximal nail fold allows rough estimation of when the inciting event occurred, given the relatively predictable rate of nail plate growth. Splinter hemorrhages, thin, linear, red to brown streaks running in the direction of nail growth, reflect small hemorrhages from the longitudinally oriented vessels of the nail bed and, while most commonly caused by simple trauma, particularly when confined to the distal nail plate, warrant consideration of infective endocarditis, vasculitis, or a coagulopathy when multiple nails are affected, when they are not clearly related to trauma, or when accompanied by other systemic symptoms. Half-and-half nails, also termed Lindsay nails, in which the proximal portion of the nail bed appears white or pale and the distal portion appears pink to brown with a sharp demarcating line, are classically associated with chronic kidney disease, believed to reflect altered nail bed vascularity or edema related to the underlying renal dysfunction.

KEY POINT: Nail findings rarely provide a standalone diagnosis but function most effectively as a prompt to consider a specific category of systemic disease in the appropriate clinical context; clubbing should prompt pulmonary and cardiac evaluation, koilonychia should prompt iron studies, splinter hemorrhages affecting multiple nails without a trauma history should prompt consideration of endocarditis or vasculitis, and half-and-half nails should prompt renal function assessment.

Leukonychia and Terry Nails

True leukonychia, whitening of the nail plate itself due to a matrix-level abnormality in keratinization, should be distinguished from apparent leukonychia, in which the nail plate is structurally normal but appears white due to an abnormality of the underlying nail bed vasculature or connective tissue visible through the translucent plate; punctate leukonychia, small white spots scattered across the nail plate, is extremely common and typically reflects minor trauma to the matrix rather than any systemic disease, and reassurance alone is generally appropriate for this frequently encountered, benign incidental finding. Terry nails, in which the nail plate appears mostly white with only a narrow band of normal pink or brown coloration retained at the distal tip, is a form of apparent leukonychia classically associated with cirrhosis, though it can also be seen in congestive heart failure, chronic kidney disease, and diabetes mellitus, and is believed to reflect increased vascularity and connective tissue changes within the nail bed rather than a primary nail plate abnormality, distinguishing its underlying mechanism from true leukonychia despite the similar white appearance.

Nail Unit Biopsy: General Principles

Nail unit biopsy requires distinct technique considerations relative to biopsy elsewhere on the skin, given the small, curved working space and the risk of permanent nail plate deformity if the procedure is performed without attention to the underlying anatomy; a digital nerve block is typically required for adequate anesthesia given the dense sensory innervation of the digit tip, and a tourniquet is frequently used to maintain a bloodless field given the rich vascularity of the nail bed and matrix. For suspected matrix pathology, such as a pigmented band requiring evaluation for possible melanoma, the biopsy specimen must include matrix tissue specifically, since a nail bed or nail plate specimen alone will not sample the site of pigment or keratin production and can produce a falsely reassuring result despite genuine matrix-level disease; the specific technique, whether a punch, shave, or elliptical matrix biopsy, is selected based on the width and location of the lesion, with narrower bands generally amenable to a punch technique and wider bands requiring a more extensive lateral longitudinal excision to adequately sample the abnormality while balancing the competing goal of minimizing permanent nail plate deformity from the procedure itself.

CAUTION: A biopsy of a suspected pigmented nail lesion that samples only the nail bed or plate rather than the matrix itself can produce a falsely reassuring negative result despite genuine matrix melanoma, since the matrix, not the bed or plate, is the site of pigment production; referral to a clinician experienced in nail unit biopsy technique is appropriate whenever this distinction is not straightforward, given the serious consequences of an inadequately sampled specimen.

Benign Nail Unit Tumors

Digital myxoid (mucous) cysts present as translucent, dome-shaped nodules typically located at the distal interphalangeal joint or the proximal nail fold, often associated with an underlying osteoarthritic joint and connected to the joint space through a small stalk that allows synovial fluid to track into the cyst, and when located over the matrix, can produce a longitudinal groove or depression in the nail plate from direct pressure effect on the underlying matrix; treatment ranges from simple aspiration, which carries a high recurrence rate given the persistent connection to the joint space, to more definitive surgical excision addressing the underlying joint connection when recurrence or nail deformity is a significant concern. Glomus tumor, a benign neoplasm arising from the glomus body, a specialized arteriovenous structure involved in thermoregulation and normally concentrated in the digits, presents classically as a small, subungual, reddish-blue nodule causing severe, disproportionate pain to light touch or cold exposure, a symptom triad, pain, point tenderness, and cold sensitivity, sufficiently distinctive that it should prompt strong consideration of this diagnosis even before imaging confirmation; magnetic resonance imaging can help localize small lesions preoperatively, and surgical excision is curative.

Subungual Exostosis and Onychopapilloma

Subungual exostosis, a benign bony proliferation typically arising from the distal phalanx of the great toe, often following minor trauma, presents as a firm, slowly enlarging subungual mass that elevates and can eventually distort or split the overlying nail plate, and radiography readily confirms the diagnosis by demonstrating the characteristic bony outgrowth, distinguishing it from other subungual masses that would not show this finding; surgical excision of the bony lesion is generally curative when the mass is symptomatic or causing significant nail deformity. Onychopapilloma, a benign, localized proliferation of the nail bed epithelium, typically presents as a solitary longitudinal band of erythema, longitudinal melanonychia, or leukonychia (whitening), often accompanied by a subtle longitudinal ridge in the nail plate and, distinctively, a wedge of subungual hyperkeratosis or splinter hemorrhage visible at the free edge of the nail, and while entirely benign, its longitudinal band appearance means it enters the differential diagnosis alongside longitudinal melanonychia and warrants biopsy when the diagnosis is not clinically certain given the overlapping presentation with potentially concerning pigmented lesions.

Onychogryphosis and Median Canaliform Dystrophy

Onychogryphosis produces markedly thickened, curved, ram's horn-like overgrowth of the nail plate, most commonly affecting the great toenail of older adults with longstanding neglect of routine nail care, often compounded by reduced mobility or visual impairment limiting the patient's ability to perform self-care, and management involves mechanical debulking, typically requiring repeated professional trimming given the difficulty patients often have managing the grossly thickened plate themselves, alongside attention to footwear that accommodates the altered nail contour without causing additional pressure injury. Median canaliform dystrophy produces a distinctive longitudinal split or groove down the center of the nail plate, most classically the thumbnail, with a characteristic fir-tree or feathered pattern of smaller cracks branching off the central defect, and while its exact cause remains debated, repetitive trauma to the proximal nail fold, such as from a habitual tic of pushing back the cuticle, is a commonly implicated contributing factor in at least a subset of cases; management centers on identifying and interrupting any repetitive trauma behavior, since the nail plate defect generally improves once the inciting trauma is eliminated, though improvement can take many months given the slow rate of nail plate growth.

Complications, Special Populations, and Patient Education

Onychocryptosis, the ingrown toenail, most commonly affecting the great toe, results from the nail plate margin penetrating the adjacent lateral nail fold soft tissue, producing pain, erythema, and often secondary infection with granulation tissue formation at the site of penetration; contributing factors include improper nail trimming, particularly cutting the nail too short or with rounded rather than straight edges, tight-fitting footwear, and, in some individuals, an inherently excessive nail plate curvature. Patient education on proper trimming technique, cutting the nail straight across rather than curved to match the toe contour and avoiding overly short trims that encourage the lateral nail fold tissue to grow over the plate margin, is a simple, low-cost preventive measure that meaningfully reduces recurrence risk once an acute episode has been treated. Conservative management, including proper trimming technique, temporary packing or splinting to lift the offending nail edge away from the soft tissue, and appropriate footwear, is effective for mild, early cases, while more severe or recurrent cases benefit from partial or complete matricectomy, a procedure that permanently narrows the nail plate at the affected margin by destroying the corresponding portion of the nail matrix, most commonly performed chemically with phenol given its high efficacy and relatively straightforward technique. Diabetic patients and those with peripheral vascular disease warrant particular caution with any nail procedure, including the ingrown toenail interventions discussed above, given impaired wound healing and elevated infection risk in this population, and a lower threshold for referral to podiatry for routine nail care is appropriate in patients with significant neuropathy or vascular compromise, given the disproportionate consequences of even a minor nail-related infection in this setting.

PATIENT EDUCATION: Patients with chronic paronychia should be counseled explicitly that antifungal or antibacterial treatment alone is unlikely to resolve their condition without also addressing the underlying moisture and irritant exposure driving the disease, and practical, specific guidance, such as glove use during dishwashing or other wet work, is often more impactful than any prescribed topical medication alone. Patients with a new pigmented nail band should be counseled that most such bands are benign, particularly in darker skin phototypes where multiple nail involvement is common and reassuring, but that any single, new, widening, or rapidly changing band warrants prompt evaluation rather than a wait-and-see approach given the serious consequences of a delayed subungual melanoma diagnosis.

Older adults with limited mobility, visual impairment, or difficulty reaching their feet for routine care are at particular risk for neglected nail conditions such as onychogryphosis and onychocryptosis, and proactive referral for regular professional foot and nail care should be considered a component of comprehensive geriatric care rather than an optional cosmetic service, particularly in patients with additional risk factors such as diabetes or peripheral vascular disease where neglected nail pathology carries a meaningfully elevated risk of progressing to a serious infection.

Clinical Case: A Widening Pigmented Band on the Thumbnail

A 58-year-old man presented for evaluation of a pigmented band on his left thumbnail that his wife had noticed had grown noticeably wider over the preceding four months, though he himself had not paid it much attention, attributing it to a minor injury from yard work several months earlier that he could not clearly recall. Examination revealed a brown to black, irregularly bordered longitudinal band occupying approximately half the width of the nail plate, with subtle extension of brown discoloration onto the adjacent proximal nail fold skin, a positive Hutchinson sign. He had no personal or family history of melanoma. Dermoscopy of the nail plate showed disruption of the normal parallel-line pattern with irregular spacing and color variation within the band, findings inconsistent with a benign process.

Given the combination of a solitary, widening band with irregular borders, a positive Hutchinson sign, and concerning dermoscopic findings, urgent referral for a nail matrix biopsy was arranged rather than a period of observation, and biopsy confirmed subungual melanoma in situ. He underwent definitive surgical management with clear margins and was referred to oncology for staging evaluation and ongoing surveillance given the diagnosis, and was counseled extensively that the delay in seeking evaluation, though understandable given his attribution of the finding to prior trauma, illustrated precisely why any pigmented nail band without a clear, corroborated trauma history and expected pattern of distal growth and resolution warrants prompt professional evaluation rather than assumption of a benign traumatic cause. His case was also used as an opportunity to counsel his wife, who had first noticed the finding, that her attentiveness had been the decisive factor in achieving an early-stage diagnosis, reinforcing the broader value of involving family members in monitoring changes to skin and nail findings that patients themselves may not closely track.

Clinical Case: Painful Nail Fold Swelling in a Frequent Hand-Washer

A 41-year-old woman working as a hospital nurse presented with several months of intermittent swelling, mild tenderness, and redness affecting the proximal nail folds of several fingers on her dominant hand, with progressive loss of the cuticle in the affected areas and mild secondary ridging of the nail plates; she had been treating the area with an over-the-counter antifungal cream without improvement after several weeks. She reported extremely frequent hand hygiene given her occupational requirements, often more than twenty times per shift, along with regular use of alcohol-based hand sanitizer. Examination confirmed erythematous, boggy swelling of the proximal nail folds on the second and third digits bilaterally, with absent cuticles and mild transverse ridging of the underlying nail plates, without evidence of a discrete abscess or acute purulent process.

The gradual onset, absence of acute abscess formation, cuticle loss, and clear relationship to her occupational moisture exposure were recognized as classic for chronic paronychia rather than a primarily fungal or acute bacterial process, and she was counseled that her prior antifungal treatment, while a reasonable initial attempt, was unlikely to succeed given that the underlying driver of her condition was barrier disruption from repeated moisture exposure rather than a primary fungal infection requiring eradication. She was started on a mid-potency topical corticosteroid applied to the affected nail folds and counseled on practical barrier protection strategies, including glove use during any additional wet work outside of required clinical hand hygiene and a moisturizing regimen to support barrier recovery between hand hygiene episodes, and at six-week follow-up her nail fold swelling and erythema had substantially improved with early cuticle regrowth visible on close examination. She was advised to continue the barrier protection measures indefinitely given her ongoing occupational exposure, since discontinuing these practical modifications once symptoms improved would likely lead to prompt recurrence of the same underlying process.

THE MORPHOLOGY-TO-MANAGEMENT SYSTEM — Reading Structure to Localize Nail Disease

Pattern Introduced This Chapter: Matrix-signature findings (pitting, ridging, Beau lines) versus nail bed-signature findings (onycholysis, oil drop sign, splinter hemorrhages), and the ABCDEF framework for distinguishing benign melanonychia from subungual melanoma.

Cross-Cutting Anchor: Localizing a nail finding to the matrix, nail bed, or surrounding folds is the anchor step that directs the differential diagnosis and the treatment approach across every condition in this chapter, from paronychia to psoriatic nail disease to pigmented nail bands.

Summary and Key Concepts

The nail matrix generates the plate and produces surface texture changes when diseased, while the nail bed governs adherence and color visible through the plate, producing onycholysis and discoloration when diseased.

Acute paronychia is typically bacterial and may require incision and drainage, while chronic paronychia reflects barrier disruption from repeated moisture exposure and responds best to irritant avoidance and topical corticosteroid therapy rather than antimicrobial therapy alone.

Psoriatic nail disease produces pitting (matrix) and the oil drop sign, onycholysis, and subungual hyperkeratosis (nail bed), and nail involvement correlates with an increased likelihood of psoriatic arthritis.

The ABCDEF criteria and the Hutchinson sign help distinguish benign longitudinal melanonychia from subungual melanoma, and any new, solitary, widening, or irregularly bordered band warrants biopsy.

Clubbing, koilonychia, Beau lines, splinter hemorrhages, and half-and-half nails each carry distinct systemic disease associations spanning pulmonary, cardiac, hematologic, infectious, and renal conditions.

Digital myxoid cysts, glomus tumors, subungual exostosis, and onychopapilloma are benign nail unit tumors, each with a distinctive presentation guiding diagnosis and, when needed, surgical management.

CHAPTER 17: BENIGN CUTANEOUS NEOPLASMS AND CYSTS

Learning Objectives

1. Recognize seborrheic keratosis and distinguish it confidently from melanocytic and malignant pigmented lesions.
2. Differentiate epidermoid and pilar cysts from other subcutaneous nodules and select an appropriate management approach for each.
3. Recognize dermatofibroma using the dimple sign and distinguish it from its more concerning mimics.
4. Classify benign melanocytic nevi by their clinical and dermoscopic growth pattern and identify features warranting biopsy.
5. Recognize pyogenic granuloma and construct an appropriate diagnostic and treatment approach given its potential to mimic amelanotic melanoma.
6. Distinguish keloid from hypertrophic scar and select a treatment approach matched to each.

Benign cutaneous neoplasms account for the overwhelming majority of skin lesions encountered in everyday clinical practice, and the essential skill this chapter builds is not merely recognizing each entity in isolation but confidently distinguishing it from its more consequential malignant mimics, since the clinical value of correctly identifying a benign lesion lies precisely in the reassurance and avoided unnecessary intervention that follows. A small number of simple bedside techniques, the dimple sign for dermatofibroma, the stuck-on appearance and pseudocysts of seborrheic keratosis, the central punctum of an epidermoid cyst, do most of the diagnostic work in this chapter, and mastering them is what allows a busy clinician to manage the large volume of benign lesion presentations efficiently while still maintaining a low threshold to biopsy when a finding does not fit its expected benign pattern. The chapters that follow in this part of the text build directly on the diagnostic instincts developed here, since the malignant and premalignant entities discussed there are most reliably recognized by contrast against the benign baseline established in this chapter.

Seborrheic Keratosis

Seborrheic keratosis is among the most common benign skin growths encountered in adults, increasing in number with age, and presents as a well-demarcated, waxy to verrucous papule or plaque with a characteristic stuck-on appearance, as though the lesion had been pasted onto the skin surface rather than arising from within it, ranging in color from tan to dark brown or black; this stuck-on quality, along with a friable, greasy surface texture and visible horn pseudocysts, small, round, keratin-filled structures visible on close or dermoscopic examination, are the key features that support a confident clinical diagnosis without the need for biopsy in the majority of cases. Seborrheic keratoses can occur anywhere on the body except the palms, soles, and mucous membranes, and while they are entirely benign, their sometimes irregular, dark, and asymmetric appearance means they are among the most common benign lesions submitted for biopsy specifically to exclude melanoma, particularly when a lesion is inflamed, irritated, or has recently changed in a way that raises clinical concern.

Dermoscopy and the Sign of Leser-Trelat

Dermoscopic examination of seborrheic keratosis characteristically reveals multiple milia-like cysts, comedo-like openings, and a sharply demarcated border, sometimes described as looking as though the lesion has been dropped onto the skin from above, findings that reliably distinguish it from melanoma even when the clinical appearance alone raises some uncertainty, making dermoscopy a valuable and often decisive tool before proceeding to an unnecessary biopsy. The sign of Leser-Trelat, the abrupt eruption of numerous new seborrheic keratoses over a short period, is a recognized, though rare, paraneoplastic phenomenon most often associated with gastrointestinal adenocarcinoma, and while the overwhelming majority of seborrheic keratoses, even multiple ones, reflect nothing more than the ordinary accumulation of these common lesions with age, a genuinely abrupt, dramatic eruption of many new lesions in a short time frame, particularly accompanied by other systemic symptoms, warrants consideration of an underlying malignancy evaluation.

THE MORPHOLOGY-TO-MANAGEMENT SYSTEM — The Stuck-On Waxy Papule

The Pattern: A well-demarcated, waxy, verrucous papule or plaque with a stuck-on appearance, greasy surface, and visible horn pseudocysts on close examination.

Presentation Variance: Color ranges from light tan to deep black; lesions can be single or, more commonly with age, numerous, and irritated or traumatized lesions can become inflamed and tender, sometimes prompting concern for a different process.

Trap Logic: A darkly pigmented, irregular seborrheic keratosis can superficially resemble melanoma; dermoscopic confirmation of milia-like cysts, comedo-like openings, and a sharply demarcated border distinguishes the two, and any lesion where this distinction remains uncertain after dermoscopy should be biopsied rather than presumed benign.

Management Pivot: Confirm the diagnosis clinically or with dermoscopy; treatment is not medically necessary but can be offered for irritated, symptomatic, or cosmetically bothersome lesions using cryotherapy, curettage, or shave removal, selected based on lesion thickness and location.

Pattern Anchor: Stuck-on appearance plus dermoscopic milia-like cysts and comedo-like openings equals seborrheic keratosis; any departure from this pattern, particularly asymmetry, irregular pigment network, or atypical vascular structures on dermoscopy, should prompt biopsy rather than reassurance.

Epidermoid and Pilar Cysts

Epidermoid cysts, often loosely referred to as sebaceous cysts despite arising from the infundibular portion of the hair follicle rather than sebaceous glands, present as firm, mobile, subcutaneous nodules, most commonly on the face, neck, and trunk, frequently with a visible central punctum, a small, dark, dilated follicular opening at the apex of the lesion, from which a foul-smelling, cheesy keratinaceous material can sometimes be expressed; this central punctum is the single most useful bedside finding distinguishing an epidermoid cyst from other subcutaneous nodules such as a lipoma, which lacks a punctum and typically has a softer, more diffusely mobile consistency without a discrete overlying skin change. Ultrasound imaging, while not routinely necessary for a classic, superficial, mobile cystic lesion, can be a useful adjunct for larger, deeper, or diagnostically uncertain lesions, helping to confirm cystic versus solid composition and delineate the lesion's relationship to surrounding structures before proceeding to excision. Epidermoid cysts can become acutely inflamed or secondarily infected, presenting with rapid enlargement, erythema, and tenderness that can be difficult to distinguish clinically from a true bacterial abscess, though the inflammatory response in an uninfected, ruptured epidermoid cyst is often a foreign body reaction to extruded keratin rather than a true infection, a distinction with direct treatment implications since antibiotics alone will not resolve an inflamed cyst if the primary process is a foreign body reaction rather than bacterial infection.

Pilar Cysts and Management Approach

Pilar cysts, also called trichilemmal cysts, arise from the outer root sheath of the hair follicle and occur predominantly on the scalp, presenting similarly to epidermoid cysts as firm, mobile subcutaneous nodules but typically without a visible central punctum, and often multiple lesions occur in the same patient given a recognized hereditary predisposition; their firm, cheesy contents are more readily and completely enucleated during excision compared to epidermoid cysts, given a distinct cyst wall composition, making complete surgical removal technically somewhat more straightforward. Definitive treatment for either cyst type requires complete surgical excision of the cyst wall, since incision and drainage alone, while providing prompt relief of an acutely inflamed or infected cyst, leaves the cyst wall in place and is followed by a high rate of recurrence; elective excision is best performed when the cyst is quiescent rather than acutely inflamed, given the more straightforward dissection and lower recurrence rate achieved under non-inflamed conditions, though incision and drainage remains appropriate as an initial step for an acutely painful, fluctuant, inflamed cyst, with definitive excision deferred to a later, quiescent interval.

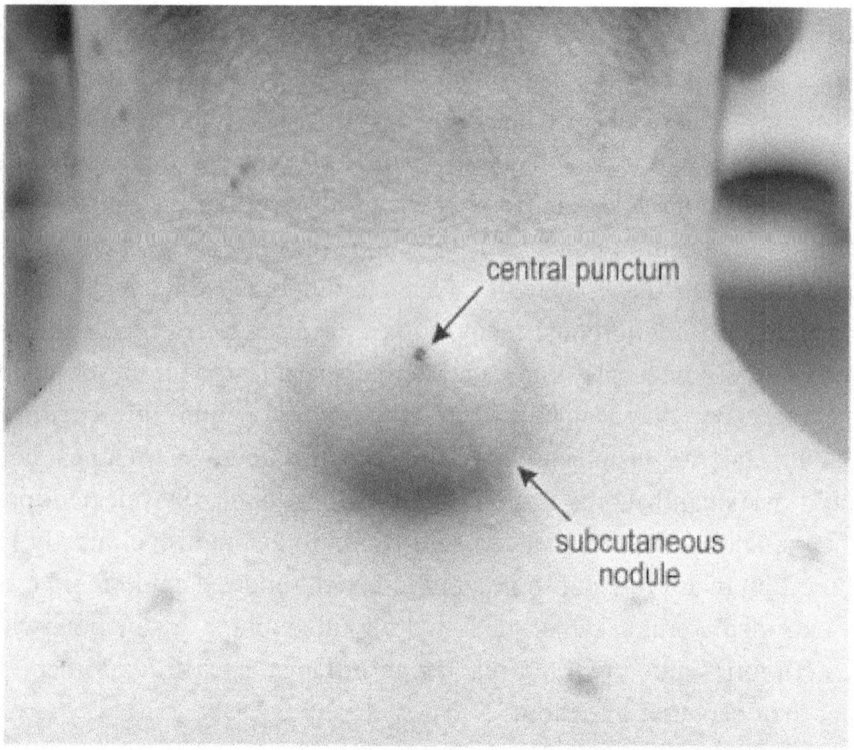

Figure 17.1 — Clinical Photography: Epidermoid Cyst With Visible Central Punctum.

Dermatofibroma

Dermatofibroma is a common, benign fibrohistiocytic proliferation presenting as a firm, well-circumscribed papule or nodule, most often on the lower extremities, frequently with a history of minor preceding trauma such as an insect bite, though many patients cannot recall a specific inciting event, and typically ranging in color from pink to tan to brown depending on the degree of associated hemosiderin deposition and overlying epidermal hyperpigmentation. The dimple sign, also called the Fitzpatrick sign, elicited by applying lateral compression to the lesion between the thumb and forefinger and observing a central dimpling or dell as the overlying skin is drawn inward, reflects the tethering of the fibrous proliferation to the overlying dermis and is a highly characteristic and reliable bedside finding that, when positive, supports the diagnosis with a high degree of confidence, distinguishing dermatofibroma from other firm dermal or subcutaneous nodules that would not demonstrate this specific tethering behavior on compression.

KEY POINT: A positive dimple sign, central dimpling of the lesion on lateral compression, is one of the most reliable bedside diagnostic maneuvers in dermatology, allowing confident clinical diagnosis of dermatofibroma without biopsy in the large majority of typical-appearing lesions; a negative dimple sign, or an atypical clinical or dermoscopic appearance, should prompt reconsideration of the diagnosis and, where malignancy cannot be confidently excluded, biopsy.

Dermatofibrosarcoma protuberans, a low-grade but locally aggressive soft tissue sarcoma, is the most important entity to distinguish from ordinary dermatofibroma, since it can present initially as a similarly firm, slow-growing dermal nodule but progressively enlarges into a larger, multinodular, protuberant plaque with a tendency toward deep local infiltration that makes complete surgical excision considerably more complex than for benign dermatofibroma; any firm dermal nodule that continues to enlarge progressively over months to years, becomes multinodular, or reaches a size atypical for ordinary dermatofibroma warrants biopsy to exclude this diagnosis given the substantially different management implications, including the frequent need for Mohs micrographic surgery or wide local excision with careful margin assessment given the tumor's tendency toward subclinical infiltrative extension well beyond its visible clinical margins.

Benign Melanocytic Nevi

Benign melanocytic nevi are classified by the location of nevomelanocytes within the skin and follow a generally predictable pattern of evolution over a person's lifetime: junctional nevi, with melanocytes confined to the dermal-epidermal junction, present as flat, evenly pigmented macules, typically arising in childhood; compound nevi, with melanocytes present at both the junction and within the underlying dermis, present as slightly raised, evenly pigmented papules, typically developing as junctional nevi mature over years; and intradermal nevi, with melanocytes confined entirely to the dermis with loss of the junctional component, present as soft, often skin-colored to tan, dome-shaped or papillomatous papules with little to no pigmentation, typically representing the most mature stage of this natural evolutionary sequence, most often appearing in mid-to-late adulthood. This natural progression from flat and pigmented to raised and pale over decades is itself a reassuring pattern, and understanding it allows a clinician to recognize an individual nevus's evolution as expected biological maturation rather than a concerning change.

Recognizing Features That Depart From Expected Nevus Evolution

The ABCDE criteria, Asymmetry, Border irregularity, Color variegation, Diameter greater than six millimeters, and Evolution or change over time, remain a useful screening framework for identifying pigmented lesions that depart from the typical, orderly nevus evolution described above and therefore warrant closer evaluation or biopsy, though these criteria should be applied as a gestalt assessment of overall lesion behavior rather than a rigid checklist, since some benign nevi, particularly congenital and Spitz nevi, can display features overlapping with these criteria despite being entirely benign, just as some early melanomas can be small, symmetric, and evenly colored, particularly nodular melanoma, which often lacks the classic ABCDE features and instead should be recognized by rapid growth and firm, elevated character (sometimes summarized as the EFG criteria: Elevated, Firm, Growing). Dermoscopy substantially improves diagnostic accuracy beyond the naked eye alone across this entire category of lesions, and any clinician managing a substantial volume of pigmented lesions benefits considerably from dermoscopic training and consistent use of this tool in practice.

Nevus Type	Melanocyte Location	Clinical Appearance	Typical Age Pattern
Junctional	Dermal-epidermal junction	Flat, evenly pigmented macule	Childhood
Compound	Junction and dermis	Slightly raised, pigmented papule	Adolescence to adulthood
Intradermal	Dermis only	Soft, dome-shaped, often skin-colored papule	Mid-to-late adulthood

Congenital and Atypical (Dysplastic) Nevi

Congenital melanocytic nevi, present at birth or appearing within the first weeks to months of life, are classified by projected adult size, small (under 1.5 centimeters), medium, large, and giant (generally defined as 20 centimeters or greater in projected adult size), a classification that carries direct prognostic significance since the lifetime melanoma risk rises meaningfully with increasing nevus size, remaining low for small and medium congenital nevi but reaching a clinically significant, though still overall modest, cumulative risk for giant congenital nevi, which also carry an associated risk of neurocutaneous melanosis when there is extensive or multiple satellite nevi involvement, warranting baseline neuroimaging in appropriate cases. Management of small to medium congenital nevi generally consists of routine monitoring given their low absolute melanoma risk, while giant congenital nevi warrant discussion of prophylactic excision, when anatomically and surgically feasible, alongside long-term dermatologic surveillance regardless of whether excision is pursued, given that excision does not eliminate risk entirely when nevus cells extend into deeper tissue planes beyond the reach of surgery.

Atypical, or dysplastic, nevi present as larger, often greater than five to six millimeters, more irregularly bordered and variably pigmented moles that can display some features overlapping with the ABCDE criteria while remaining entirely benign on histology, and patients with numerous atypical nevi, particularly in the setting of a strong family history of melanoma, meet criteria for the dysplastic nevus syndrome (familial atypical multiple mole and melanoma syndrome), a condition carrying a substantially elevated lifetime melanoma risk that warrants regular total body skin examination, often at more frequent intervals than the general population, along with baseline and serial total body photography to facilitate detection of new or changing lesions against a backdrop of numerous baseline atypical-appearing nevi that would otherwise make subtle change difficult to detect through memory or single-visit assessment alone.

KEY POINT: Total body photography is a particularly valuable tool in patients with numerous atypical nevi, since it provides an objective baseline against which new lesions or changes to existing lesions can be reliably detected at follow-up visits, addressing the genuine clinical challenge of tracking subtle change across dozens or even hundreds of nevi that would otherwise be difficult to monitor by memory or clinical impression alone.

Pyogenic Granuloma

Pyogenic granuloma, a misnomer reflecting an outdated understanding of its pathogenesis since it is neither purulent nor a true granuloma but rather a benign, rapidly growing lobular capillary hemangioma, presents as a friable, bright red to violaceous papule or nodule that bleeds readily and often profusely with even minor trauma, frequently developing over days to a few weeks following a minor injury, and with a particular predilection for the fingers, lips, and gingiva, the latter especially during pregnancy given the hormonal influence on this lesion's development in a subset of cases (sometimes termed a pregnancy tumor or granuloma gravidarum in this context). Its rapid growth, friability, and tendency to bleed with minimal provocation are its most characteristic and clinically useful features, and while the diagnosis is often apparent clinically given this distinctive rapid growth pattern and history, the differential diagnosis, most importantly amelanotic melanoma, which can present as a similarly rapidly growing, vascular-appearing, non-pigmented nodule, means that biopsy for histologic confirmation is generally recommended for any lesion fitting this description, both to confirm the diagnosis and to exclude this more serious mimic.

CAUTION: A rapidly growing, friable, bleeding red nodule should never be assumed to be a pyogenic granuloma without histologic confirmation, since amelanotic melanoma can present with a strikingly similar clinical appearance; the consequence of missing an amelanotic melanoma by presuming a benign pyogenic granuloma without biopsy is far more serious than the minor additional step of sending an excised or shave-removed specimen for pathologic confirmation.

Treatment of pyogenic granuloma typically involves shave removal with base cauterization or curettage and electrodesiccation, both of which provide the tissue needed for histologic confirmation while also treating the lesion, and recurrence is not uncommon, particularly if the base is inadequately treated, given the lesion's inherent tendency toward proliferative vascular growth; recurrent or deeply based lesions may require full excision for more definitive treatment. Pregnancy-associated lesions frequently, though not universally, regress at least partially following delivery as the hormonal influence driving their growth resolves, and this natural history can be discussed with pregnant patients considering whether to pursue removal during pregnancy versus deferring treatment until the postpartum period for lesions that are not significantly symptomatic or bleeding.

Cherry Angioma and Other Common Vascular Proliferations

Cherry angioma, also termed a Campbell de Morgan spot, is an extremely common, benign vascular proliferation presenting as a small, smooth, bright red to violaceous papule, most often on the trunk, increasing in number with age to the point that most older adults have numerous such lesions, and requiring no treatment beyond reassurance given their universally benign nature, though laser therapy or light electrodesiccation can be offered for cosmetically bothersome lesions. Venous lakes, soft, compressible, dark blue to violaceous papules most commonly occurring on the lips, ears, and face of older adults with a history of significant cumulative sun exposure, represent dilated venous channels rather than a true neoplastic proliferation, and their compressibility, blanching partially or completely with firm, sustained pressure, is a useful distinguishing bedside feature from a pigmented lesion such as melanoma, which will not blanch with compression given its solid, non-vascular composition.

Skin Tags and Sebaceous Hyperplasia

Acrochordons, commonly known as skin tags, are extremely common, benign, soft, pedunculated papules most often occurring in areas of friction, the neck, axillae, and groin, increasing in prevalence with age, obesity, and insulin resistance, and while overwhelmingly benign, their presence in large numbers, particularly in a younger patient, can serve as a cutaneous clue prompting consideration of underlying metabolic syndrome or, less commonly, acromegaly, given recognized associations between these conditions and increased skin tag burden, an association that parallels the acanthosis nigricans discussion in the preceding chapter as another example of a common, seemingly minor cutaneous finding carrying genuine systemic screening value. Treatment is not medically necessary but is commonly requested for cosmetic reasons or because a tag has become irritated or caught on clothing or jewelry, and simple removal by scissor excision, cryotherapy, or light electrodesiccation is quick, well-tolerated, and definitive given the superficial, pedunculated nature of these lesions.

Sebaceous Hyperplasia

Sebaceous hyperplasia is one of the most common benign facial growths seen in clinical practice and presents as small, soft, yellowish papules with a characteristic central dell or umbilication, most commonly on the forehead and cheeks of middle-aged and older adults, reflecting benign enlargement of sebaceous glands around a central hair follicle, and its dermoscopic appearance, showing peripheral crown vessels arranged around the central umbilication in a pattern sometimes likened to a wreath, is distinctive enough to reliably distinguish it from basal cell carcinoma, an important mimic given that both conditions can present as a pearly or translucent papule on sun-exposed facial skin; when the distinction remains uncertain despite dermoscopic examination, biopsy should be pursued given the substantially different management implications of a missed basal cell carcinoma. Treatment, again not medically necessary, can include light electrodesiccation, shave removal, or topical or oral agents that reduce sebaceous gland activity for patients bothered by numerous or cosmetically prominent lesions.

Keloid Versus Hypertrophic Scar

Hypertrophic scars are raised, firm scars that remain confined to the boundaries of the original wound or incision and typically develop within weeks of the inciting injury, often improving gradually over months to a couple of years as the scar matures and remodels, whereas keloids extend beyond the original wound margins, invading adjacent normal skin in a manner hypertrophic scars do not, can develop months after the inciting injury rather than immediately, and do not regress spontaneously over time, instead often continuing to enlarge; this distinction, extension beyond the original wound boundary being the single most reliable differentiating feature, carries direct treatment implications since the two conditions, despite their superficial similarity, differ meaningfully in expected treatment response and recurrence risk. Both conditions can also be pruritic or tender, particularly in their early, actively growing phase, and this symptomatic component, while secondary to the cosmetic concern for most patients, should be addressed directly as part of the treatment plan rather than overlooked in favor of appearance alone. Keloids show a strong predisposition in individuals with darker skin phototypes and a meaningful genetic and familial component, and characteristic high-risk anatomic sites, including the earlobes, anterior chest, shoulders, and upper back, reflect areas of greater skin tension and mechanical stress that appear to promote the aberrant fibroblast response underlying keloid formation.

Treatment Approaches

Intralesional corticosteroid injection is first-line therapy for both hypertrophic scars and keloids, softening and flattening the lesion by suppressing the excessive collagen production driving the fibrotic process, though keloids generally require more prolonged and repeated treatment courses given their more aggressive underlying fibroproliferative behavior; silicone sheeting or gel, applied consistently over the maturing scar, is a useful, low-risk adjunct particularly valuable for prevention in patients with a known predisposition to abnormal scarring, ideally initiated as soon as the wound has re-epithelialized. Surgical excision of a keloid carries a high recurrence rate, frequently resulting in a keloid larger than the original lesion, when performed as monotherapy without adjunctive treatment, and is therefore generally combined with immediate postoperative intralesional corticosteroid injection or another adjunctive modality such as radiation therapy or pressure therapy to reduce this substantial recurrence risk; patients with a known personal or strong family history of keloid formation should be counseled explicitly about this elevated risk before undergoing any elective procedure at a high-risk anatomic site, allowing a shared decision about whether to proceed and what preventive measures to implement from the outset.

PATIENT EDUCATION: Patients with a personal history of keloid formation should be counseled to disclose this history before any future elective skin procedure, including ear piercing, cosmetic surgery, or even routine biopsy at a high-risk site such as the chest or shoulder, so that preventive measures, such as intralesional corticosteroid injection at the time of the procedure or careful site selection when elective, can be planned proactively rather than only after a new keloid has already formed.

Patients with numerous benign lesions of any type discussed in this chapter benefit from an annual full-body skin examination as a baseline standard of care, both to reassess existing lesions for any departure from their expected stable, benign appearance and to identify any new lesion warranting closer attention, and this practice should be routinely offered and encouraged rather than reserved only for patients who specifically request it or who carry a known elevated melanoma risk.

Spitz Nevus and Nevus Sebaceus

Spitz nevus presents as a rapidly growing, often solitary, pink to reddish-brown, dome-shaped papule most commonly on the face or extremities of children and young adults, with a dermoscopic pattern showing a distinctive starburst pattern of symmetric, radially arranged pigment streaks at the periphery, and while classically and overwhelmingly benign, its rapid growth and, in some cases, histologic overlap with spitzoid melanoma make it a genuinely challenging diagnostic category, particularly in older patients or when histologic features are ambiguous even to an experienced dermatopathologist; complete excisional biopsy, rather than a partial shave or punch sample, is generally recommended for suspected Spitz nevi given the diagnostic importance of assessing the complete architecture of the lesion, and some atypical or histologically ambiguous cases are managed with complete excision and close clinical follow-up given genuine uncertainty even after full pathologic review.

Nevus Sebaceus

Nevus sebaceus is a congenital hamartoma composed of an overgrowth of sebaceous glands, hair follicles, and apocrine glands, typically presenting at birth as a smooth, yellow-orange, hairless plaque on the scalp or face that becomes more verrucous and thickened around puberty under hormonal influence, and while historically associated with a meaningful risk of secondary neoplasm development within the lesion later in life, most commonly trichoblastoma and, less commonly, basal cell carcinoma, more recent evidence suggests this risk was previously overestimated and that the large majority of secondary growths arising within a nevus sebaceus are themselves benign; current practice generally favors clinical monitoring for new nodularity or change within the lesion over routine prophylactic excision, reserving surgical removal for lesions that are symptomatic, cosmetically bothersome, or that develop a new, concerning growth warranting biopsy.

Complications, Special Populations, and Patient Education

Milia, small, firm, white to yellow superficial keratin-filled cysts most commonly seen on the face, can occur spontaneously in neonates, where they resolve without intervention within the first few weeks of life, or develop in adults, either spontaneously or secondary to skin trauma, blistering conditions, or certain topical products, and are managed conservatively with simple extraction using a sterile blade or needle when cosmetically bothersome, a straightforward in-office procedure with minimal risk. Neurofibromas, benign peripheral nerve sheath tumors presenting as soft, compressible, skin-colored papules or nodules that classically demonstrate a distinctive "buttonhole" sign, invaginating readily beneath a palpating finger with a springy return, occur sporadically as solitary lesions in the general population but should prompt evaluation for neurofibromatosis type 1 when multiple, given the syndrome's associated diagnostic criteria discussed in the preceding chapter on pigmentary disorders. Lipomas, soft, mobile, subcutaneous nodules composed of mature adipocytes, are exceedingly common and benign, generally requiring treatment only when symptomatic or cosmetically bothersome, though rapidly growing, deep, large, or painful lesions warrant consideration of imaging and, in appropriate cases, referral to exclude the rare but more concerning liposarcoma. Children and adolescents presenting with a changing or new pigmented lesion warrant the same careful evaluation applied to adults, since although melanoma is rare in this age group, delayed diagnosis when it does occur is a recognized problem, often because both patients, families, and clinicians are inclined to presume any pigmented lesion in a child is benign; a lesion in a child that fails to follow the expected slow, orderly evolution described earlier in this chapter still warrants the same biopsy threshold as it would in an adult.

Clinical Case: A Firm Lower Leg Papule With a Reassuring Bedside Sign

A 32-year-old woman presented for evaluation of a firm, brownish papule on her lower leg that she had noticed approximately eight months earlier, recalling a possible insect bite in the same area around that time, and had become increasingly worried about after reading online about skin cancer warning signs. Examination revealed a five-millimeter, firm, tan-brown papule with a slightly raised, dome-shaped contour, and lateral compression between the thumb and forefinger produced a clear, central dimpling of the lesion, a positive dimple sign. Dermoscopic examination showed a central white patch (representing the fibrotic core) surrounded by a delicate pigment network at the periphery, a pattern characteristic of and consistent with dermatofibroma.

Given the classic history of possible preceding minor trauma, the positive dimple sign, and the reassuring, typical dermoscopic pattern, she was confidently reassured that the lesion represented a benign dermatofibroma without need for biopsy, and the mechanism and typical natural history of the lesion, including its tendency to remain stable in size over years, were explained to address her specific cancer-related anxiety directly rather than simply offering reassurance without explanation. She was counseled on the specific features, rapid growth, changing color, new bleeding, or loss of the dimple sign response, that would warrant a return visit for reevaluation, empowering her to monitor the lesion appropriately herself going forward rather than requiring routine repeat visits for a lesion with such a classic, reassuring presentation. She was also encouraged to schedule a baseline full-body skin examination given that she had never previously had one performed, an opportunity to establish a documented starting point for any future comparison.

Clinical Case: A Rapidly Growing Bleeding Nodule on the Finger

A 26-year-old man presented with a two-week history of a rapidly growing, bright red nodule on his index finger that had developed at the site of a minor cut from yard work, describing that it bled easily and profusely with even minimal contact, to the point that he had begun wrapping the finger to avoid staining his clothing. Examination revealed a friable, moist-appearing, bright red, dome-shaped nodule approximately eight millimeters in diameter at the base of the fingernail, with a thin collarette of scale at its base and no evidence of pigmentation or irregular vascular pattern beyond what would be expected for a vascular proliferation.

Given the classic history of rapid growth following minor trauma, the friable, bleeding character, and the typical clinical appearance, a diagnosis of pyogenic granuloma was suspected, but given the recognized potential for amelanotic melanoma to mimic this presentation, shave removal with base cauterization was performed rather than accepting the clinical diagnosis alone, and the specimen was sent for histopathologic confirmation, which returned consistent with lobular capillary hemangioma (pyogenic granuloma), confirming the benign diagnosis. He was counseled about the modest but recognized risk of recurrence at the treated site, given the lesion's proliferative vascular nature, and advised to return promptly if a new area of rapid growth or bleeding developed at or near the treatment site, both to address recurrence early and, given the importance of confirming the benign nature of any new growth in this location, to ensure any recurrence was appropriately re-biopsied rather than presumptively re-treated without pathologic confirmation. He was also reassured that the histologic confirmation obtained at this visit meant that, should a similar-appearing lesion recur at the same site, the prior established diagnosis would inform, though not entirely replace, the need for careful reassessment at that time.

THE MORPHOLOGY-TO-MANAGEMENT SYSTEM — Bedside Signs That Confirm a Benign Diagnosis

Pattern Introduced This Chapter: The stuck-on appearance of seborrheic keratosis, the central punctum of an epidermoid cyst, the dimple sign of dermatofibroma, and the natural junctional-to-intradermal evolution of melanocytic nevi as reliable bedside patterns confirming a benign diagnosis.

Cross-Cutting Anchor: Every benign lesion in this chapter has a specific, learnable bedside sign or evolutionary pattern that supports confident clinical diagnosis without biopsy; any lesion that departs from its expected sign or pattern, whether a dermatofibroma with a negative dimple sign or a nevus with atypical evolution, is the anchor trigger for biopsy rather than reassurance.

Summary and Key Concepts

Seborrheic keratosis presents with a stuck-on appearance and characteristic dermoscopic milia-like cysts and comedo-like openings, reliably distinguishing it from melanoma in the large majority of cases.

Epidermoid cysts show a central punctum and require complete surgical excision of the cyst wall for definitive treatment, since incision and drainage alone carries a high recurrence rate.

A positive dimple sign on lateral compression reliably identifies dermatofibroma, while progressive, multinodular enlargement should prompt biopsy to exclude dermatofibrosarcoma protuberans.

Benign melanocytic nevi evolve predictably from flat, pigmented junctional nevi to raised, pale intradermal nevi over decades, and the ABCDE criteria help identify lesions departing from this expected pattern.

Pyogenic granuloma presents as a rapidly growing, friable, bleeding vascular nodule that should be biopsied to exclude amelanotic melanoma given the overlapping clinical presentation.

Keloids extend beyond the original wound margin and do not spontaneously regress, distinguishing them from hypertrophic scars, and both are treated with intralesional corticosteroid injection, with surgical excision of keloids requiring adjunctive therapy to reduce high recurrence risk.

CHAPTER 18: ACTINIC DAMAGE AND KERATINOCYTE CARCINOMA

Learning Objectives

1. Recognize actinic keratosis and explain the concept of field cancerization and its implications for treatment planning.
2. Distinguish the major clinical subtypes of basal cell carcinoma and correlate each with its expected growth behavior and appropriate treatment approach.
3. Recognize squamous cell carcinoma and its precursor lesions and identify high-risk features that influence treatment selection.
4. Differentiate keratoacanthoma from well-differentiated squamous cell carcinoma and understand why the two are managed similarly despite differing natural histories.
5. Select the appropriate treatment modality, from topical field therapy through Mohs micrographic surgery, for a given keratinocyte carcinoma presentation.
6. Construct an evidence-based photoprotection and surveillance plan for patients at elevated risk of keratinocyte carcinoma.

Keratinocyte carcinomas, basal cell carcinoma and squamous cell carcinoma, together represent the most common malignancy in humans, far outnumbering all other cancer types combined in aggregate incidence, occurring so frequently in fair-skinned, chronically sun-exposed populations that a large proportion of clinical practice in this area is devoted less to esoteric diagnosis and more to efficient, high-volume recognition, biopsy, and treatment selection matched appropriately to tumor risk. Because cumulative ultraviolet exposure is the dominant shared driver of both this chapter's malignancies and the actinic keratoses that frequently precede them, this chapter treats photodamage as a continuum, from field-level subclinical change through actinic keratosis to invasive carcinoma, an organizing framework that shapes both diagnostic vigilance and the increasingly field-directed nature of modern treatment.

Actinic Keratosis and Field Cancerization

Actinic keratosis presents as a rough, scaly, erythematous to skin-colored papule or macule on chronically sun-exposed skin, the face, scalp in balding individuals, ears, dorsal forearms, and hands, often more easily felt than seen given its characteristic sandpaper-like texture, and represents a proliferation of atypical keratinocytes confined to the epidermis that is widely regarded as a precursor lesion on the pathway to squamous cell carcinoma, though the absolute risk of any individual actinic keratosis progressing to invasive carcinoma is low, estimated at well under one percent per lesion per year; the clinical significance of actinic keratosis lies less in any single lesion's individual risk and more in what its presence signals about the surrounding field of chronically sun-damaged skin, since a patient with numerous actinic keratoses has, by definition, sustained widespread subclinical photodamage extending well beyond the visible, palpable lesions themselves.

The Field Cancerization Concept

Field cancerization describes the phenomenon in which an entire region of chronically sun-exposed skin harbors widespread subclinical genetic and cellular alterations from cumulative ultraviolet damage, such that visible actinic keratoses represent only the most clinically apparent tip of a much larger area of abnormal, at-risk epidermis, with additional lesions likely to continue emerging over time from the same damaged field even after existing visible lesions are treated. This concept has direct, practical treatment implications: field-directed therapies, addressing the entire affected area rather than only individually visible lesions, are increasingly favored over lesion-directed treatment alone in patients with extensive photodamage and numerous actinic keratoses, since treating only the currently visible lesions leaves the remaining damaged field untreated and predictably productive of new lesions over subsequent months to years.

Treatment Approach	Examples	Best Suited For
Lesion-directed	Cryotherapy, curettage	Few, isolated, well-defined lesions
Field-directed topical	5-fluorouracil, imiquimod, ingenol mebutate/diclofenac	Numerous lesions across a broadly photodamaged field
Field-directed procedural	Photodynamic therapy, chemical peel	Extensive field damage, often combined with topical field therapy

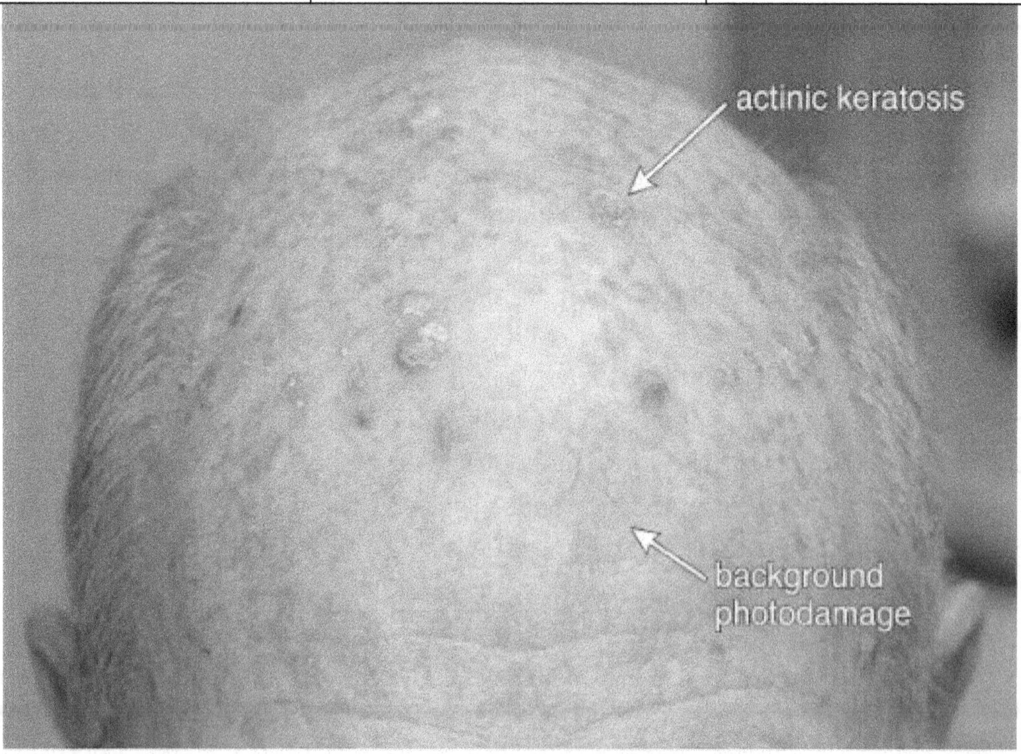

Figure 18.1 — Clinical Photography: Multiple Actinic Keratoses on the Photodamaged Scalp.

Treatment of Actinic Keratosis

Cryotherapy with liquid nitrogen remains the most commonly used lesion-directed treatment for individual or a limited number of actinic keratoses, providing rapid, effective destruction of the treated lesion with minimal downtime, though it treats only the clinically visible lesion and does nothing for the surrounding subclinically damaged field. Topical 5-fluorouracil, an antimetabolite that preferentially targets rapidly dividing atypical keratinocytes, is a well-established field-directed therapy applied over a defined course, typically two to four weeks depending on concentration and formulation, producing an expected, often dramatic inflammatory reaction, erythema, erosion, and crusting, that reflects the treatment working as intended by unmasking and destroying subclinical lesions throughout the treated field; patients require thorough counseling about this expected reaction in advance, since an unprepared patient may otherwise discontinue an effective treatment prematurely, mistaking the expected inflammatory response for an adverse reaction or infection.

Additional Field-Directed Options

Topical imiquimod, an immune response modifier that stimulates local innate and cell-mediated immune activity through toll-like receptor 7 agonism, offers an alternative field-directed option with a similarly expected inflammatory reaction during treatment, generally applied over a longer intermittent course than 5-fluorouracil given its different mechanism and tolerability profile. Photodynamic therapy, involving application of a photosensitizing agent, most commonly aminolevulinic acid, followed by exposure to a specific wavelength of light that activates the agent and generates reactive oxygen species selectively within the more metabolically active, photodamaged keratinocytes, offers an effective procedural field-directed option, particularly valuable for larger or cosmetically sensitive areas such as the face, where it can achieve good cosmetic outcomes alongside meaningful field clearance. Combining a field-directed topical or procedural therapy with targeted lesion-directed cryotherapy for any particularly thick or persistent individual lesions is a common and often effective combined approach in patients with extensive photodamage.

PATIENT EDUCATION: Patients starting a field-directed topical therapy for actinic keratosis should be shown photographs of the expected inflammatory reaction in advance and counseled explicitly that redness, erosion, and crusting during treatment reflect the medication working correctly by exposing and treating subclinical lesions throughout the field, not an infection or an adverse reaction requiring early discontinuation; this proactive counseling meaningfully improves treatment completion rates.

Basal Cell Carcinoma: Clinical Subtypes

Basal cell carcinoma is the single most common malignancy overall in fair-skinned populations, arising from cells of the basal layer of the epidermis and outer root sheath of the hair follicle, and its extraordinarily low but non-zero metastatic potential relative to its high incidence is precisely what allows the wide range of treatment intensities discussed later in this chapter, since even a locally destructive, longstanding tumor is very unlikely to threaten life, a reassurance that is nonetheless balanced against the genuine risk of substantial local tissue destruction, particularly on the face, if treatment is delayed for years. Nodular basal cell carcinoma, the most common subtype, presents as a pearly, translucent papule or nodule with rolled, well-defined borders and prominent, arborizing (branching) telangiectasias coursing across its surface, frequently developing a central depression or ulceration with a rolled, pearly border as the lesion enlarges, a presentation sometimes termed a rodent ulcer in older literature; this subtype grows slowly and, while capable of significant local tissue destruction if neglected for years, only rarely metastasizes, reflecting the generally indolent biological behavior characteristic of basal cell carcinoma as a category. Superficial basal cell carcinoma presents as a thin, pink to red, scaly patch or minimally elevated plaque, often on the trunk, that can closely resemble a patch of eczema or superficial fungal infection, making biopsy essential whenever a persistent, non-resolving scaly patch fails to respond to appropriate treatment for these more common inflammatory or infectious mimics.

Morpheaform and Pigmented Basal Cell Carcinoma

Morpheaform (also termed infiltrative or sclerosing) basal cell carcinoma presents as a subtle, ill-defined, whitish to skin-colored, scar-like plaque without the classic pearly, rolled border of the nodular subtype, and this deceptively unremarkable clinical appearance, combined with a biologically more aggressive, infiltrative growth pattern that extends well beyond the visible clinical margins in strands and columns of tumor cells, makes this subtype particularly prone to underestimation of true extent based on clinical examination alone, a mismatch between innocuous appearance and aggressive subclinical extension that has direct implications for treatment margin selection. Pigmented basal cell carcinoma, most common in patients with darker skin phototypes, shows the same rolled, pearly border and telangiectasia as nodular basal cell carcinoma but with brown to black pigmentation throughout the lesion, creating a diagnostic overlap with melanoma that makes dermoscopic examination, revealing arborizing vessels and blue-gray ovoid nests characteristic of basal cell carcinoma rather than the pigment network typical of melanocytic lesions, a valuable tool for narrowing the differential before biopsy confirmation.

THE MORPHOLOGY-TO-MANAGEMENT SYSTEM — Pearly Papule Versus Ill-Defined Scar-Like Plaque

---

The Pattern: A pearly, translucent papule or nodule with rolled borders and arborizing telangiectasia (nodular) versus a subtle, ill-defined, scar-like plaque without these classic features (morpheaform).

Presentation Variance: Superficial basal cell carcinoma presents as a thin, scaly, erythematous patch resembling eczema or tinea; pigmented basal cell carcinoma shows the classic nodular architecture but with brown to black color overlap with melanocytic lesions.

Trap Logic: Sebaceous hyperplasia can mimic a small nodular basal cell carcinoma but shows a central dell and crown vessels rather than a rolled border with arborizing vessels on dermoscopy; a persistent scaly patch unresponsive to eczema or antifungal treatment should prompt biopsy to exclude superficial basal cell carcinoma rather than continued empiric treatment.

Management Pivot: Biopsy any suspicious lesion for histologic confirmation and subtype determination, since subtype (particularly morpheaform versus nodular) directly informs the appropriate treatment modality and expected surgical margin given differing infiltrative behavior.

Pattern Anchor: Rolled, pearly border with arborizing telangiectasia equals classic nodular basal cell carcinoma; an innocuous, scar-like, ill-defined plaque should never be dismissed without biopsy, since this appearance is characteristic of the more aggressively infiltrative morpheaform subtype.

Squamous Cell Carcinoma and Its Precursors

Squamous cell carcinoma in situ (Bowen disease) presents as a well-demarcated, erythematous, scaly patch or thin plaque, often larger, more persistent, and more sharply demarcated than a typical actinic keratosis, representing full-thickness epidermal atypia that has not yet breached the basement membrane to become invasive; when involving the glans penis, this same in situ process is termed erythroplasia of Queyrat, and its potential for progression to invasive disease, along with its frequent association with human papillomavirus infection at this specific anatomic site, warrants particular attention and prompt treatment when identified in this location. Invasive squamous cell carcinoma presents as a firm, hyperkeratotic, often tender papule, plaque, or nodule, frequently with overlying scale, crusting, or ulceration, arising most commonly on chronically sun-exposed skin, though it can also arise within chronic wounds, burn scars, or areas of chronic inflammation (Marjolin ulcer) after a notably long latency period, sometimes decades, from the original injury.

High-Risk Features and Metastatic Potential

Unlike basal cell carcinoma, squamous cell carcinoma carries a meaningful, though still overall modest, risk of regional lymph node and distant metastasis, and this risk is substantially higher for tumors displaying recognized high-risk features: tumor diameter greater than two centimeters, depth of invasion beyond a defined threshold, perineural invasion, poor histologic differentiation, location on the ear or lip, and origin within a chronic wound, scar, or area of prior radiation, all of which should prompt consideration of a more aggressive treatment approach, closer surveillance, and, in select high-risk cases, nodal basin imaging or sentinel lymph node evaluation. Immunosuppressed patients, particularly solid organ transplant recipients maintained on chronic immunosuppressive therapy, develop squamous cell carcinoma at a dramatically increased rate compared to the general population, with lesions that behave more aggressively and recur more frequently, making this population a distinct, higher-vigilance surveillance group requiring more frequent skin examination and a correspondingly lower threshold for biopsy and treatment of any new or changing lesion.

CAUTION: Solid organ transplant recipients and other chronically immunosuppressed patients develop squamous cell carcinoma at rates many times higher than the general population, with tumors that behave more aggressively, recur more often, and carry higher metastatic risk; this population warrants dedicated, more frequent dermatologic surveillance beginning early after transplantation, ideally established proactively in coordination with the transplant team rather than initiated reactively after a first skin cancer has already developed. Chronic lymphocytic leukemia and other hematologic malignancies similarly predispose to more aggressive keratinocyte carcinoma behavior, reflecting a shared theme of impaired tumor immune surveillance across these otherwise distinct immunocompromising conditions.

Risk Stratification of Squamous Cell Carcinoma

Formal risk stratification systems, most notably the tumor staging framework developed at Brigham and Women's Hospital and the American Joint Committee on Cancer staging system, incorporate the high-risk features discussed above into a structured scoring approach that more reliably predicts the likelihood of nodal metastasis, local recurrence, and disease-specific death than clinical gestalt alone, and increasingly inform decisions about adjuvant imaging, sentinel lymph node biopsy consideration, and the intensity of post-treatment surveillance. Under these frameworks, tumors accumulating multiple high-risk features, larger size, deeper invasion, perineural invasion of a named or large-caliber nerve, poor differentiation, and high-risk anatomic location, are classified into progressively higher risk tiers, with the highest tier carrying a nodal metastasis risk high enough to warrant multidisciplinary tumor board discussion, imaging of the regional nodal basin, and consideration of adjuvant radiation therapy following surgical treatment, a markedly more intensive management pathway than the single excision typically sufficient for a low-risk tumor.

KEY POINT: Perineural invasion, tumor cells tracking along a nerve, deserves particular attention as a high-risk feature: invasion of a small, unnamed nerve branch identified incidentally on pathology carries a different, generally lower-risk implication than invasion of a large-caliber, named nerve, which is associated with a substantially higher risk of local recurrence and perineural spread and often changes the management approach to include radiation therapy or more extensive imaging to assess for proximal extension along the nerve.

Etiology and Risk Factors Across Keratinocyte Carcinoma

Cumulative ultraviolet radiation exposure is the dominant shared risk factor across actinic keratosis, basal cell carcinoma, and squamous cell carcinoma, with both cumulative lifetime sun exposure and, for basal cell carcinoma specifically, a history of intense, intermittent sun exposure and blistering sunburns, particularly in childhood, showing strong epidemiologic association, while squamous cell carcinoma correlates more closely with cumulative total lifetime ultraviolet dose. Fair skin phototype, red or blond hair, light eye color, and a tendency to burn rather than tan are well-established host risk factors reflecting reduced melanin-based photoprotection, and indoor tanning bed use has been independently and consistently associated with increased risk of both basal cell and squamous cell carcinoma, an entirely modifiable exposure that deserves explicit discouragement during any photoprotection counseling conversation. Arsenic exposure, historically from contaminated well water or certain medicinal tonics and now more commonly from occupational exposure in specific industries, is a recognized cause of multiple squamous cell carcinomas and Bowen disease, often with a distinctive pattern of associated arsenical keratoses on the palms and soles, and human papillomavirus infection, particularly at genital and periungual sites, is an important cofactor in a meaningful subset of squamous cell carcinoma and Bowen disease arising outside the classic chronically sun-exposed distribution.

Keratoacanthoma

Keratoacanthoma presents as a rapidly growing, dome-shaped nodule with a characteristic central keratin-filled crater, typically reaching its full size within weeks, considerably faster than the growth rate typical of most squamous cell carcinomas, and has long been recognized to have the potential, in at least some cases, to regress spontaneously over months if simply observed; despite this potential for spontaneous involution, keratoacanthoma is now widely regarded histologically and clinically as a well-differentiated variant of squamous cell carcinoma rather than a truly distinct, reliably self-limited entity, and current practice generally favors treating keratoacanthoma with the same surgical approach used for squamous cell carcinoma rather than relying on observation for spontaneous regression, given the inability to reliably predict in advance which individual lesions will regress spontaneously versus which will continue to grow and behave in a locally destructive manner indistinguishable from conventional invasive squamous cell carcinoma.

KEY POINT: Although keratoacanthoma can regress spontaneously, this behavior cannot be reliably predicted for any individual lesion at initial presentation, and the current histologic consensus regards it as a well-differentiated form of squamous cell carcinoma; treating a keratoacanthoma with the same surgical rigor applied to conventional squamous cell carcinoma, rather than choosing observation in hopes of spontaneous regression, is the safer and currently preferred approach in most clinical circumstances.

Multiple keratoacanthomas occurring in the same patient, particularly in a distinctive eruptive pattern, can rarely reflect an underlying genetic syndrome or be triggered by certain medications, most notably some targeted anticancer therapies, and this pattern warrants consideration of these less common associations rather than assuming each lesion represents an isolated, unrelated event.

Treatment Selection for Keratinocyte Carcinoma

Standard surgical excision with predetermined margins, typically four millimeters for low-risk basal cell carcinoma and four to six millimeters for low-risk squamous cell carcinoma, remains an effective, widely available treatment for the large majority of low-risk keratinocyte carcinomas on the trunk and extremities, providing tissue for margin confirmation via standard postoperative pathology processing. Mohs micrographic surgery, in which the surgeon serves simultaneously as both surgeon and pathologist, examining complete margins of excised tissue in real time through frozen section processing and re-excising only the specific areas where residual tumor is identified, offers the highest cure rate of any treatment modality alongside maximal preservation of normal surrounding tissue, making it the preferred approach for tumors in cosmetically and functionally critical areas such as the central face, periorbital region, nose, and ears, for high-risk histologic subtypes such as morpheaform basal cell carcinoma, for recurrent tumors, and for tumors with poorly defined clinical margins where standard excision risks either incomplete removal or excessive, unnecessarily wide margins.

Non-Surgical and Adjunctive Options

Electrodesiccation and curettage offers a rapid, cost-effective treatment option for select low-risk, superficial or small nodular basal cell carcinomas on the trunk and extremities in appropriately selected patients, though it is generally avoided on the face and in high-risk histologic subtypes given comparatively lower cure rates and inferior cosmetic outcomes relative to surgical excision or Mohs surgery in these settings. Topical therapies, including imiquimod and 5-fluorouracil, and photodynamic therapy carry an approved or reasonable off-label role for select cases of superficial basal cell carcinoma and squamous cell carcinoma in situ in patients who are poor surgical candidates or who prefer a non-surgical approach, though these modalities carry lower cure rates than surgical treatment and are generally reserved for low-risk lesions where the trade-off between cure rate and treatment invasiveness favors the non-surgical option. Radiation therapy offers a valuable option for patients who are not surgical candidates given age, comorbidity, or lesion location, and hedgehog pathway inhibitors, targeting the specific molecular signaling pathway characteristically dysregulated in basal cell carcinoma, provide a systemic treatment option for locally advanced or metastatic basal cell carcinoma not amenable to surgery or radiation, representing an important advance for the small subset of patients with basal cell carcinoma too extensive or inaccessible for these more standard local treatment approaches.

Treatment Modality	Best Suited For	Key Consideration
Standard surgical excision	Low-risk BCC/SCC on trunk and extremities	Predetermined margins; postoperative margin confirmation
Mohs micrographic surgery	High-risk histology, cosmetically sensitive sites, recurrent tumors	Highest cure rate; maximal tissue preservation
Electrodesiccation and curettage	Select low-risk, superficial/small nodular BCC on trunk/extremities	Avoid on face and in high-risk subtypes
Topical therapy/photodynamic therapy	Superficial BCC, SCC in situ in select patients	Lower cure rate; reserved for low-risk lesions or poor surgical candidates
Radiation therapy	Poor surgical candidates, select anatomic sites	Alternative primary treatment or adjuvant therapy
Hedgehog pathway inhibitors	Locally advanced or metastatic BCC	Systemic therapy for disease not amenable to surgery/radiation

Photoprotection: Practical Counseling Points

Broad-spectrum sunscreen, providing protection against both ultraviolet B, the primary driver of sunburn and a major contributor to keratinocyte carcinoma risk, and ultraviolet A, which penetrates more deeply and contributes to photoaging and skin cancer risk through a distinct mechanism, should be recommended with a sun protection factor of at least thirty, applied generously and reapplied at least every two hours during sustained outdoor exposure or after swimming or sweating, since the protection offered by any sunscreen degrades with time and physical removal regardless of its labeled sun protection factor. Mineral (physical) sunscreens containing zinc oxide or titanium dioxide reflect and scatter ultraviolet radiation and are generally well tolerated even in sensitive skin, while chemical sunscreens absorb ultraviolet radiation and convert it to heat, offering a lighter, more cosmetically elegant texture preferred by many patients, and either category, used correctly and consistently, provides meaningful protection; the best sunscreen for any given patient is ultimately the one that patient will actually apply consistently and in adequate quantity, making patient preference and cosmetic tolerability legitimate and important considerations in this recommendation rather than a secondary concern to formulation chemistry alone.

Beyond Sunscreen: Comprehensive Photoprotection

Sunscreen alone is an incomplete photoprotection strategy, and comprehensive counseling should include behavioral measures with an evidence base at least as strong as sunscreen itself: seeking shade, particularly during peak ultraviolet intensity hours in the late morning through mid-afternoon, wearing wide-brimmed hats and sun-protective clothing, ideally with a labeled ultraviolet protection factor, and wearing UV-blocking sunglasses to protect the periocular skin and eyes, a frequently overlooked site for both photoaging and, as discussed elsewhere in this text, ocular surface disease from chronic ultraviolet exposure. Patients should also be counseled that ultraviolet exposure continues on cloudy days, given that a substantial proportion of ultraviolet radiation penetrates cloud cover, and that reflected ultraviolet exposure from surfaces such as snow, sand, and water can meaningfully increase total exposure beyond what direct overhead sun alone would suggest, both counterintuitive points that patients frequently underestimate when assessing their own sun exposure risk on a given day.

Post-Treatment Surveillance

Patients treated for any keratinocyte carcinoma require structured, ongoing surveillance given both the risk of local recurrence at the treated site and, more commonly, the development of an entirely new lesion elsewhere within the same chronically photodamaged field, reflecting the field cancerization concept discussed earlier in this chapter; a patient who has developed one basal cell or squamous cell carcinoma carries a substantially elevated risk of developing additional lesions over subsequent years compared to a patient with no prior history, justifying more frequent skin examinations, typically every six to twelve months depending on individual risk factors, than would be offered to an average-risk patient with no such history. Surveillance visits should include careful examination of the treated site for recurrence, evidenced by new nodularity, ulceration, or a firm scar developing atypical features, alongside a complete skin examination for new lesions elsewhere, and patients should be taught simple self-examination techniques and the warning signs, a sore that does not heal, a new or changing growth, to prompt earlier presentation between scheduled surveillance visits rather than waiting for the next appointment when a concerning new finding develops.

Complications, Special Populations, and Photoprotection

Actinic cheilitis, the actinic keratosis equivalent affecting the lower lip, presents as persistent dryness, scaling, and blurring of the normally sharp vermilion border, and deserves particular vigilance since squamous cell carcinoma arising on the lip, particularly the lower lip given its greater relative sun exposure compared to the upper lip, carries a higher risk of metastasis than similar tumors arising on most other cutaneous sites; persistent, treatment-resistant lip scaling or a new nodule or ulceration at this site should prompt a low threshold for biopsy given these stakes. Erythroplasia of Queyrat, the genital variant of squamous cell carcinoma in situ discussed earlier, similarly warrants prompt treatment given both its malignant potential and its frequent human papillomavirus association, and evaluation and treatment of this condition is often best coordinated with urology or gynecology given the anatomic considerations involved. Basal cell nevus syndrome (Gorlin syndrome), an autosomal dominant condition resulting from mutations in the same hedgehog signaling pathway targeted therapeutically in advanced basal cell carcinoma, produces numerous basal cell carcinomas beginning at an unusually young age, alongside characteristic extracutaneous findings including odontogenic keratocysts of the jaw, palmar and plantar pitting, and skeletal abnormalities; recognition of this syndrome in a young patient presenting with multiple basal cell carcinomas is important both for the patient's own long-term surveillance planning and for offering genetic counseling and evaluation to at-risk family members. Xeroderma pigmentosum, a rare autosomal recessive disorder of defective nucleotide excision repair of ultraviolet-induced DNA damage, produces an extreme, life-threatening sensitivity to sun exposure with markedly elevated rates of skin cancer, including keratinocyte carcinoma and melanoma, at a young age, and affected patients require rigorous, near-total sun avoidance alongside intensive dermatologic surveillance from early childhood, often necessitating specialized ultraviolet-protective clothing, window films, and significant lifestyle accommodation given the severity of photosensitivity involved.

PATIENT EDUCATION: All patients with a history of keratinocyte carcinoma, and particularly those with multiple prior skin cancers or significant cumulative sun exposure, benefit from a structured, lifelong surveillance schedule, rigorous daily broad-spectrum photoprotection, and, in select high-risk patients, consideration of oral nicotinamide, which has demonstrated a modest but statistically significant reduction in new keratinocyte carcinoma and actinic keratosis development in this population when taken consistently as a chemopreventive measure.

Oral retinoids, most commonly acitretin, offer an additional chemopreventive option for select very high-risk patients, particularly solid organ transplant recipients with a demonstrated pattern of numerous or aggressive keratinocyte carcinomas, though their use requires careful discussion of side effects, including mucocutaneous dryness, hyperlipidemia, and, for women of childbearing potential, the mandatory pregnancy avoidance given teratogenicity that persists for an extended period after discontinuation of certain agents in this drug class, factors that must be weighed against the chemopreventive benefit on an individualized basis in coordination with the patient's other treating physicians.

Clinical Case: A Non-Healing Facial Papule

A 68-year-old man presented with a small papule near his left nasal ala that he reported had been present for over a year, occasionally bleeding with minor trauma such as facial washing before scabbing over and appearing to heal, only to reopen again within a few weeks in a recurring cycle he described as "never quite healing." He had a lifetime history of significant outdoor sun exposure from decades working as a landscaper and reported rarely using sunscreen consistently until recent years. Examination revealed a four-millimeter, pearly, translucent papule with a rolled border and several fine, arborizing telangiectasias visible on its surface, with a small central area of superficial erosion. Dermoscopy confirmed arborizing vessels and blue-gray ovoid structures without a pigment network, and a shave biopsy confirmed nodular basal cell carcinoma.

Given the tumor's location near the nasal ala, a cosmetically and functionally sensitive site where tissue conservation is particularly important, he was referred for Mohs micrographic surgery rather than standard excision, allowing complete margin confirmation while sparing as much surrounding normal tissue as possible in a location where even a small amount of unnecessary tissue removal could have a disproportionate cosmetic and functional impact. The procedure achieved clear margins after a single stage, and the resulting defect was repaired with a local flap by the Mohs surgeon; he was counseled on the recurring, "heals-then-reopens" pattern he had described as a classic history for basal cell carcinoma that many patients initially attribute to a slow-healing pimple or minor injury, and was scheduled for regular skin surveillance given his demonstrated risk for developing additional lesions. Given his extensive occupational sun exposure history, a full-body skin examination was also performed at this visit, identifying several actinic keratoses on his forearms and scalp that were treated with cryotherapy, and he was counseled at length on daily broad-spectrum sunscreen use and protective clothing going forward, changes he had not previously prioritized despite his occupational exposure history.

Clinical Case: A Rapidly Growing Nodule in a Transplant Recipient

A 61-year-old man with a kidney transplant six years earlier, maintained on chronic immunosuppressive therapy, presented with a firm, tender nodule on his forearm that had grown rapidly over approximately three weeks, developing a central keratin-filled crater. Given his transplant history and the recognized dramatically elevated risk of aggressive squamous cell carcinoma in this population, the lesion was biopsied promptly rather than observed for potential spontaneous regression despite its clinical appearance being consistent with keratoacanthoma, and histopathology confirmed a well-differentiated squamous cell carcinoma with keratoacanthoma-type features. A review of his history revealed this was his fourth biopsy-confirmed keratinocyte carcinoma in the six years since transplantation, a pattern consistent with the well-documented, markedly accelerated skin cancer burden observed in long-term solid organ transplant recipients relative to the general population.

Given his immunosuppressed status and the elevated aggressive potential of keratinocyte carcinoma in transplant recipients, standard surgical excision with adequate margins was performed rather than observation or a more conservative approach, and his transplant team was informed of the diagnosis to coordinate discussion of his immunosuppressive regimen, since reduction of immunosuppression intensity, when feasible without jeopardizing graft function, is a recognized strategy for reducing future skin cancer risk in transplant recipients with demonstrated aggressive cutaneous malignancy. He was transitioned to a dedicated, more frequent dermatologic surveillance schedule reflecting his elevated risk category, with explicit counseling on rigorous daily photoprotection and self-examination between visits, given the established pattern of recurrent and multiple keratinocyte carcinomas in transplant recipients who develop one such lesion. Given the multiple risk factors now present, his prior lesion count, immunosuppressed status, and this newly confirmed aggressive-behaving tumor, a discussion of oral chemoprevention with acitretin was also initiated in coordination with his transplant physicians, weighing the anticipated reduction in future lesion burden against his individual side effect profile and the coordination required across his multiple treating specialists.

THE MORPHOLOGY-TO-MANAGEMENT SYSTEM — Reading Photodamage Along a Continuum

Pattern Introduced This Chapter: The rough, sandpaper-textured actinic keratosis as a marker of field cancerization, the pearly rolled border of nodular basal cell carcinoma versus the deceptively subtle scar-like morpheaform subtype, and the rapid growth and central crater of keratoacanthoma understood as a variant of squamous cell carcinoma.

Cross-Cutting Anchor: Every lesion in this chapter exists on a shared continuum driven by cumulative ultraviolet exposure, and treatment selection across the entire chapter is anchored on matching modality intensity, from field-directed topical therapy through Mohs micrographic surgery, to the tumor's individual risk profile: subtype, location, size, and host immune status.

Summary and Key Concepts

Actinic keratosis represents the clinically visible tip of a broader field of subclinical ultraviolet-induced photodamage, and field-directed therapy is increasingly favored over lesion-directed treatment alone in patients with extensive actinic damage.

Basal cell carcinoma subtypes carry distinct clinical appearances and growth behavior: nodular shows a classic pearly, rolled border, superficial resembles an eczematous patch, and morpheaform presents deceptively as a subtle, scar-like plaque with more aggressive infiltrative behavior.

Squamous cell carcinoma carries meaningful metastatic potential, particularly with high-risk features including large size, poor differentiation, perineural invasion, high-risk location, and origin in a chronic wound or in an immunosuppressed host.

Keratoacanthoma, despite potential for spontaneous regression, is now managed as a well-differentiated variant of squamous cell carcinoma given the inability to reliably predict which lesions will regress versus progress.

Mohs micrographic surgery offers the highest cure rate and maximal tissue preservation for high-risk tumors and cosmetically sensitive locations, while standard excision, electrodesiccation and curettage, and non-surgical options remain appropriate for select low-risk presentations.

Immunosuppressed patients, particularly solid organ transplant recipients, develop keratinocyte carcinoma at markedly elevated rates with more aggressive behavior, warranting dedicated, more frequent surveillance.

CHAPTER 19: MELANOMA AND PIGMENTED LESION ASSESSMENT

Learning Objectives

1. Recognize the four major clinical subtypes of melanoma and correlate each with its characteristic growth pattern and typical anatomic distribution.
2. Apply dermoscopic pattern analysis to distinguish melanoma from its benign melanocytic mimics.
3. Construct an appropriate biopsy technique for a suspected melanoma and explain why technique selection matters for accurate staging.
4. Explain the components of melanoma staging, including Breslow depth, ulceration, and mitotic rate, and their prognostic significance.
5. Select an appropriate surgical margin and determine sentinel lymph node biopsy candidacy based on tumor stage.
6. Recognize the major systemic treatment classes for advanced melanoma and construct a risk-based surveillance and prevention plan.

Melanoma represents a small minority of all skin cancers by incidence yet accounts for the large majority of skin cancer deaths, a disproportion that defines the entire clinical approach to this chapter: early detection, while the primary lesion is thin and confined to the skin, converts melanoma into a highly curable disease, while delayed recognition allows a tumor with genuine metastatic capability, unlike the keratinocyte carcinomas of the preceding chapter, to progress toward a systemic disease with markedly worse prognosis. Every diagnostic technique in this chapter, from the ABCDE criteria through dermoscopy to biopsy technique selection, exists in service of this single overriding goal: catching melanoma while it remains thin. The dramatic difference in prognosis between thin, localized melanoma and advanced metastatic disease, a difference far starker than for most other solid tumor types, is precisely what makes early detection education, both for clinicians and for the general public, one of the highest-yield interventions available in all of oncology.

Superficial Spreading and Nodular Melanoma

Superficial spreading melanoma, the most common subtype in fair-skinned populations, typically arises on intermittently sun-exposed skin, the trunk in men and the lower legs in women, and characteristically displays a radial growth phase lasting months to years during which the tumor spreads laterally within the epidermis before invading the dermis, producing the asymmetric, irregularly bordered, variably colored, enlarging pigmented lesion captured by the ABCDE criteria; this relatively prolonged radial growth phase is precisely what gives careful surveillance and early biopsy the opportunity to catch the tumor while it remains thin and highly curable, before it transitions to a vertical, invasive growth phase. Nodular melanoma, in sharp contrast, lacks this prolonged radial growth phase, instead invading vertically from the outset, and therefore fails to display the classic ABCDE asymmetry and border irregularity that patients and clinicians are trained to look for, presenting instead as a rapidly growing, firm, often symmetric and evenly colored papule or nodule, sometimes amelanotic (lacking visible pigment altogether); this subtype is more reliably recognized using the EFG criteria, Elevated, Firm, and Growing, than the traditional ABCDE framework, and its lack of a prolonged radial growth phase before invasion contributes to its disproportionately worse average prognosis at diagnosis relative to superficial spreading melanoma.

CAUTION: Nodular melanoma is the subtype most likely to be missed using the ABCDE criteria alone, since it frequently lacks asymmetry, irregular borders, and color variegation, presenting instead as a symmetric, evenly colored, firm, rapidly growing papule or nodule that can be amelanotic; any elevated, firm, and growing lesion, pigmented or not, warrants biopsy regardless of how reassuringly symmetric or evenly colored it may appear by traditional ABCDE assessment.

Lentigo Maligna and Acral Lentiginous Melanoma

Lentigo maligna, the in situ precursor of lentigo maligna melanoma, arises on chronically sun-damaged facial and scalp skin of older adults, presenting as a slowly enlarging, irregularly pigmented macule or patch that can be present for years to decades before invasive transformation, closely resembling and sometimes indistinguishable from a benign solar lentigo at early stages, a diagnostic challenge compounded by the frequent presence of numerous other pigmented and pigment-irregular lesions on the same chronically photodamaged facial skin; dermoscopy, revealing asymmetric pigmented follicular openings and a gray-blue pseudonetwork pattern, is particularly valuable for this subtype given the difficulty of distinguishing early lentigo maligna from benign photodamage-related pigmentation on clinical grounds alone. Acral lentiginous melanoma arises on the palms, soles, and nail unit and is notable both for occurring at similar absolute rates across all skin phototypes, unlike the other subtypes discussed in this chapter which show strong fair-skin predominance, and for representing a disproportionately larger share of melanoma among patients with darker skin phototypes given the comparatively lower incidence of other subtypes in this population; this subtype is frequently diagnosed at a more advanced stage than other melanoma subtypes, in part because these anatomic sites are less routinely examined by patients and clinicians alike and in part because delayed recognition, sometimes including prior misattribution to trauma as discussed for subungual melanoma in the preceding chapter on nail disorders, remains a persistent and correctable problem.

Subtype	Typical Site	Growth Pattern	Key Recognition Point
Superficial spreading	Trunk (men), legs (women)	Prolonged radial growth phase before invasion	Classic ABCDE presentation
Nodular	Any site	Vertical growth from outset, no radial phase	EFG criteria; often lacks classic ABCDE features
Lentigo maligna	Chronically sun-damaged face/scalp	Slow radial growth over years to decades	Resembles solar lentigo; dermoscopy essential

Acral lentiginous	Palms, soles, nail unit	Variable; often diagnosed later	Occurs across all skin phototypes; frequent diagnostic delay

Figure 19.1 — Clinical Photography: Asymmetric Pigmented Plaque of Superficial Spreading Melanoma

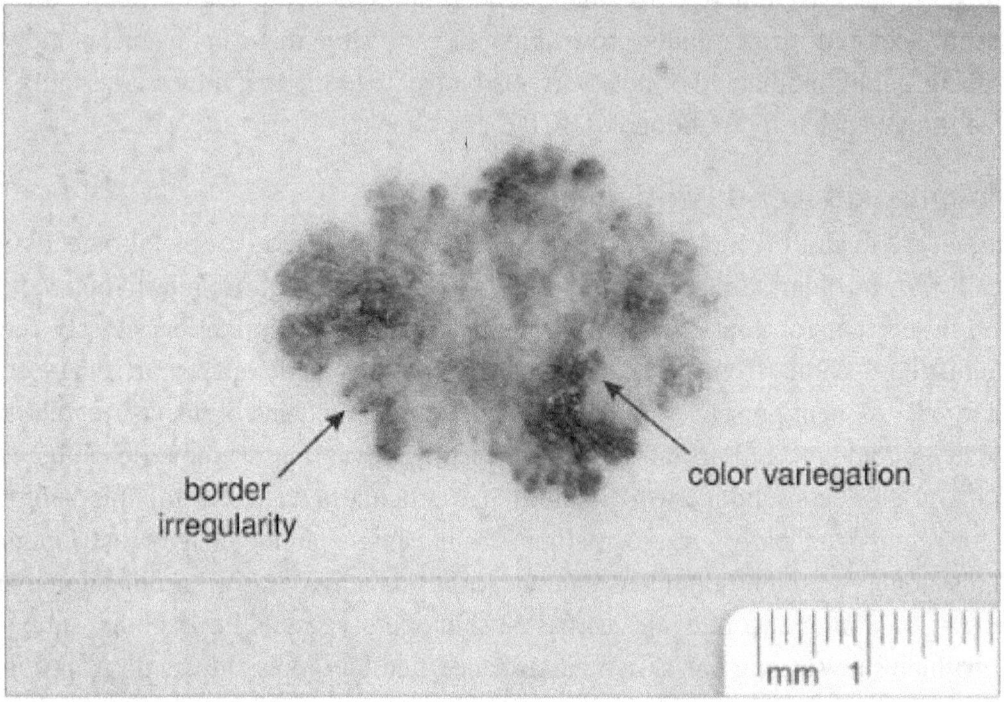

Epidemiology and Risk Factors

Understanding melanoma epidemiology and its modifiable and non-modifiable risk factors informs both individual patient counseling and broader public health prevention efforts. Cumulative and, for several subtypes, intermittent intense ultraviolet exposure remains the dominant modifiable risk factor for melanoma, though the relationship differs meaningfully by subtype: superficial spreading and nodular melanoma correlate more strongly with a history of intense, intermittent exposure and blistering sunburns, particularly in childhood and adolescence, while lentigo maligna correlates more directly with cumulative lifetime sun exposure on chronically exposed skin. A high total nevus count and, in particular, the presence of numerous atypical (dysplastic) nevi, discussed in the preceding chapter, are independent risk factors for melanoma development, both because these patients have a higher probability that any individual nevus will undergo malignant transformation and because a substantial proportion of melanomas, particularly in these high-nevus-count patients, arise de novo in otherwise normal skin rather than within a preexisting nevus, meaning that a low threshold for evaluating any new or changing lesion, not only preexisting nevi, remains essential even in this high-risk population. A personal or family history of melanoma, discussed further below, and a history of significant immunosuppression, including solid organ transplantation, both meaningfully elevate melanoma risk and warrant intensified surveillance.

Indoor Tanning and Additional Modifiable Exposures

Indoor tanning bed use, particularly when initiated before age thirty-five and with greater cumulative sessions over a patient's lifetime, has been consistently and independently associated with significantly increased melanoma risk across multiple large epidemiologic studies, an association strong enough that several jurisdictions have enacted age restrictions or outright bans on tanning bed use by minors, and this remains one of the most directly modifiable risk factors available for patient counseling given that, unlike ambient sun exposure accumulated through ordinary daily life and outdoor activity, indoor tanning is an entirely elective, avoidable exposure with no corresponding health benefit to offset its documented carcinogenic risk.

Distant Metastasis, Additional Staging Considerations, and Uncommon Subtypes

A comprehensive staging evaluation, once a high-risk primary tumor or nodal involvement has been confirmed, typically incorporates cross-sectional imaging to assess for distant disease before finalizing the treatment plan. Beyond the primary tumor and regional nodal staging discussed above, the presence of distant metastatic disease, most commonly to skin and soft tissue, lung, liver, brain, and bone, defines the most advanced stage category and carries the most significant prognostic implications; serum lactate dehydrogenase level at the time of distant metastatic disease diagnosis provides additional independent prognostic information within this most advanced stage category, with an elevated level correlating with a less favorable prognosis. Desmoplastic melanoma, an uncommon histologic variant most often arising on chronically sun-damaged skin of older adults, frequently presents as a firm, scar-like, often amelanotic or minimally pigmented lesion that can be easily overlooked or mistaken for a benign fibrous process, and carries a distinctive biological behavior pattern, including a relatively lower rate of nodal metastasis relative to its Breslow depth but a comparatively higher rate of local recurrence and perineural invasion, considerations that meaningfully influence both surgical margin planning and the sentinel lymph node biopsy discussion for this particular variant relative to conventional melanoma of similar depth.

Adjuvant Systemic Therapy

The decision to pursue adjuvant therapy following surgical resection represents one of the more consequential shared decision-making conversations in modern melanoma management. Following complete surgical resection of high-risk stage melanoma, most notably stage III disease with confirmed nodal involvement and select high-risk stage II disease without nodal involvement, adjuvant systemic therapy with immune checkpoint inhibitor therapy or, for BRAF-mutated tumors, targeted BRAF/MEK inhibitor combination therapy has been shown to meaningfully reduce the risk of disease recurrence compared to observation alone, representing a substantial shift in the management of resected high-risk melanoma over the past several years; this adjuvant treatment decision is made collaboratively between the patient and a multidisciplinary oncology team, weighing the demonstrated recurrence-risk reduction against the potential toxicity of prolonged systemic immunotherapy or targeted therapy, which, while generally more tolerable than traditional cytotoxic chemotherapy, still carries a meaningful risk of immune-related adverse effects, including endocrinopathies, colitis, and pneumonitis, that require ongoing monitoring throughout the treatment course.

Dermoscopy of Pigmented Lesions

Dermoscopic pattern analysis substantially improves diagnostic accuracy for pigmented lesions beyond naked-eye examination alone, meaningfully increasing sensitivity for melanoma detection while simultaneously reducing the number of unnecessary biopsies performed on benign lesions when used by an appropriately trained examiner, and a structured approach, often beginning with a determination of overall pattern symmetry versus asymmetry across both structure and color, forms the foundation of dermoscopic assessment. Features favoring melanoma include an atypical, irregular pigment network with thickened, branching lines of variable thickness distributed asymmetrically, rather than the regular, uniform network typical of a benign nevus; irregular, asymmetrically distributed streaks or pseudopods at the lesion periphery, reflecting asymmetric radial growth; blue-white veil, a structureless, irregular area of blue-white pigmentation reflecting compact orthokeratosis overlying dermal melanin, considered one of the more specific though not universally present dermoscopic melanoma indicators; irregular dots and globules of varying size and distribution rather than the regular, evenly distributed pattern of a benign nevus; and atypical vascular patterns, including irregular linear or dotted vessels, particularly valuable for assessing amelanotic or hypomelanotic lesions where pigment-based criteria cannot be applied.

The Seven-Point Checklist and Pattern Analysis

The seven-point dermoscopic checklist offers a structured, semi-quantitative scoring system assigning weighted points to specific major criteria, atypical pigment network, blue-white veil, and atypical vascular pattern, each worth two points, and minor criteria, irregular streaks, irregular dots and globules, irregular blotches, and regression structures, each worth one point, with a total score of three or more supporting a recommendation for biopsy; this structured approach is particularly valuable for clinicians developing dermoscopic proficiency, offering a more reproducible framework than pure pattern-recognition gestalt alone, though experienced dermoscopists often rely on a more holistic pattern analysis approach once sufficient experience has been accumulated. Regardless of which specific structured framework is used, the overarching principle remains consistent: any degree of genuine dermoscopic asymmetry in structure or color that cannot be confidently attributed to a specific benign process should lower the threshold for biopsy rather than be explained away, since the clinical cost of a missed melanoma substantially outweighs the cost of an unnecessary but appropriately performed biopsy of a lesion that proves benign.

THE MORPHOLOGY-TO-MANAGEMENT SYSTEM — Structural Asymmetry Across Color and Pattern

The Pattern: Asymmetry of structure and color on dermoscopy, atypical pigment network, blue-white veil, irregular streaks, dots, and vascular structures, distributed unevenly across the lesion rather than in the ordered, symmetric pattern of a benign nevus.

Presentation Variance: Superficial spreading melanoma shows classic ABCDE features with dermoscopic asymmetry; nodular melanoma lacks this classic pattern, requiring the EFG approach instead; lentigo maligna shows subtle asymmetric follicular pigmentation against a background of diffuse photodamage.

Trap Logic: Benign nevi can show some dermoscopic features overlapping with melanoma criteria, particularly Spitz nevi with their starburst pattern and some congenital or traumatized nevi; the overall gestalt of asymmetry across the whole lesion, rather than any single isolated criterion, should guide the biopsy decision.

Management Pivot: Any lesion with genuine dermoscopic asymmetry that cannot be confidently attributed to a specific benign process warrants biopsy; select the biopsy technique (excisional preferred) that preserves accurate Breslow depth measurement rather than one that risks incomplete or non-representative sampling.

Pattern Anchor: Structural and color asymmetry on dermoscopy is the anchor finding across every melanoma subtype in this chapter, even when the specific clinical presentation, nodular, acral, or lentiginous, departs from the classic ABCDE picture taught for superficial spreading melanoma.

Reflectance Confocal Microscopy and Total Body Photography

Beyond standard dermoscopy, several additional imaging modalities have emerged to further refine pigmented lesion assessment in specific clinical scenarios. Reflectance confocal microscopy, a noninvasive imaging technique that provides near-histologic resolution of the epidermis and superficial dermis in real time at the bedside, offers an additional diagnostic layer beyond standard dermoscopy for select equivocal pigmented lesions, particularly valuable for lentigo maligna, where it can help delineate the often subtle and poorly defined margins of this subtype both for initial diagnosis and for margin assessment prior to definitive treatment, though its availability remains limited to specialized academic and referral centers rather than routine general practice. Total body photography and sequential digital dermoscopic monitoring, discussed briefly in the preceding chapter in the context of atypical nevus syndrome, are particularly valuable adjuncts in patients with numerous nevi, allowing detection of new lesions and subtle interval change in existing lesions against an objective, reproducible baseline that would otherwise be extremely difficult to track reliably across dozens or hundreds of nevi through unaided clinical impression alone; a lesion that shows any degree of interval change on sequential imaging, even if it would not independently meet biopsy criteria on a single isolated assessment, warrants biopsy given the demonstrated change itself as a concerning finding in its own right.

Biopsy Technique for Suspected Melanoma

Biopsy technique selection for a suspected melanoma is a decision with direct downstream consequences for staging accuracy and should never be treated as an afterthought once the decision to biopsy has been made. Complete excisional biopsy with narrow margins, typically one to three millimeters of clinically normal skin around the visible lesion, extending to a depth adequate to include the full thickness of the dermis, is the preferred biopsy technique for a suspected melanoma whenever anatomically and technically feasible, since accurate measurement of Breslow depth, the single most important prognostic factor in melanoma staging, requires that the entire vertical extent of the tumor be captured in the specimen; a partial biopsy that samples only a portion of the lesion risks either understaging a deeper component that was not included in the sample or, if a superficial shave inadvertently transects the deepest portion of an invasive tumor, an artifactually and unreliably measured Breslow depth that can meaningfully mislead subsequent management decisions. When complete excisional biopsy is not feasible given lesion size or anatomic location, such as a large facial lentigo maligna, a full-thickness incisional or punch biopsy of the most clinically concerning or dermoscopically atypical area, rather than a superficial shave biopsy, is preferred to preserve depth information.

CAUTION: A shave biopsy that transects the base of an invasive melanoma produces an unreliable Breslow depth measurement that can understage the tumor and lead to inadequate initial treatment planning, including an insufficiently wide surgical margin or a missed indication for sentinel lymph node biopsy; when melanoma is a genuine diagnostic consideration, biopsy technique should be selected specifically to preserve full-thickness tissue architecture rather than defaulting reflexively to the shave technique commonly used for other, more superficial lesions.

Melanoma Staging: Breslow Depth, Ulceration, and Mitotic Rate

Formal melanoma staging integrates several histopathologic variables from the primary tumor with clinical and pathologic assessment of regional and distant disease to arrive at an overall prognostic stage that informs both treatment intensity and surveillance planning. Breslow depth, the vertical measurement in millimeters from the granular layer of the epidermis to the deepest identifiable tumor cell, is the single most powerful independent prognostic factor in melanoma and forms the foundation of the current American Joint Committee on Cancer staging system, with prognosis worsening in a graded, continuous fashion as depth increases rather than through discrete threshold effects alone, though specific depth thresholds are used to define staging categories for practical clinical decision-making regarding surgical margins and sentinel lymph node biopsy candidacy. Ulceration, the histologic absence of an intact epidermis overlying the invasive tumor, is an independent adverse prognostic factor at any given Breslow depth, reflecting more aggressive tumor biology, and upstages a tumor within its depth category accordingly; mitotic rate, the number of mitotic figures identified per square millimeter of tumor, provides additional prognostic information particularly relevant for thin melanomas, where an elevated mitotic rate can influence the sentinel lymph node biopsy discussion even when Breslow depth alone would not clearly indicate this procedure.

Sentinel Lymph Node Biopsy

Once distant metastatic disease has been excluded through appropriate staging workup, attention turns to regional nodal assessment. Sentinel lymph node biopsy, identifying and pathologically examining the first lymph node or nodes draining the primary tumor site using a combination of radioactive tracer and blue dye injected around the biopsy site, provides critical staging information by determining whether microscopic nodal metastasis is present, information that carries substantial prognostic weight and informs decisions about adjuvant systemic therapy candidacy, even though the procedure itself has not been definitively shown to improve overall survival directly. Current guidelines generally recommend discussing sentinel lymph node biopsy for melanomas with a Breslow depth of 0.8 millimeters or greater, or for thinner melanomas with ulceration or an elevated mitotic rate, reflecting an increased likelihood of occult nodal involvement at these thresholds, while very thin melanomas without these additional adverse features carry a low enough likelihood of nodal involvement that the procedure's modest incremental staging value is generally felt not to outweigh its associated risks and costs in this lower-risk population.

Surgical Margins and Systemic Therapy for Advanced Disease

Wide local excision margins for confirmed melanoma are determined by Breslow depth, with melanoma in situ generally requiring a 0.5 to 1 centimeter margin, invasive melanoma up to 1 millimeter in depth generally requiring a 1 centimeter margin, and progressively wider margins, up to 2 centimeters, recommended for thicker tumors, reflecting an evidence-based balance between adequate local tumor control and minimizing unnecessary additional tissue removal and its associated cosmetic and functional consequences, particularly in anatomically constrained locations such as the face, hands, and feet. Mohs micrographic surgery or a staged excision technique with complete margin assessment, sometimes termed the "slow Mohs" approach when melanocytic immunostains are required for margin interpretation, is increasingly used for melanoma in situ and lentigo maligna specifically, given the often poorly defined clinical margins of these lesions on background photodamaged skin and the value of complete margin confirmation in anatomically constrained, cosmetically sensitive facial locations where these subtypes most commonly arise. For advanced, unresectable, or metastatic melanoma, systemic therapy has been transformed over the past decade by the introduction of immune checkpoint inhibitors, most notably antibodies targeting programmed cell death protein 1 and cytotoxic T-lymphocyte-associated protein 4, which restore the capacity of the patient's own immune system to recognize and attack tumor cells, achieving durable, and in some cases apparently curative, responses in a meaningful proportion of patients with advanced disease that would have been considered almost uniformly fatal within a relatively short time frame prior to the availability of these therapies.

EVIDENCE: The introduction of immune checkpoint inhibitor therapy has produced a dramatic and well-documented improvement in survival for patients with advanced, metastatic melanoma over the past decade, transforming a disease with historically dismal median survival once metastatic into one in which a meaningful proportion of treated patients now achieve long-term, durable disease control, representing one of the most significant therapeutic advances across the whole of oncology in this period, not merely within dermatology, and reshaping expectations for what a stage IV melanoma diagnosis means for a patient today compared to only a decade or so ago.

Molecular testing for actionable mutations is now a routine component of the workup for advanced or metastatic melanoma, guiding selection among the systemic therapy options discussed in this section. For melanomas harboring a BRAF V600 mutation, present in a substantial proportion of cutaneous melanomas, particularly those arising on intermittently sun-exposed skin, targeted therapy combining a BRAF inhibitor with a MEK inhibitor offers an additional, often rapidly effective treatment option, particularly valuable for patients with a high burden of symptomatic disease requiring a faster initial response than immunotherapy typically provides, though these targeted agents are generally used in combination with, sequentially with, or as an alternative to immunotherapy depending on the specific clinical scenario, tumor burden, and mutation status, decisions that are increasingly individualized within a multidisciplinary oncology framework given the expanding and evolving array of treatment sequencing strategies now available for this disease.

Complications, Special Populations, and Prevention

Patients with a personal history of melanoma carry a substantially elevated risk of developing a second primary melanoma compared to the general population, warranting lifelong, structured dermatologic surveillance, typically every three to twelve months depending on stage and individual risk factors, along with rigorous ongoing photoprotection and patient education in skin self-examination technique. Familial melanoma, associated with CDKN2A and, less commonly, CDK4 mutations, should be considered in patients with multiple first-degree relatives affected by melanoma or with a personal history of multiple primary melanomas, and genetic counseling and testing, along with consideration of associated pancreatic cancer surveillance given the recognized CDKN2A-associated pancreatic cancer risk, is appropriate in this population. Identification of a pathogenic CDKN2A mutation carries implications extending beyond the individual patient, since at-risk first-degree relatives can be offered predictive genetic testing and, if found to carry the mutation, enrolled in an intensified surveillance program beginning at a younger age than would otherwise apply, making genetic counseling referral, rather than testing performed in clinical isolation without this broader family counseling context, an essential component of care in suspected familial melanoma. Pregnant patients with melanoma present a particularly sensitive management scenario, since pregnancy does not appear to independently worsen melanoma prognosis when treatment is not unnecessarily delayed, but does raise unique considerations regarding the safety and timing of both surgical and, particularly, systemic therapy, warranting close, individualized coordination between dermatology, oncology, and maternal-fetal medicine. Melanoma is also one of the malignancies capable of crossing the placenta to the fetus, an exceedingly rare but recognized event that, while not altering standard management for most pregnant patients with melanoma, underscores the importance of placental pathology examination following delivery when the mother carries an advanced-stage diagnosis.

Melanoma in Children and Adolescents

Melanoma is rare in the pediatric population, accounting for only a small fraction of childhood malignancy, but poses a distinctive diagnostic challenge given that it frequently fails to display the classic ABCDE pattern relied upon in adults, more often presenting as an amelanotic or minimally pigmented, symmetric, uniformly colored papule or nodule that can closely mimic a pyogenic granuloma, wart, or other common benign pediatric skin finding, a diagnostic overlap that has been termed the need for modified ABCD criteria in this population, emphasizing Amelanotic or Bump-like presentation, Bleeding or bumps, Color uniformity, and De novo development in a child without a preexisting nevus at the site, in contrast to the asymmetric, irregularly bordered, variegated presentation taught for adult melanoma. Any rapidly growing, bleeding, or persistently changing nodule in a child, particularly one that does not fit the profile of a more common benign pediatric lesion or that fails to resolve as such a lesion would be expected to, warrants a low threshold for biopsy despite the rarity of melanoma at this age, given the well-documented pattern of diagnostic delay contributing to more advanced stage at diagnosis in the small number of pediatric melanoma cases that do occur.

Multidisciplinary Management of Advanced Disease

The treatment paradigm for the most advanced stage of disease reflects this same principle of matching intensity to risk that has governed every decision point earlier in this chapter. Management of stage IV metastatic melanoma has evolved into a genuinely multidisciplinary undertaking, incorporating medical oncology for systemic therapy selection and sequencing, radiation oncology for symptomatic or oligometastatic disease, particularly brain metastases where stereotactic radiosurgery has become a mainstay of management given melanoma's relatively high propensity for central nervous system spread, and surgical oncology for selected cases of oligometastatic disease amenable to metastasectomy, which can offer meaningful survival benefit in carefully selected patients with limited, resectable metastatic burden, particularly when combined with effective systemic therapy. Regular multidisciplinary tumor board discussion for patients with advanced or recurrent melanoma allows integration of these various treatment modalities and specialist perspectives into a coordinated plan rather than a series of sequential, siloed specialist encounters, and has been associated with improved adherence to evidence-based treatment pathways and, in several published studies, meaningfully improved outcomes for patients managed through this collaborative model compared to more fragmented, less coordinated care.

PATIENT EDUCATION: Patients should be taught the ABCDE criteria and, importantly, the EFG criteria for nodular melanoma, and encouraged to perform monthly self-skin examinations using a full-length mirror and a hand mirror for hard-to-see areas, enlisting a partner or family member to help examine the back, scalp, and other difficult-to-visualize sites; the message that any new or changing lesion, regardless of whether it fits the classic ABCDE pattern, warrants prompt evaluation is at least as important as memorization of the criteria themselves, given the diagnostic pitfalls of nodular and acral melanoma discussed throughout this chapter.

Population-level screening for melanoma through routine total body skin examination in asymptomatic, average-risk individuals remains an area of ongoing evidence development, with current major screening guidelines generally recommending a risk-stratified approach, more frequent professional skin examinations for patients with recognized elevated risk factors, fair skin phototype, high nevus count, family history, or prior melanoma, rather than universal population-wide screening at fixed intervals regardless of individual risk profile; this risk-stratified approach reflects an effort to concentrate the genuine benefits of early detection among those most likely to develop the disease, while avoiding the costs, both financial and in terms of unnecessary biopsies of benign lesions, that would accompany indiscriminate universal screening of a population whose overwhelming majority will never develop melanoma.

Clinical Case: A Rapidly Growing Nodule Mistaken for a Blood Blister

A 55-year-old man with fair skin and a self-described history of significant sunburns in his youth presented at his wife's insistence for evaluation of a dark, raised lesion on his upper back that he had assumed was a blood blister from a minor injury while moving furniture approximately six weeks earlier, expecting it would resolve on its own, but which had instead continued to grow steadily and had recently begun to bleed with minimal contact. Examination revealed a firm, dome-shaped, deeply pigmented nodule measuring approximately nine millimeters, notably symmetric with fairly even coloration throughout, features that his wife's own online research had led her to believe were reassuring given the classic ABCDE teaching she had encountered, but which the clinician recognized instead as consistent with the EFG pattern, elevated, firm, and growing, characteristic of nodular melanoma rather than a benign process. Dermoscopy showed a structureless blue-black area without a discernible pigment network, and given the high clinical suspicion, a complete excisional biopsy with narrow margins was performed.

Pathology confirmed nodular melanoma with a Breslow depth of 2.1 millimeters without ulceration and a mitotic rate within an unremarkable range, and given this depth, sentinel lymph node biopsy was recommended and performed concurrently with the wide local excision, which returned negative for nodal metastasis, information that carried substantial favorable prognostic weight for the patient and informed the decision against adjuvant systemic therapy at this stage. He and his wife were both counseled at length about the EFG criteria specifically, given that this case exemplified precisely why nodular melanoma is so often initially dismissed as a benign process, a bruise, blood blister, or other traumatic lesion, by patients who have understandably learned to look for the classic ABCDE asymmetry and irregular borders rather than the elevated, firm, rapidly growing pattern that this particular subtype actually presents with; he was scheduled for structured long-term surveillance given his confirmed melanoma diagnosis and elevated risk of a subsequent primary lesion. A baseline total body photography session was arranged at his first surveillance visit to establish an objective reference point for his numerous other nevi, and his wife was specifically thanked for her role in prompting the initial evaluation, reinforcing to both of them the broader value of a second set of eyes in monitoring skin changes, particularly on anatomic sites such as the back that patients cannot easily examine themselves.

THE MORPHOLOGY-TO-MANAGEMENT SYSTEM — Reading Melanoma Beyond the Classic ABCDE Picture

Pattern Introduced This Chapter: The prolonged radial growth phase of superficial spreading melanoma fitting classic ABCDE criteria, contrasted with the vertical-growth-from-outset pattern of nodular melanoma requiring the EFG criteria, and the diagnostic challenge of lentigo maligna and acral lentiginous melanoma against their respective backgrounds of photodamage or low clinical suspicion.

Cross-Cutting Anchor: Dermoscopic structural and color asymmetry, and, when this is absent or atypical, the EFG behavioral criteria, are the anchor findings that should trigger biopsy across every melanoma subtype in this chapter, and biopsy technique must be selected to preserve accurate Breslow depth measurement, the single most powerful prognostic anchor in melanoma staging.

Summary and Key Concepts

Superficial spreading melanoma displays a prolonged radial growth phase and classic ABCDE features, while nodular melanoma invades vertically from the outset and is more reliably recognized using the EFG criteria (Elevated, Firm, Growing).

Lentigo maligna arises on chronically photodamaged facial skin and can be difficult to distinguish from a benign solar lentigo, while acral lentiginous melanoma occurs at similar rates across all skin phototypes and is frequently diagnosed at a more advanced stage.

Dermoscopic assessment of structural and color asymmetry, atypical pigment network, blue-white veil, and irregular vascular patterns substantially improves diagnostic accuracy for pigmented lesions.

Complete excisional biopsy is the preferred technique for a suspected melanoma to preserve accurate Breslow depth measurement, the single most important independent prognostic factor in melanoma staging.

Sentinel lymph node biopsy is generally discussed for melanomas 0.8 millimeters or deeper, or thinner melanomas with ulceration or an elevated mitotic rate, given increased likelihood of occult nodal involvement at these thresholds.

Immune checkpoint inhibitors and BRAF/MEK-targeted therapy have transformed outcomes for advanced, metastatic melanoma, and patients with a personal melanoma history require lifelong structured surveillance given elevated risk of a second primary tumor.

CHAPTER 20: CUTANEOUS LYMPHOMA AND RARE CUTANEOUS MALIGNANCIES

Learning Objectives

1. Recognize the clinical stages of mycosis fungoides and understand why prolonged diagnostic delay is common in this disease.
2. Distinguish Sezary syndrome from mycosis fungoides and identify its distinguishing clinical and laboratory features.
3. Recognize Merkel cell carcinoma using the AEIOU mnemonic and explain why this tumor warrants urgent, aggressive management.
4. Distinguish primary cutaneous B-cell lymphoma from cutaneous involvement by systemic lymphoma.
5. Recognize extramammary Paget disease and construct an appropriate evaluation for an associated underlying malignancy.
6. Identify the major rare cutaneous sarcomas discussed in this chapter and understand the role of specialized surgical and multidisciplinary management in each.

This chapter addresses a group of cutaneous malignancies that, while individually rare, share a common clinical trap: each can closely mimic a far more common, benign inflammatory or infectious dermatosis for months to years before the correct diagnosis is finally established, and this diagnostic delay is itself a well-documented, recurring theme across every condition discussed here. The unifying clinical lesson of this chapter is therefore less about memorizing a long list of rare tumor names and more about recognizing the specific pattern of treatment-resistance, in which a presumed eczema, psoriasis, or dermatitis simply never responds as expected to appropriate standard therapy, that should prompt biopsy and reconsideration of the working diagnosis.

Epidemiology and Risk Factors of Cutaneous Lymphoma

Cutaneous lymphomas as a group are considerably less common than the keratinocyte carcinomas and melanoma discussed in the preceding chapters, but they carry an outsized clinical importance because of the diagnostic delay that so frequently accompanies them and the highly specialized, stage-directed treatment pathways they require once correctly identified. Cutaneous T-cell lymphomas, of which mycosis fungoides is by far the most common subtype, account for the large majority of primary cutaneous lymphomas overall, with an incidence that rises steadily with age and a modest male predominance; Black patients in the United States are diagnosed with mycosis fungoides at a younger age on average and, in some studies, experience a more aggressive disease course, a disparity whose underlying biological and access-to-care contributors remain incompletely understood and an area of active investigation. Primary cutaneous B-cell lymphomas are considerably rarer than their T-cell counterparts and, as discussed later in this chapter, span a spectrum from highly indolent subtypes managed with skin-directed therapy alone to an aggressive subtype requiring systemic chemoimmunotherapy, making accurate subtyping essential before any treatment discussion with the patient begins. No single modifiable risk factor has been definitively established for most cutaneous lymphomas, in contrast to the well-defined ultraviolet exposure relationship that drives keratinocyte carcinoma risk, though chronic antigenic stimulation and immune dysregulation are believed to contribute to lymphomagenesis in at least some cases, and a minority of patients with long-standing, severe chronic dermatitis are ultimately found, after repeated biopsies over time, to have evolved or unmasked an underlying cutaneous lymphoma rather than a purely inflammatory process.

Mycosis Fungoides: Clinical Stages

Mycosis fungoides, the most common form of cutaneous T-cell lymphoma, typically follows an indolent, slowly progressive course through recognizable clinical stages, beginning with the patch stage, presenting as scaly, erythematous to slightly hyperpigmented or hypopigmented patches favoring non-sun-exposed skin, classically the buttocks, groin, and other areas not typically exposed to the sun (sometimes described by the mnemonic "bathing trunk" distribution), a presentation so frequently mistaken for eczema, psoriasis, or a nonspecific dermatitis that a diagnostic delay of several years between initial presentation and confirmed diagnosis is common and well documented in the literature. As the disease progresses, patches evolve into the plaque stage, with more infiltrated, palpable, often irregularly shaped and annular plaques, and ultimately, in a minority of patients, to the tumor stage, with frank nodules and tumors that can ulcerate, reflecting deeper dermal invasion by the malignant T-cell infiltrate.

Why Diagnostic Delay Is So Common

Several factors converge to make mycosis fungoides one of the most commonly delayed diagnoses in dermatology: the disease frequently improves, at least partially and temporarily, with topical corticosteroids, the very treatment also used for its common inflammatory mimics, creating a false reassurance of correct diagnosis; early lesions can show subtle or nonspecific histologic findings on biopsy that fail to meet full diagnostic criteria at initial biopsy, sometimes requiring multiple biopsies over time before a confirmatory pattern emerges; and the disease's characteristically slow, patch-stage progression over years means that neither patient nor clinician may perceive the gradual change as concerning at any single visit, in a manner analogous to trying to detect gradual change in a slowly growing photograph one frame at a time. Any patient with a persistent, scaly, erythematous eruption, particularly in a bathing trunk distribution, that fails to respond fully and durably to appropriate treatment for the presumed diagnosis, or that recurs promptly after treatment discontinuation, warrants biopsy, and repeat biopsy over time should be pursued for persistently suspicious lesions even when an initial biopsy was non-diagnostic, given the well-recognized pattern of evolving histologic findings in early disease.

CAUTION: A presumed eczema or psoriasis diagnosis that transiently improves with topical corticosteroids but reliably recurs, often in the same distribution, once treatment is tapered or discontinued, particularly in a bathing trunk distribution, should prompt reconsideration of mycosis fungoides; this deceptively partial treatment response is one of the most consistently described contributors to the extended diagnostic delay characteristic of this disease.

Diagnostic Workup and Staging of Mycosis Fungoides

Skin biopsy remains the cornerstone of diagnosis, though as noted above, early-stage disease can show subtle histologic findings requiring clinicopathologic correlation and, at times, repeat biopsy over time; characteristic findings when present include epidermotropism, atypical lymphocytes infiltrating the epidermis without accompanying spongiosis (a discordance termed "epidermotropism without spongiosis" that is a useful distinguishing feature from spongiotic inflammatory dermatoses), and Pautrier microabscesses, small, well-defined intraepidermal collections of atypical lymphocytes considered a more specific, though not universally present, diagnostic finding. T-cell receptor gene rearrangement studies, demonstrating a clonal population of T lymphocytes, provide valuable supportive evidence of a malignant rather than reactive process, particularly useful when routine histology alone is equivocal, though a clonal result should always be interpreted within the complete clinical and histologic context rather than treated as independently diagnostic, since some benign inflammatory conditions can rarely show clonal or pseudoclonal populations as well.

Staging and Treatment Approach

Staging incorporates the extent of skin involvement (patch/plaque versus tumor stage, and percentage of body surface area involved), lymph node involvement, evidence of blood involvement, and visceral organ involvement, with early-stage, skin-limited disease carrying a generally favorable prognosis and often a near-normal life expectancy, while advanced-stage disease with nodal, blood, or visceral involvement carries a substantially worse prognosis. Treatment for early-stage, skin-limited disease centers on skin-directed therapies, including topical corticosteroids, topical nitrogen mustard, phototherapy (both narrowband ultraviolet B and psoralen plus ultraviolet A), and localized radiation for isolated, treatment-resistant plaques or tumors, while more advanced or refractory disease incorporates systemic therapies, including oral retinoids, histone deacetylase inhibitors, and, for the most advanced or treatment-resistant cases, monoclonal antibody therapy and, in appropriate candidates, allogeneic stem cell transplantation, reflecting a treatment escalation pathway that closely mirrors disease stage and treatment response.

Folliculotropic and Other Clinical Variants of Mycosis Fungoides

Beyond the classic patch-plaque-tumor progression described above, several recognized clinical variants of mycosis fungoides can further complicate and delay diagnosis. Folliculotropic mycosis fungoides, the most clinically significant variant, preferentially involves the hair follicle epithelium rather than the interfollicular epidermis, producing grouped follicular papules, alopecia, and, classically, comedo-like or cyst-like lesions concentrated on the head and neck; because the malignant infiltrate is centered on the follicle rather than the surface epidermis, this variant is more prone to a falsely reassuring, non-diagnostic superficial shave biopsy and generally requires a deeper punch biopsy extending into the subcutis to adequately sample the follicular infiltrate, and it also tends to respond less completely to skin-directed phototherapy than classic mycosis fungoides given the relative difficulty of ultraviolet light penetrating to the depth of the affected follicle. Other recognized variants include pagetoid reticulosis, a localized, slowly progressive form typically confined to a single limb, and granulomatous slack skin, an exceedingly rare variant producing pendulous, redundant folds of lax skin in the axillae and groin; while individually uncommon, awareness of these variants is important because each can present in a manner that diverges substantially from the classic bathing trunk patch presentation, further reinforcing this chapter's central lesson that an atypical, treatment-resistant eruption of almost any morphology warrants consideration of an underlying lymphoproliferative process once more common explanations have been excluded.

Sezary Syndrome

Sezary syndrome is a distinct, leukemic variant of cutaneous T-cell lymphoma characterized by the triad of diffuse erythroderma, generalized lymphadenopathy, and the presence of circulating Sezary cells, malignant T lymphocytes with a characteristic cerebriform (convoluted, brain-like) nuclear morphology, identified on peripheral blood smear or flow cytometry above a defined diagnostic threshold; unlike mycosis fungoides, which typically begins with localized patches and plaques and may never progress beyond skin-limited disease, Sezary syndrome presents from the outset, or evolves relatively rapidly, with diffuse erythroderma affecting the large majority of the body surface, intense pruritus that is often the most distressing and functionally limiting symptom for affected patients, and a range of associated findings including palmoplantar keratoderma, ectropion from chronic facial skin tightening and edema, and lymphadenopathy reflecting nodal involvement by the malignant clone.

KEY POINT: Sezary syndrome should be considered in the differential diagnosis of any patient presenting with erythroderma of unclear etiology, alongside the other causes of erythroderma discussed in the chapter on dermatologic emergencies later in this text; peripheral blood flow cytometry for a Sezary cell count, alongside T-cell receptor gene rearrangement studies on both skin and blood, is an essential component of the workup for erythroderma that does not have another readily apparent explanation.

Treatment of Sezary syndrome typically involves systemic therapy from the outset given its inherently more advanced, blood-involving nature at presentation, with extracorporeal photopheresis, a treatment in which the patient's blood is processed to expose circulating lymphocytes to a photosensitizing agent and ultraviolet light before being returned to the patient, serving as a well-established, relatively well-tolerated first-line option, often combined with other systemic agents including oral retinoids, histone deacetylase inhibitors, or monoclonal antibody therapy directed against specific T-cell surface antigens; management of the intense, often debilitating pruritus that frequently accompanies this condition is itself an important and sometimes challenging component of overall symptom-directed care, given its substantial impact on patient quality of life independent of disease-directed treatment.

Lymphomatoid Papulosis and CD30-Positive Lymphoproliferative Disorders

Lymphomatoid papulosis occupies an unusual position within this chapter as a chronic, recurrent, self-healing condition that is nonetheless classified within the spectrum of cutaneous CD30-positive lymphoproliferative disorders, a classification that reflects its underlying clonal T-cell population rather than its outwardly benign, self-limited clinical behavior. Patients present with recurrent crops of papules and small nodules, often numbering from a few to dozens of lesions, that characteristically progress through a papule-to-necrotic-ulceration-to-spontaneous-resolution cycle over a period of weeks, leaving behind small hypopigmented or hyperpigmented scars, with new crops continuing to appear over months to years in a relapsing, remitting pattern that can persist indefinitely. The diagnosis is confirmed by biopsy of an active lesion, which characteristically shows a wedge-shaped infiltrate of large, atypical, CD30-positive lymphocytes, and while the disease itself typically requires no more than symptomatic management or, for more extensive or bothersome disease, low-dose methotrexate or phototherapy, patients with lymphomatoid papulosis carry a modestly elevated lifetime risk of developing a second lymphoma, most often mycosis fungoides or primary cutaneous anaplastic large cell lymphoma, warranting long-term dermatologic follow-up even during periods when the disease itself is behaving in its characteristically indolent fashion.

Primary cutaneous anaplastic large cell lymphoma, the more aggressive relative within this same CD30-positive spectrum, typically presents as a solitary or localized cluster of larger nodules or tumors that, unlike lymphomatoid papulosis, do not spontaneously regress and instead persist and enlarge, though the overall prognosis remains favorable with radiation therapy or surgical excision for the substantial majority of patients whose disease remains confined to the skin at diagnosis. Distinguishing lymphomatoid papulosis from primary cutaneous anaplastic large cell lymphoma, and both from a systemic anaplastic large cell lymphoma with secondary cutaneous involvement, again depends on a combination of clinical course, extent of disease, and histopathologic and immunophenotypic assessment, reinforcing the recurring theme across this chapter that dermatopathology subspecialty input is indispensable whenever a cutaneous lymphoma is suspected or confirmed.

KEY POINT: A recurrent, self-healing eruption of papules that ulcerate and resolve over a period of weeks, leaving small residual scars, should raise suspicion for lymphomatoid papulosis; although the disease itself typically follows a benign, chronic course, the associated modestly elevated lifetime risk of a second lymphoma warrants sustained long-term dermatologic surveillance.

Merkel Cell Carcinoma

Merkel cell carcinoma is a rare but aggressive neuroendocrine skin cancer, most commonly arising on chronically sun-exposed skin of older, often immunosuppressed adults, and driven in the large majority of cases by clonal integration of Merkel cell polyomavirus into the tumor genome, with a smaller proportion of cases, more common in areas of intense cumulative ultraviolet exposure, driven instead by ultraviolet-induced mutations independent of viral integration. The AEIOU mnemonic captures the characteristic clinical presentation and risk factors: Asymptomatic (the lesion itself is typically painless despite its aggressive behavior, a deceptive feature that can delay presentation), Expanding rapidly (often over weeks), Immunosuppressed (a well-documented risk factor, particularly in solid organ transplant recipients and patients with chronic lymphocytic leukemia), Older than fifty years, and Ultraviolet-exposed site; a lesion meeting most or all of these criteria, typically presenting as a firm, red to violaceous, dome-shaped nodule, should prompt urgent biopsy given the tumor's aggressive natural history and disproportionately poor prognosis relative to its unremarkable, easily overlooked clinical appearance.

THE MORPHOLOGY-TO-MANAGEMENT SYSTEM — The Deceptively Innocuous Rapidly Growing Nodule

The Pattern: A firm, painless, red to violaceous, rapidly growing dome-shaped nodule on chronically sun-exposed skin of an older or immunosuppressed adult, meeting most of the AEIOU criteria.

Presentation Variance: The lesion's painless nature and unremarkable clinical appearance frequently lead both patients and clinicians to underestimate its significance relative to its markedly aggressive underlying biological behavior.

Trap Logic: This presentation can be mistaken for a cyst, an insect bite reaction, or a benign vascular lesion; the AEIOU criteria and the tumor's disproportionately rapid growth rate relative to these benign mimics should prompt urgent biopsy rather than a period of watchful observation.

Management Pivot: Biopsy promptly given the tumor's aggressive natural history; once confirmed, pursue sentinel lymph node biopsy given the high rate of nodal micrometastasis even in clinically node-negative disease, and coordinate wide local excision or Mohs micrographic surgery with radiation oncology and medical oncology given frequent need for adjuvant radiation and, in advanced disease, immunotherapy.

Pattern Anchor: Meeting most of the AEIOU criteria on a rapidly growing nodule should prompt urgent, expedited biopsy and workup regardless of how benign the lesion appears on casual inspection, since Merkel cell carcinoma's aggressive behavior is markedly discordant with its deceptively unremarkable clinical appearance.

Merkel cell carcinoma carries a substantially higher rate of regional lymph node metastasis at diagnosis than either basal cell or squamous cell carcinoma, making sentinel lymph node biopsy a routine component of initial staging even in clinically node-negative disease, and management typically combines wide local excision or Mohs micrographic surgery with adjuvant radiation therapy to the primary site and, frequently, the draining nodal basin given the tumor's marked propensity for local and regional recurrence. For advanced or metastatic disease, immune checkpoint inhibitor therapy has produced meaningful and durable responses in a substantial proportion of patients, representing a similarly transformative advance for this disease as for melanoma discussed in the preceding chapter, reflecting the immunogenic nature of Merkel cell polyomavirus-driven tumors in particular.

Primary Cutaneous B-Cell Lymphoma

Primary cutaneous B-cell lymphomas, considerably less common than cutaneous T-cell lymphomas, present as firm, erythematous to violaceous papules, plaques, or nodules, most commonly on the scalp, forehead, or trunk, and are subdivided into distinct subtypes with markedly different prognoses: primary cutaneous follicle center lymphoma and primary cutaneous marginal zone lymphoma both carry an excellent prognosis with skin-directed therapy alone, including local radiation or intralesional or systemic rituximab, and only rarely progress to systemic involvement, while primary cutaneous diffuse large B-cell lymphoma, leg type, most commonly affecting the lower extremities of older women, behaves considerably more aggressively, with a higher rate of systemic dissemination and a correspondingly worse prognosis, typically requiring systemic combination chemoimmunotherapy analogous to that used for systemic diffuse large B-cell lymphoma rather than skin-directed therapy alone.

KEY POINT: Distinguishing the specific subtype of primary cutaneous B-cell lymphoma is essential before finalizing a treatment plan, since the indolent follicle center and marginal zone subtypes are managed very differently, and with a far more favorable prognosis, than the aggressive diffuse large B-cell lymphoma, leg type; this distinction relies on specific histologic and immunohistochemical features rather than clinical appearance alone, underscoring the importance of dermatopathology subspecialty input for any suspected cutaneous lymphoma.

Treatment Approach by Primary Cutaneous B-Cell Lymphoma Subtype

For primary cutaneous follicle center lymphoma and primary cutaneous marginal zone lymphoma presenting as a solitary or small number of localized lesions, local radiation therapy alone frequently achieves durable clinical clearance and is generally preferred as first-line treatment given its excellent efficacy and favorable side-effect profile for skin-limited disease; intralesional or systemic rituximab is a reasonable alternative for patients with more widespread cutaneous involvement, multiple recurrent lesions, or a preference to avoid radiation, and surgical excision may be considered for a truly solitary, easily accessible lesion. Because both indolent subtypes only rarely progress to systemic involvement, extensive systemic staging beyond a thorough skin examination and basic laboratory evaluation is generally not required, in contrast to the comprehensive systemic staging warranted for primary cutaneous diffuse large B-cell lymphoma, leg type, which is managed following protocols essentially identical to those used for nodal diffuse large B-cell lymphoma, typically incorporating rituximab in combination with systemic chemotherapy, most commonly following a cyclophosphamide, doxorubicin, vincristine, and prednisone-based regimen, given this subtype's meaningfully higher risk of systemic dissemination and correspondingly less favorable prognosis relative to its indolent counterparts.

Extramammary Paget Disease

Extramammary Paget disease presents as a persistent, well-demarcated, erythematous, eczematous-appearing plaque, most commonly affecting the vulva, scrotum, or perianal skin, and represents an intraepidermal adenocarcinoma, most often originating from apocrine gland-bearing skin at these sites; its clinical resemblance to a simple, treatment-resistant eczema or intertrigo is the recurring diagnostic trap for this condition, entirely analogous to the diagnostic delay theme running throughout this chapter, and any persistent, well-demarcated genital or perianal eczematous plaque unresponsive to appropriate topical treatment over several weeks warrants biopsy to exclude this diagnosis before a longer course of ultimately ineffective empiric treatment is pursued. A meaningful proportion of extramammary Paget disease cases, though not the majority, are associated with an underlying visceral adenocarcinoma, most commonly of the gastrointestinal or genitourinary tract depending on the specific anatomic location of the cutaneous lesion, making age-appropriate malignancy screening, guided by the anatomic site involved, an essential component of the initial workup once the diagnosis is confirmed.

CAUTION: A persistent, treatment-resistant, well-demarcated eczematous plaque in the vulvar, scrotal, or perianal region should prompt biopsy rather than an escalating sequence of empiric topical treatments; the diagnosis of extramammary Paget disease is easily and commonly delayed precisely because its clinical appearance so closely mimics far more common, benign inflammatory conditions in this anatomic region.

Diagnostic Workup Once Extramammary Paget Disease Is Confirmed

Once biopsy confirms extramammary Paget disease, the initial workup should focus on distinguishing primary cutaneous disease, arising directly from adjacent apocrine-bearing epidermis without an associated internal malignancy, from secondary extramammary Paget disease, in which the epidermal involvement represents extension from an underlying visceral adenocarcinoma, since this distinction meaningfully alters both prognosis and the required extent of additional evaluation; immunohistochemical staining patterns on the biopsy specimen can help suggest the likely site of origin when secondary disease is suspected. Age-appropriate colonoscopy and, depending on the anatomic site and patient sex, gynecologic or urologic evaluation should be pursued, and any patient with vulvar or perianal extramammary Paget disease and a personal history suggestive of an underlying gastrointestinal or genitourinary malignancy warrants a correspondingly lower threshold for more extensive imaging. Treatment of the cutaneous disease itself, once secondary disease has been excluded or the associated malignancy addressed, most commonly involves wide local excision, though the disease's characteristic pattern of subclinical extension well beyond the visible clinical margins, similar in principle to the challenge described for dermatofibrosarcoma protuberans, makes Mohs micrographic surgery an increasingly favored approach at experienced centers, with topical imiquimod or photodynamic therapy reserved as alternatives for patients who are poor surgical candidates or who have extensive disease not amenable to complete surgical clearance.

Angiosarcoma and Atypical Fibroxanthoma

Cutaneous angiosarcoma is a rare, aggressive vascular malignancy that classically presents in one of two distinct clinical contexts: as an ill-defined, bruise-like, violaceous patch or plaque on the scalp or face of an older adult, a presentation that is very frequently and understandably mistaken for a simple bruise or hematoma, particularly given the patient's often advanced age and correspondingly higher likelihood of incidental minor trauma, or as a lymphedema-associated angiosarcoma (Stewart-Treves syndrome) arising within a limb affected by chronic lymphedema, most classically following axillary lymph node dissection for breast cancer treatment, presenting as violaceous nodules or plaques within the chronically lymphedematous limb. Given the tumor's tendency toward extensive subclinical spread well beyond its visible clinical margins and its overall poor prognosis, wide surgical excision, when feasible, combined with radiation therapy, and multidisciplinary oncologic management are generally required, and any bruise-like facial or scalp lesion in an older adult that fails to resolve over the expected timeframe for a traumatic bruise, or that continues to enlarge, warrants biopsy given this diagnostic possibility.

Atypical Fibroxanthoma and Dermatofibrosarcoma Protuberans Revisited

Atypical fibroxanthoma presents as a rapidly growing, often ulcerated, dome-shaped nodule on chronically sun-damaged skin of older adults, most commonly the head and neck, and is generally considered a low-grade cutaneous sarcoma with a relatively favorable prognosis following complete surgical excision, in contrast to its deeper, more aggressive histologic relative, pleomorphic dermal sarcoma, which shows similar histologic features but with deeper tissue invasion and a correspondingly higher risk of local recurrence and, rarely, metastasis; distinguishing between the two requires careful histologic assessment of the depth and extent of invasion, underscoring again the value of adequate biopsy depth and dermatopathology expertise for any lesion in this category. Dermatofibrosarcoma protuberans, introduced in the preceding chapter as an important mimic of benign dermatofibroma, is most definitively treated with Mohs micrographic surgery or wide local excision with careful, often specialized margin assessment given its characteristic pattern of finger-like subclinical extension well beyond visible tumor margins, a feature that makes standard excision with conventional margins more prone to incomplete removal and subsequent local recurrence than for most other cutaneous malignancies discussed in this text.

Complications, Special Populations, and Patient Education

Patients with any cutaneous lymphoma or rare cutaneous malignancy discussed in this chapter benefit enormously from care coordinated through a specialized multidisciplinary center with dermato-oncology, hematology-oncology, and dermatopathology expertise specific to these uncommon conditions, given both the diagnostic complexity involved and the evolving, increasingly specialized treatment landscape for several of these diseases; referral to such a center should be considered proactively rather than only after standard, more generalized treatment approaches have failed. Immunosuppressed patients, particularly organ transplant recipients, carry meaningfully elevated risk for several conditions in this chapter, most notably Merkel cell carcinoma, underscoring the theme, recurring throughout the malignancy-focused chapters of this text, that immunosuppressed patients require a fundamentally different, more vigilant threshold for biopsy and a correspondingly more frequent surveillance schedule than the general population.

Special Populations: Pediatric, Pregnant, and Older Adult Considerations

Cutaneous lymphoma is uncommon in children, but mycosis fungoides does occur in the pediatric population and, in this age group, more frequently presents with a hypopigmented rather than the classically erythematous patch morphology described earlier in this chapter, a presentation that is itself commonly mistaken for pityriasis alba or vitiligo and that consequently carries its own well-documented pattern of diagnostic delay distinct from, though conceptually parallel to, the delay described for adult-onset disease; children with mycosis fungoides generally have an excellent long-term prognosis, and treatment follows the same stage-directed, skin-directed-therapy-first approach used in adults. Pregnancy meaningfully complicates management planning for any of the conditions in this chapter given the need to defer or modify systemic therapies, radiation, and certain phototherapy regimens, making close coordination between dermatology, maternal-fetal medicine, and oncology essential whenever a new diagnosis arises during pregnancy or when an established diagnosis requires treatment modification to protect the pregnancy. Older adults, who constitute the large majority of patients with Merkel cell carcinoma, angiosarcoma, and atypical fibroxanthoma discussed in this chapter, frequently carry additional comorbidities and reduced physiologic reserve that must be weighed carefully against the generally more aggressive treatment approaches these malignancies require, underscoring the importance of a comprehensive geriatric assessment and multidisciplinary discussion of goals of care alongside the oncologic treatment plan itself.

Long-term surveillance frequency for patients treated for any diagnosis in this chapter should be individualized to the specific disease, its stage at diagnosis, and the treatment received, but as a general principle, patients with early-stage, skin-limited mycosis fungoides or an indolent primary cutaneous B-cell lymphoma subtype are typically followed at intervals of every three to six months, while patients with Sezary syndrome, Merkel cell carcinoma, or any of the aggressive cutaneous sarcomas discussed in this chapter warrant more frequent surveillance, often monthly to every three months during the initial one to two years following treatment, given the correspondingly higher recurrence risk associated with these more aggressive diagnoses.

PATIENT EDUCATION: Patients with a persistent skin condition that has not responded as expected to appropriate standard treatment over a reasonable trial period should be encouraged to return for reevaluation and possible biopsy rather than continuing an ineffective treatment indefinitely or assuming the lack of response reflects their own inadequate adherence; this message, applicable across nearly every diagnosis discussed in this chapter, empowers patients to be active participants in recognizing when a presumed benign or common diagnosis warrants reconsideration.

Clinical Case: A Persistent Rash Finally Explained

A 61-year-old man presented with a four-year history of scaly, mildly itchy, erythematous patches on his buttocks and lower back that had been treated intermittently by several different clinicians as eczema, with topical corticosteroids providing partial, temporary improvement each time but the eruption reliably recurring within weeks of tapering treatment. He had never been biopsied given the presumed straightforward diagnosis. Examination revealed several irregularly shaped, scaly, erythematous to slightly hyperpigmented patches with a somewhat atrophic, wrinkled surface texture in a bathing trunk distribution, findings that prompted consideration of a diagnosis beyond simple eczema given the atypical surface texture and the years-long, treatment-resistant course.

A skin biopsy showed epidermotropism of atypical lymphocytes without accompanying spongiosis, and T-cell receptor gene rearrangement studies confirmed a clonal T-cell population, together supporting a diagnosis of patch-stage mycosis fungoides. Staging workup, including a complete skin examination for additional involvement and laboratory evaluation, confirmed disease limited to the skin without nodal, blood, or visceral involvement, corresponding to early-stage disease with a generally favorable prognosis. He was started on topical corticosteroid therapy combined with narrowband ultraviolet B phototherapy, and was counseled extensively that although his diagnosis had taken years to establish, a pattern he learned was unfortunately common for this specific disease given its frequent early resemblance to ordinary eczema, his current early stage carried a favorable long-term prognosis with appropriate skin-directed treatment and ongoing surveillance for any evidence of disease progression.

Clinical Case: A Painless Nodule That Grew Too Fast to Ignore

A 74-year-old man with a history of chronic lymphocytic leukemia presented with a firm, red, dome-shaped nodule on his right temple that his wife had first noticed approximately three weeks earlier as a small bump, now grown to nearly one centimeter, entirely painless throughout its rapid growth. Examination confirmed a firm, well-vascularized, violaceous-red nodule with a smooth, shiny surface, and given his age, immunosuppressed status from his underlying hematologic malignancy, the tumor's sun-exposed location, and its notably rapid, painless growth, meeting the large majority of the AEIOU criteria, Merkel cell carcinoma was strongly suspected and an urgent biopsy was arranged rather than a period of observation.

Biopsy confirmed Merkel cell carcinoma, and given the tumor's well-documented propensity for regional nodal metastasis even in clinically node-negative disease, sentinel lymph node biopsy was performed concurrently with wide local excision, which unfortunately confirmed microscopic nodal involvement not otherwise clinically apparent on examination or imaging. Given this nodal positivity, he was referred urgently to a multidisciplinary tumor board for coordinated planning of adjuvant radiation therapy to both the primary site and the involved nodal basin, and his case was flagged for close ongoing surveillance given both his confirmed nodal disease and his underlying chronic immunosuppression from his leukemia, a combination placing him at meaningfully elevated risk for recurrence relative to an immunocompetent patient with a similarly staged tumor.

THE MORPHOLOGY-TO-MANAGEMENT SYSTEM — Recognizing the Malignancy Hiding Behind a Benign Mimic

Pattern Introduced This Chapter: The treatment-resistant, partially steroid-responsive patch of mycosis fungoides, the deceptively painless rapidly growing nodule of Merkel cell carcinoma, and the persistent eczematous genital plaque of extramammary Paget disease, each a rare malignancy disguised as a common benign process.

Cross-Cutting Anchor: Treatment resistance, and specifically a pattern of partial or temporary improvement followed by reliable recurrence despite appropriate standard therapy for the presumed benign diagnosis, is the anchor finding that should trigger biopsy and reconsideration across every condition in this chapter, regardless of how convincingly each individually mimics a far more common process.

Summary and Key Concepts

Mycosis fungoides progresses through patch, plaque, and tumor stages, and its frequent partial, temporary response to topical corticosteroids is a well-documented contributor to often years-long diagnostic delay.

Sezary syndrome is a leukemic variant of cutaneous T-cell lymphoma presenting with erythroderma, lymphadenopathy, and circulating Sezary cells, and should be considered in any patient with erythroderma of unclear cause.

Merkel cell carcinoma, recognized using the AEIOU criteria, is an aggressive neuroendocrine skin cancer requiring urgent biopsy, sentinel lymph node biopsy, and multidisciplinary treatment despite its often deceptively unremarkable clinical appearance.

Primary cutaneous B-cell lymphoma subtypes carry markedly different prognoses, with follicle center and marginal zone subtypes behaving indolently and diffuse large B-cell lymphoma, leg type behaving aggressively.

Extramammary Paget disease mimics genital eczema and warrants biopsy of any persistent, treatment-resistant plaque in this location, along with screening for an associated underlying visceral malignancy.

Angiosarcoma, atypical fibroxanthoma, and dermatofibrosarcoma protuberans are rare cutaneous sarcomas each requiring specialized surgical management given their patterns of subclinical extension and, for angiosarcoma, aggressive systemic behavior.

CHAPTER 21: PEDIATRIC DERMATOLOGY

Learning Objectives

1. Distinguish common, self-limited neonatal skin eruptions from findings that warrant further evaluation.
2. Classify infantile hemangiomas and vascular malformations and identify features that warrant early specialist referral.
3. Construct an evidence-based approach to diaper dermatitis, including recognition of its common mimics and complications.
4. Recognize the major pediatric viral exanthems and distinguish them from one another using their characteristic clinical timelines.
5. Identify the clinical features of the major genodermatoses discussed in this chapter and understand the role of early multidisciplinary care.
6. Apply pediatric-specific safety considerations to topical and systemic dermatologic therapy, including dosing adjustments and formulation choices.

Pediatric dermatology requires a distinct clinical framework from adult dermatology, not simply because children present with a different spectrum of disease, but because the skin itself behaves differently across developmental stages, from the physiologically immature epidermal barrier of the neonate to the markedly higher surface-area-to-body-mass ratio of the infant and young child, a difference with direct and clinically important implications for topical medication absorption and systemic toxicity risk. This chapter addresses the conditions that are either unique to childhood or that present and are managed in a meaningfully different way in pediatric patients than in the adult populations discussed elsewhere in this text, along with the practical safety considerations that should inform every prescribing decision in this age group.

Transient Neonatal Skin Findings

A substantial proportion of neonates develop one or more benign, self-limited cutaneous eruptions within the first days to weeks of life, and confident recognition of these entities spares both families and clinicians unnecessary anxiety, testing, and treatment. Erythema toxicum neonatorum, despite its alarming name, is an entirely benign condition affecting a large proportion of term neonates, presenting as erythematous macules and papules that rapidly evolve into pustules, characteristically sparing the palms and soles, appearing within the first few days of life and resolving spontaneously within one to two weeks; a Wright-stained smear of pustule contents, when diagnostic uncertainty exists, shows a predominance of eosinophils, distinguishing it from the more clinically concerning entities discussed below. Transient neonatal pustular melanosis, more common in infants with darker skin tones, presents with pustules present at birth that rupture within hours to days, leaving a characteristic collarette of scale and a hyperpigmented macule that can persist for several weeks to months; a Wright-stained smear here shows predominantly neutrophils rather than eosinophils, and no treatment is required beyond reassurance regarding the expected gradual fading of the residual pigmentation.

Milia, tiny, firm, white to yellow papules resulting from retained keratin within the pilosebaceous follicle, are extremely common on the face of neonates and resolve spontaneously within the first few weeks to months of life without intervention. Neonatal acne, presenting as inflammatory papules and pustules on the cheeks and forehead, typically emerges around two to four weeks of life, is thought to relate to maternal and neonatal androgen stimulation of sebaceous glands, and generally resolves spontaneously within several months; persistent or unusually severe facial pustulosis beyond the expected timeframe, particularly if accompanied by other signs of hyperandrogenism, should prompt consideration of an underlying endocrinologic evaluation rather than a default assumption of ordinary neonatal acne.

KEY POINT: The distribution, timing, and morphology of a neonatal eruption, together with a simple bedside Wright-stained smear when needed, are usually sufficient to distinguish the common benign transient neonatal eruptions from one another and from more concerning diagnoses; extensive laboratory workup is rarely necessary for a neonate who otherwise appears well and whose eruption fits a recognized benign pattern.

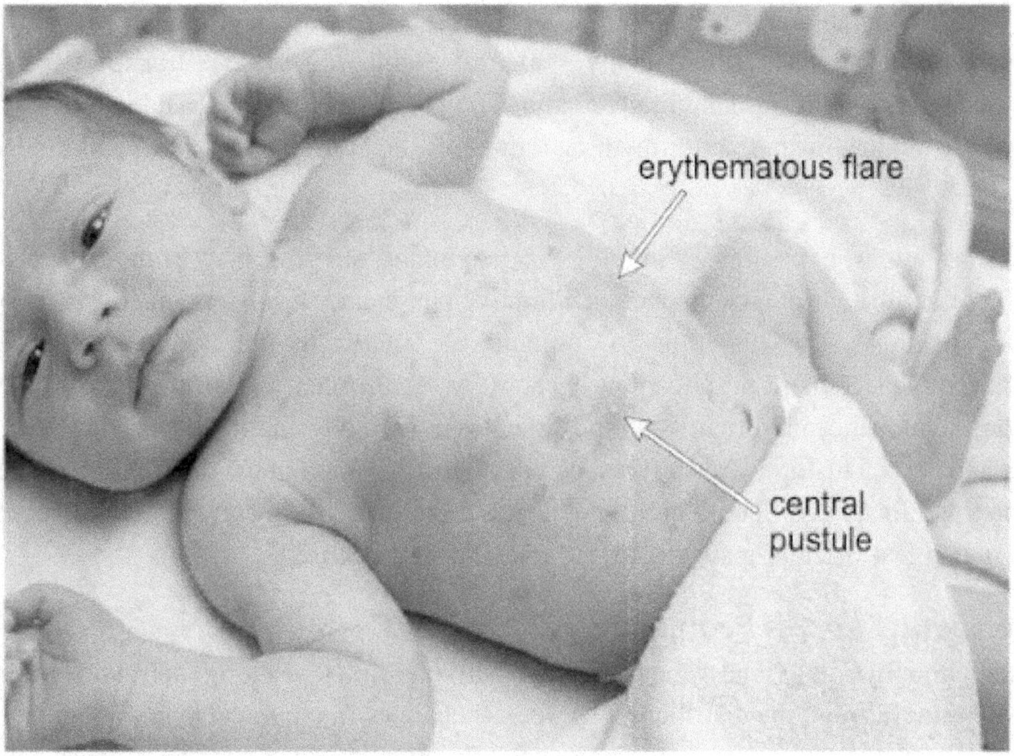

Figure 21.1 — Erythema Toxicum Neonatorum on a newborn's trunk.

Infantile Hemangiomas and Vascular Anomalies

Infantile hemangiomas, the most common vascular tumor of infancy, follow a highly characteristic and clinically important natural history: absent or only subtly present at birth, they undergo a proliferative phase over the first several months of life, often growing rapidly during this period, followed by a slower involuting phase extending over several years, during which the lesion gradually flattens and lightens in color. Superficial hemangiomas present as bright red, lobulated papules or plaques, while deeper hemangiomas present as a bluish, compressible subcutaneous nodule with less distinct overlying color change, and many lesions show a mixed superficial and deep component. Most infantile hemangiomas require no treatment beyond observation given their generally favorable natural involution, but specific features warrant early specialist referral and, in many cases, treatment with oral propranolol, now the well-established first-line systemic therapy: periocular hemangiomas that risk visual axis obstruction or astigmatism, hemangiomas involving the airway or overlying the lumbosacral spine (a location raising concern for underlying spinal dysraphism), ulcerated hemangiomas causing pain and risk of infection or scarring, and multiple cutaneous hemangiomas, which raise concern for associated visceral hemangiomas, most notably hepatic, warranting screening ultrasound.

CAUTION: A rapidly proliferating hemangioma near the eye, over the airway, or in a segmental beard distribution on the face warrants urgent specialist referral rather than routine observation, given the risk of amblyopia, airway compromise, and, in the beard distribution, coexisting airway hemangioma that may not yet be clinically apparent.

The GLUT1 immunohistochemical stain provides a useful adjunctive diagnostic tool when the clinical distinction between an infantile hemangioma and a vascular malformation remains uncertain, since infantile hemangiomas characteristically express this glucose transporter protein on immunohistochemistry while vascular malformations do not, though in the considerable majority of cases the characteristic clinical history and growth pattern alone are sufficient for confident diagnosis without biopsy.

Vascular malformations, in contrast to infantile hemangiomas, are present at birth, grow proportionately with the child rather than through a distinct proliferative phase, and never spontaneously involute, a set of distinguishing features that is essential to communicate clearly to families given the very different prognosis and management implications; capillary malformations (port-wine stains), venous malformations, lymphatic malformations, and arteriovenous malformations each have distinct clinical appearances and natural histories, and a facial capillary malformation in the distribution of the ophthalmic branch of the trigeminal nerve should prompt evaluation for Sturge-Weber syndrome, given its associated risk of leptomeningeal vascular malformation, glaucoma, and seizures.

Atopic Dermatitis Across Pediatric Age Groups

Although the pathophysiology and general management principles of atopic dermatitis are addressed in detail elsewhere in this text, the distribution of disease changes in a clinically important and highly age-dependent way across childhood that warrants specific attention in a pediatric-focused discussion. In infancy, atopic dermatitis characteristically involves the cheeks, scalp, and extensor surfaces of the extremities, a distribution that reflects the greater surface area exposed to friction from crawling and the relative sparing of the diaper area, which benefits from the occlusive, hydrating effect of the diaper itself; this infantile distribution can make the eruption resemble seborrheic dermatitis, and the two conditions can in fact coexist or overlap in early infancy, occasionally requiring an empiric treatment trial to clarify the dominant process. As children begin walking and the classic flexural distribution emerges, atopic dermatitis characteristically shifts to involve the antecubital and popliteal fossae, the wrists, and the ankles, a transition that generally occurs by early childhood and that persists, with some further evolution toward hand and eyelid involvement, into adolescence and adulthood.

Two practical pediatric-specific considerations deserve emphasis. First, food allergy testing is not recommended as a routine, reflexive component of pediatric atopic dermatitis evaluation in a child without a clear history suggesting an immediate hypersensitivity reaction, such as urticaria, angioedema, or respiratory symptoms temporally linked to a specific food, since broad, untargeted food allergen panel testing carries a high rate of clinically irrelevant false-positive results that can lead to unnecessary and potentially nutritionally harmful dietary restriction. Second, growth parameters should be monitored over time in children with moderate to severe atopic dermatitis maintained on prolonged courses of topical corticosteroids, and any concern for growth deceleration should prompt reassessment of the treatment regimen and consideration of non-corticosteroid alternatives, including topical calcineurin inhibitors or, for more severe disease, the systemic biologic and small-molecule therapies increasingly available for pediatric patients.

Molluscum Contagiosum and Cutaneous Warts in Children

Molluscum contagiosum, caused by a poxvirus and transmitted through direct skin contact or fomites, presents as small, firm, dome-shaped, umbilicated papules that can appear anywhere on the body but are especially common in the axillae, antecubital fossae, and groin in children, spreading readily through autoinoculation from scratching; the condition is self-limited in immunocompetent children, typically resolving over a period of months to a few years without treatment, and this natural history should be discussed explicitly with families, since many caregivers understandably expect and request active treatment given the lesions' visible and sometimes cosmetically bothersome nature. When treatment is desired, options include cantharidin applied in-office, cryotherapy, topical retinoids, and, for extensive or persistent disease, curettage, with the choice guided by lesion number, location, and the child's tolerance for a given procedure; an inflammatory, eczematous reaction developing around individual molluscum lesions, sometimes termed a molluscum dermatitis or "BOTE sign" (Beginning Of The End), is a reassuring sign of the host immune response mounting against the virus and typically heralds impending spontaneous resolution rather than representing a secondary bacterial infection requiring antibiotic treatment.

Plantar warts, a common subtype of cutaneous wart, are frequently mistaken for calluses given their location on weight-bearing surfaces, but characteristically show interruption of the normal skin lines and pinpoint black dots representing thrombosed capillaries when the surface hyperkeratosis is gently pared, features that reliably distinguish a plantar wart from a simple callus at the bedside.

Common cutaneous warts, caused by human papillomavirus, are similarly extremely common in school-age children and are most often managed with destructive therapies including salicylic acid and cryotherapy, with the choice and pace of treatment tailored to the child's age, the number and location of lesions, and their tolerance for the mild discomfort that cryotherapy in particular can cause; as with molluscum contagiosum, spontaneous resolution over a period of months to a few years is common, and a conservative, patience-based approach is entirely reasonable for lesions that are not causing functional impairment or significant distress, particularly in a very young child for whom repeated treatment sessions can themselves be a source of distress.

Pediatric Mastocytosis

Cutaneous mastocytosis, resulting from a clonal proliferation of mast cells within the skin, most commonly presents in infancy as one of several recognized patterns: solitary mastocytoma, a single tan-brown to reddish-brown plaque or nodule; urticaria pigmentosa, multiple tan-brown macules and papules distributed across the trunk and extremities; or, least commonly, diffuse cutaneous mastocytosis, with widespread skin thickening and infiltration. A characteristic and clinically useful bedside finding across all forms is the Darier sign, in which firm stroking of an individual lesion provokes localized urtication and erythema within minutes, reflecting mast cell degranulation triggered by the mechanical stimulus; eliciting this sign at the bedside is often sufficient to support the clinical diagnosis without biopsy in a classic-appearing case. The considerable majority of pediatric cutaneous mastocytosis, particularly solitary mastocytoma and urticaria pigmentosa presenting in infancy, follows a benign course with a strong tendency toward spontaneous improvement or resolution by adolescence, and management centers on avoidance of recognized mast cell degranulation triggers, including certain medications, temperature extremes, and vigorous friction to the skin, together with antihistamines for symptomatic pruritus or flushing; systemic mastocytosis with bone marrow involvement is far more characteristic of adult-onset disease, and extensive systemic workup is generally not required for a child with a classic, limited cutaneous presentation and no systemic symptoms.

KEY POINT: A positive Darier sign, localized urtication provoked by firmly stroking a tan-brown macule or plaque, strongly supports a diagnosis of cutaneous mastocytosis at the bedside; the considerable majority of pediatric cases follow a benign, self-limited course with spontaneous improvement expected well before adulthood.

Diaper Dermatitis

Irritant diaper dermatitis, by far the most common cause of diaper-area eruption, results from prolonged contact with urine and feces in a warm, occluded environment, producing erythema that characteristically spares the deep inguinal folds, a distribution feature that helps distinguish it from candidal diaper dermatitis, in which the eruption characteristically does involve the inguinal folds and is accompanied by satellite pustules beyond the main area of erythema. Management of irritant diaper dermatitis centers on frequent diaper changes, gentle cleansing, liberal application of a barrier ointment such as zinc oxide or petrolatum at every diaper change, and, for more inflamed cases, a brief course of a low-potency topical corticosteroid; candidal diaper dermatitis requires the addition of a topical antifungal, and persistent or recurrent candidal involvement should prompt consideration of concurrent oral thrush or, in a child with recent antibiotic exposure, the disruption of normal cutaneous flora as a contributing factor.

Several less common but clinically important mimics of ordinary diaper dermatitis warrant specific recognition. Allergic contact dermatitis to a component of the diaper itself or to a topical product applied to the area should be considered when the eruption has a sharply demarcated distribution corresponding to contact with a specific material rather than the diffuse pattern typical of irritant dermatitis. Psoriasis can present in the diaper area with well-demarcated, minimally scaly erythematous plaques that fail to respond as expected to standard irritant dermatitis management, and Langerhans cell histiocytosis, though rare, should be considered for a persistent, treatment-resistant, petechial or erosive diaper-area eruption, particularly when accompanied by other systemic findings, given its potential for multisystem involvement and the importance of prompt recognition and appropriate hematology-oncology referral.

Pediatric Viral Exanthems

The classically described childhood viral exanthems each follow a sufficiently characteristic clinical timeline and morphology to allow confident bedside diagnosis in the large majority of cases. Roseola infantum, caused by human herpesvirus 6, presents with several days of high fever in an otherwise well-appearing infant, followed by an abrupt defervescence coinciding with the appearance of a diffuse, blanching, rose-pink macular or maculopapular eruption on the trunk, a fever-then-rash sequence that is itself the key diagnostic clue and that distinguishes it from exanthems in which fever and rash occur concurrently. Erythema infectiosum (fifth disease), caused by parvovirus B19, classically begins with a bright red "slapped cheek" facial erythema, followed several days later by a lacy, reticulated erythematous eruption on the trunk and extremities that can recur intermittently over subsequent weeks with heat, sun, or physical exertion; parvovirus B19 infection acquired during pregnancy carries a risk of fetal hydrops, making documentation of exposure and maternal immune status an important consideration whenever a pregnant contact is identified.

Hand-foot-mouth disease, most commonly caused by coxsackievirus, presents with painful oral erosions together with vesicular lesions on the palms, soles, and buttocks, and is generally managed supportively, though attention to hydration is important given the discomfort oral lesions can cause with feeding; a distinct and more severe coxsackievirus A6 strain has been increasingly recognized in recent years, producing a more widespread, sometimes bullous eruption extending beyond the classically described hand-foot-mouth distribution, with subsequent onychomadesis (nail shedding) occurring several weeks after the acute illness in some affected children, a delayed finding that can otherwise cause unnecessary parental concern if its connection to the preceding viral illness is not recognized and explained.

KEY POINT: The temporal relationship between fever and rash onset is one of the most useful bedside clues for differentiating pediatric viral exanthems: a rash that appears as the fever resolves suggests roseola, while a rash that appears concurrently with or before fever onset points toward a different diagnosis; combined with the characteristic morphology and distribution of each exanthem, this timeline usually allows confident clinical diagnosis without additional testing in an otherwise well-appearing child.

Varicella in the Vaccine Era

Varicella (chickenpox), caused by primary infection with varicella-zoster virus, classically presents with successive crops of pruritic vesicles on an erythematous base, described as appearing in "crops" such that lesions at multiple stages, papules, vesicles, and crusted lesions, are simultaneously present, a finding often summarized as a "dewdrop on a rose petal" appearance for the individual vesicle and a distinctly polymorphic overall eruption at any single point in the illness; widespread routine childhood vaccination has substantially reduced both the incidence and the typical severity of varicella in vaccinated populations, and breakthrough varicella in a previously vaccinated child, when it occurs, characteristically presents as a milder, more atypical illness with fewer lesions, a more macular or papular rather than vesicular predominant morphology, and a correspondingly lower, though not absent, risk of transmission to susceptible contacts, a pattern that can make clinical diagnosis more challenging than in the classic unvaccinated presentation. Complications of varicella, though now less frequently encountered given widespread vaccination, include secondary bacterial infection of scratched lesions, most often with Staphylococcus aureus or Streptococcus pyogenes, and, rarely, more serious complications including varicella pneumonia and cerebellar ataxia; aspirin should never be administered to a child with varicella or any other viral illness given the well-established association with Reye syndrome, a critical prescribing safety point that bears repeating in any pediatric-focused discussion of viral exanthem management.

Genodermatoses: Epidermolysis Bullosa and Ichthyosis

Epidermolysis bullosa comprises a group of inherited disorders of skin fragility resulting from mutations in genes encoding structural proteins that anchor the epidermis to the underlying dermis, producing blistering and erosions in response to minimal friction or trauma; the major subtypes, simplex, junctional, and dystrophic, are distinguished by the specific ultrastructural level of tissue separation and carry markedly different severity and prognosis, ranging from a relatively mild, friction-triggered blistering tendency that improves with age in simplex disease to severe, mutilating scarring, esophageal strictures, and a substantially elevated lifetime risk of aggressive cutaneous squamous cell carcinoma in the most severe dystrophic subtypes. Diagnosis in a newborn with unexplained blistering or erosions is established through skin biopsy with immunofluorescence mapping or genetic testing, and management requires a highly specialized, multidisciplinary approach centered on meticulous wound care, nutritional support given the substantial caloric demands of chronic wound healing, and proactive surveillance for the complications specific to each subtype; families benefit enormously from connection to a specialized epidermolysis bullosa center given the disease's rarity and the highly specialized nature of optimal supportive care.

The ichthyoses comprise a heterogeneous group of inherited cornification disorders producing generalized scaling that ranges in severity from the common, mild, autosomal dominant ichthyosis vulgaris, frequently associated with atopic dermatitis and a filaggrin gene mutation, to the rare, severe, autosomal recessive congenital ichthyoses presenting at birth with a taut, restrictive collodion membrane or, in the most severe form, harlequin ichthyosis, with thick, plate-like armor-like scaling requiring intensive neonatal supportive care given the risks of impaired thermoregulation, fluid loss through the compromised skin barrier, and respiratory compromise from the restrictive effect of the taut skin on chest wall excursion. Management across the ichthyosis spectrum centers on aggressive emollient therapy and, for more severe subtypes, topical or systemic retinoids, with the specific approach tailored to disease severity and the particular subtype's underlying pathophysiology.

CAUTION: A neonate presenting with unexplained blistering, erosions, or a taut, restrictive skin membrane at birth requires urgent dermatology and, where available, connection to a specialized center;

both epidermolysis bullosa and the severe congenital ichthyoses carry immediate risks related to fluid balance, thermoregulation, and infection that require expert, coordinated neonatal intensive care alongside dermatologic management.

Cutaneous Clues to Neurocutaneous Syndromes

Certain pediatric skin findings serve as important early clues to an underlying neurocutaneous syndrome, and recognizing them promptly allows timely referral for the systemic surveillance these conditions require. Neurofibromatosis type 1 should be suspected in a child with six or more café-au-lait macules exceeding a defined size threshold, together with axillary or inguinal freckling (Crowe sign), and, as the child ages, the development of cutaneous or subcutaneous neurofibromas; children meeting diagnostic criteria require ongoing surveillance for the condition's broader systemic manifestations, including optic pathway glioma, skeletal abnormalities, and, though individually uncommon, plexiform neurofibromas with a small but meaningful lifetime risk of transformation into a malignant peripheral nerve sheath tumor, underscoring the value of coordinated care through a specialized neurofibromatosis clinic. Tuberous sclerosis complex presents with a distinct constellation of cutaneous findings, including hypopigmented "ash-leaf" macules, often the earliest visible sign and best appreciated with a Wood lamp examination in a young infant, facial angiofibromas that typically become apparent in early childhood, a shagreen patch (a connective tissue nevus with a characteristic pebbled, orange-peel texture) most often on the lower back, and periungual fibromas that tend to appear later in childhood or adolescence; the cutaneous findings again serve as the visible surface marker of a multisystem condition with important renal, cardiac, and neurologic manifestations, including a well-recognized association with infantile spasms and other seizure disorders, making early recognition of the skin findings clinically consequential well beyond dermatology alone.

CAUTION: Multiple café-au-lait macules or a suspicious hypopigmented ash-leaf macule identified on routine examination of an infant or young child should prompt a systematic search for the remaining diagnostic criteria of the associated neurocutaneous syndrome and referral for appropriate systemic evaluation, since the cutaneous findings frequently precede the syndrome's more consequential neurologic, ophthalmologic, or oncologic manifestations by months to years.

Cutaneous Findings and the Recognition of Child Abuse

Dermatologists and other clinicians evaluating children have an important, sometimes underappreciated role in recognizing cutaneous findings that may reflect physical abuse, and distinguishing these findings from the numerous benign or accidental conditions that can superficially mimic them is a critical clinical skill. Bruising patterns that raise concern for abuse include bruises on the torso, ears, or neck in a child younger than four years (regions rarely bruised accidentally in a pre-mobile or early-mobile child), bruises of distinctly different ages suggesting repeated episodes of trauma, and patterned bruising reflecting the outline of an object such as a belt or cord, in contrast to the shin and forehead bruising commonly seen in mobile toddlers from ordinary accidental trauma. Cigarette burns, characteristically small, round, and uniformly deep, and immersion burns, characteristically producing a sharply demarcated "stocking" or "glove" pattern with sparing of flexural creases where the limb was held away from the hot water, are important patterns to recognize, though several benign conditions are frequently and mistakenly raised as concerns in this context and should be confidently distinguished: Mongolian spots (dermal melanocytosis), congenital blue-gray macular patches most common over the lumbosacral area in infants of darker skin tones, are occasionally mistaken for bruising by unfamiliar examiners but are present from birth, do not evolve through the color changes characteristic of a resolving bruise, and carry no clinical significance beyond correct recognition and reassurance; and cultural practices such as cupping or coining, which can produce circular ecchymoses or linear petechial streaks respectively, should be recognized as culturally rooted therapeutic practices rather than reflexively assumed to represent abuse. Any finding that raises genuine concern for non-accidental trauma warrants prompt, appropriately documented evaluation through established child protection protocols rather than either dismissal or an accusatory approach with the family.

Pediatric-Specific Safety Considerations in Topical and Systemic Therapy

Infants and young children have a substantially higher body surface-area-to-body-mass ratio than adults, meaning that a given quantity of topical medication applied per unit area of skin results in a proportionally much larger systemic dose relative to body weight, an especially important consideration for high-potency topical corticosteroids, which carry a meaningfully increased risk of systemic absorption and hypothalamic-pituitary-adrenal axis suppression when applied over large body surface areas, under occlusion, or to thin-skinned regions such as the face and diaper area in this age group; treatment plans for young children should default to the lowest effective potency, limit the treated body surface area and duration of use where possible, and specifically avoid high-potency corticosteroids in the diaper area, where the occlusive effect of the diaper itself further increases absorption. Topical calcineurin inhibitors carry a boxed warning regarding a theoretical malignancy risk that has not been substantiated by subsequent long-term surveillance data, and current guidance supports their use, with appropriate informed discussion, as a valuable non-corticosteroid option in pediatric atopic dermatitis, particularly for sensitive areas such as the face and skin folds where prolonged topical corticosteroid use carries its own recognized risks of atrophy and telangiectasia.

Systemic medication dosing throughout pediatric dermatology should be calculated on a weight-based or, for certain agents, body surface area basis rather than extrapolated from adult dosing, and several medications used commonly in adult dermatology carry specific pediatric contraindications or require particular caution, including tetracycline-class antibiotics, which are generally avoided in children younger than eight years given the risk of permanent tooth discoloration and, in very young children, potential effects on bone growth, and systemic retinoids, which require the same rigorous pregnancy-prevention counseling framework in adolescent patients of childbearing potential as in adult patients, discussed in greater detail in the chapter on acne and its therapeutic principles.

Formulation choice is itself an important pediatric-specific consideration distinct from the medication's active ingredient: ointments are generally better tolerated and less irritating than creams or lotions for young children with sensitive or already inflamed skin given their lower alcohol and preservative content, though the greasier texture and cosmetic feel of an ointment can reduce adherence in an older child or adolescent who is more sensitive to how a topical product feels and appears to peers, an adherence consideration that should be discussed directly with the patient, not only the parent, whenever developmentally appropriate. Flavored or otherwise more palatable oral formulations can meaningfully improve adherence to systemic antihistamines or antibiotics in young children who resist standard tablets or capsules, and involving the child directly, to the extent developmentally appropriate, in choosing between reasonable formulation options can improve adherence to a treatment plan that will often need to be sustained over weeks to months.

Sunscreen selection and photoprotection counseling also require pediatric-specific adjustment: mineral-based sunscreens containing zinc oxide or titanium dioxide are generally preferred over chemical sunscreen formulations for infants and young children given a lower theoretical risk of systemic absorption and irritation, and sunscreen use is not recommended at all for infants younger than six months, for whom shade, protective clothing, and avoidance of peak sun-intensity hours remain the primary recommended photoprotection strategies given the immaturity of the neonatal skin barrier at this very young age.

PATIENT EDUCATION: Parents and caregivers applying topical medications to an infant or young child should be given specific, explicit guidance on the quantity to apply, using a measure such as the fingertip unit, and the maximum frequency and duration of use, since the higher surface-area-to-body-mass ratio in this age group means that well-intentioned over-application carries a meaningfully greater risk of unwanted systemic absorption than the same practice would in an adult.

Clinical Case: A Neonate With a Rapidly Growing Facial Lesion

A 6-week-old girl was brought in by her parents for evaluation of a bright red, raised lesion on her upper eyelid that had been barely noticeable at birth but had grown substantially over the preceding four weeks, now partially obscuring her line of sight on that side. Examination revealed a well-demarcated, bright red, lobulated, compressible papule measuring approximately 1.5 centimeters, consistent with a superficial infantile hemangioma in its early proliferative phase, with partial obstruction of the visual axis on the affected side.

Given the periocular location and the risk of amblyopia and astigmatism from ongoing visual axis obstruction during this critical period of visual development, she was referred urgently to a pediatric dermatologist experienced in vascular anomalies, and oral propranolol was initiated after appropriate baseline cardiovascular screening, with close monitoring during treatment initiation given the medication's blood pressure and heart rate-lowering effects in this young and small patient population. Over the subsequent months, the hemangioma's growth halted and then began to regress, and ongoing collaboration with pediatric ophthalmology confirmed no evidence of amblyopia developing during treatment, illustrating the importance of prompt recognition and specialist referral for infantile hemangiomas in this anatomically high-risk location.

Clinical Case: A Toddler With Persistent Groin Redness Despite Treatment

A 14-month-old boy was brought in for a diaper-area eruption that had been present for nearly three weeks despite consistent use of a zinc oxide barrier ointment and a brief course of over-the-counter hydrocortisone cream recommended by his pediatrician, with his parents reporting that the eruption seemed to worsen rather than improve with the topical steroid. Examination revealed bright red, well-demarcated erythema extending into the inguinal folds themselves, accompanied by multiple small satellite pustules and papules beyond the main area of confluent erythema, a distribution and morphology distinctly different from the fold-sparing pattern expected in simple irritant diaper dermatitis.

Given the involvement of the inguinal folds and the presence of satellite lesions, a diagnosis of candidal diaper dermatitis was made, and a review of his recent history revealed a course of oral antibiotics for acute otitis media approximately three weeks earlier, providing a plausible explanation for disruption of his normal cutaneous and mucosal flora and subsequent candidal overgrowth. He was started on a topical antifungal cream in place of the hydrocortisone, with continuation of the barrier ointment and frequent diaper changes, and his parents were counseled explicitly that the topical corticosteroid, while a reasonable initial choice for uncomplicated irritant dermatitis, had likely been ineffective, and possibly mildly counterproductive, because the underlying process was candidal rather than purely irritant in nature. His eruption resolved completely within ten days of starting appropriate antifungal therapy, and this case was used as an opportunity to reinforce with the family the specific distinguishing features, fold involvement and satellite lesions, that should prompt reconsideration of a diaper dermatitis diagnosis that is not responding as expected.

THE MORPHOLOGY-TO-MANAGEMENT SYSTEM — Reading the Pediatric Eruption Through a Developmental Lens

Pattern Introduced This Chapter: The self-limited neonatal pustular eruption that mimics infection, the proliferating periocular hemangioma racing against a critical developmental window, and the diaper-area eruption that fails to respond because it was never simple irritant dermatitis to begin with.

Cross-Cutting Anchor: Every pediatric eruption in this chapter is correctly interpreted only when its timeline relative to age and developmental stage, rather than its morphology in isolation, is placed at the center of the diagnostic reasoning, since the same lesion can carry a completely different significance depending on whether it appears in the first days of life, the first months, or later childhood.

Summary and Key Concepts

Erythema toxicum neonatorum and transient neonatal pustular melanosis are benign, self-limited neonatal eruptions distinguished from one another and from more concerning diagnoses by their timing, distribution, and a bedside Wright-stained smear when needed.

Infantile hemangiomas proliferate over the first months of life before slowly involuting over years, and periocular, airway, lumbosacral, and ulcerated lesions warrant early referral and, frequently, oral propranolol therapy.

Vascular malformations are present at birth and grow proportionately with the child without spontaneous involution, a distinction from infantile hemangiomas that is essential for family counseling and management planning.

Candidal diaper dermatitis involves the inguinal folds with satellite pustules, distinguishing it from irritant diaper dermatitis, which spares the deep folds; psoriasis and Langerhans cell histiocytosis are important mimics to consider in treatment-resistant cases.

The temporal relationship between fever and rash, together with characteristic morphology, allows confident bedside diagnosis of most pediatric viral exanthems, including roseola, fifth disease, and hand-foot-mouth disease.

Pediatric topical and systemic dermatologic therapy requires specific safety adjustments given the higher surface-area-to-body-mass ratio of young children, including cautious topical corticosteroid potency selection and avoidance of tetracyclines in young children.

CHAPTER 22: DIAGNOSIS AND MANAGEMENT ACROSS SKIN TONES

Learning Objectives

1. Recognize how erythema, inflammation, and pigmentary change present differently across the range of human skin tones and adjust the clinical examination accordingly.
2. Construct an evidence-based approach to post-inflammatory hyperpigmentation and post-inflammatory hypopigmentation, including their prevention and management.
3. Identify the dermatologic conditions that occur disproportionately, or with a distinct clinical presentation, in patients with skin of color.
4. Distinguish keloid formation from hypertrophic scarring and apply an appropriate stepwise management approach.
5. Recognize the hair and scalp disorders that occur with particular frequency in patients of African descent, including central centrifugal cicatricial alopecia and traction alopecia.
6. Apply Fitzpatrick-appropriate technique modifications for laser and energy-based device procedures to reduce the risk of pigmentary complications.

Dermatologic training and reference materials have historically underrepresented the full range of human skin tones, a gap with direct clinical consequences: delayed diagnosis of common inflammatory conditions whose classic descriptions emphasize erythema that is far less visually apparent in darker skin, disproportionate rates of missed or delayed melanoma diagnosis in patients with skin of color, and a persistent undertreatment of the pigmentary sequelae that patients with skin of color consistently identify as among their most distressing dermatologic concerns. This chapter addresses the specific clinical adjustments, disease associations, and procedural modifications required to deliver equitable, accurate dermatologic care across the full spectrum of skin tones, building on the disease-specific chapters throughout this text with a dedicated focus on the recognition and management principles that most directly affect patients with more deeply pigmented skin.

Recognizing Inflammation and Erythema Across Skin Tones

The classic descriptions of erythema used throughout most of dermatologic education, bright or pink-red discoloration that blanches with pressure, apply reliably to lightly pigmented skin but become considerably less visually apparent, and at times entirely absent, in more deeply pigmented skin, where the same underlying inflammatory process instead frequently presents as violaceous, gray-brown, or simply darker discoloration relative to the surrounding uninvolved skin. This difference has direct diagnostic consequences across nearly every inflammatory and infectious condition discussed elsewhere in this text: cellulitis, for example, may show more subtle color change in darker skin, making warmth, tenderness, and the presence of associated systemic signs such as fever proportionately more important components of the clinical assessment than visual erythema alone; psoriasis plaques in darker skin tones often appear violaceous to gray-brown rather than the classic salmon-pink color emphasized in most textbook photography, with the silvery scale remaining a comparatively reliable, skin-tone-independent diagnostic clue; and atopic dermatitis in patients with skin of color more frequently presents with a follicular, papular morphology and more prominent lichenification than the primarily erythematous, eczematous plaques classically depicted, a distinction discussed in greater detail in the dedicated atopic dermatitis chapter.

Photographic documentation practices within dermatology should also be adapted for accurate representation of darker skin tones, since standard camera exposure and white-balance settings calibrated primarily for lighter skin can distort the true color and severity of a finding when applied without adjustment to darker skin, a practical concern relevant both for clinical photographic documentation used to track treatment response over time and for the broader effort to improve representation of the full range of skin tones in medical education and reference materials, an effort this text has deliberately sought to reflect throughout its visual content.

KEY POINT: When erythema is subtle or difficult to appreciate in darker skin tones, palpation for warmth and induration, careful attention to surface texture and scale, and a lower threshold to rely on associated systemic or historical features become correspondingly more important components of the clinical examination than visual inspection for redness alone.

Erythema-based clinical severity scoring tools developed and validated primarily in lightly pigmented populations, including several scales used to grade the severity of atopic dermatitis and psoriasis, have documented limitations when applied to patients with darker skin tones, given their heavy reliance on erythema intensity as a scored parameter; clinicians should be aware of this limitation and weight induration, scale, and patient-reported symptom severity more heavily when using these tools in patients for whom erythema is difficult to visually assess, and several revised scoring instruments incorporating this consideration have been developed and are increasingly used in both clinical practice and dermatologic research.

Post-Inflammatory Hyperpigmentation and Hypopigmentation

Post-inflammatory hyperpigmentation, the deposition of excess melanin at the site of a preceding inflammatory or traumatic cutaneous event, occurs with substantially greater frequency and intensity in more deeply pigmented skin, and patients with skin of color consistently and repeatedly identify this pigmentary sequela, rather than the original inflammatory condition itself, as their most bothersome and persistent dermatologic concern across numerous patient-reported outcome studies; this reality has direct treatment implications, since a management plan that successfully controls acne, eczema, or another inflammatory dermatosis but fails to specifically address the resulting pigmentary change will often leave the patient feeling that their concern was inadequately addressed. Effective management of post-inflammatory hyperpigmentation begins with early, aggressive control of the underlying inflammatory trigger, since ongoing inflammation continuously feeds the pigmentary process, combined with strict, consistent broad-spectrum photoprotection, given that ultraviolet exposure meaningfully darkens and prolongs existing post-inflammatory pigmentation; topical agents including hydroquinone, azelaic acid, topical retinoids, and tranexamic acid each have a role in accelerating resolution, and for more persistent or extensive pigmentation, chemical peels or laser and energy-based device treatment can be considered, though these procedural interventions carry their own meaningful risk of paradoxically worsening pigmentation if performed with inappropriate technique or parameters in patients with darker skin tones, discussed further below.

Post-inflammatory hypopigmentation, though less commonly the presenting concern than hyperpigmentation, occurs with several specific conditions and requires its own distinct counseling and management approach; unlike post-inflammatory hyperpigmentation, which generally responds to the pigment-lightening approaches described above, post-inflammatory hypopigmentation instead requires patience, since it generally resolves through the slow, gradual repopulation of melanocytes over a period of months, a timeline that should be explained clearly to patients to set realistic expectations, and photoprotection of the surrounding normally pigmented skin should be emphasized to avoid a widening color contrast that can make even a stable area of hypopigmentation more visually apparent over time.

Camouflage and correcting cosmetics can provide meaningful psychosocial benefit while pigment-directed medical therapy takes its expected months-long course to produce visible improvement, and clinicians should be prepared to offer specific product recommendations, including green- or yellow-based color-correcting formulations for erythematous or violaceous discoloration and appropriately shade-matched concealers for hyperpigmented or hypopigmented patches, rather than assuming this practical, immediately actionable form of support falls outside the scope of dermatologic care.

PATIENT EDUCATION: Post-inflammatory pigmentary change following an inflammatory skin condition can take considerably longer to resolve than the inflammatory condition itself, sometimes many months for hyperpigmentation and up to a year or more for hypopigmentation; setting this expectation early, and emphasizing the essential role of consistent sun protection during the resolution period, helps prevent frustration with an otherwise successfully treated underlying condition.

Keloids and Hypertrophic Scarring

Keloids, which occur with substantially greater frequency in patients with darker skin tones and carry a recognized genetic and familial predisposition, are distinguished from hypertrophic scars by their characteristic extension beyond the original wound margins and their tendency to continue growing over time rather than gradually flattening, in contrast to hypertrophic scars, which remain confined to the original wound boundaries and typically improve gradually over one to two years without specific intervention. Common anatomic sites for keloid formation include the earlobes, frequently following ear piercing, the central chest, the shoulders, and the jawline, and any elective procedure in a patient with a personal or strong family history of keloid formation warrants an explicit pre-procedural discussion of this risk, since the decision to proceed with an elective cosmetic or even medically indicated procedure in a keloid-prone patient should incorporate the patient's own assessment of this risk relative to the benefit of the procedure.

Management of established keloids follows a stepwise approach beginning with intralesional corticosteroid injection, typically triamcinolone acetonide, administered at intervals of several weeks, which remains the first-line treatment for the majority of keloids and can be combined with intralesional 5-fluorouracil for more resistant lesions; silicone gel sheeting and pressure therapy provide a lower-risk adjunctive or preventive option, particularly for patients at high risk following a planned procedure. Surgical excision alone carries a high rate of keloid recurrence, often with an even larger keloid than the original, and is generally reserved for lesions that have failed intralesional therapy, and when performed, should be combined with adjuvant treatment, most commonly immediate postoperative intralesional corticosteroid injection or radiation therapy for the highest-risk lesions, to reduce this substantial recurrence risk.

Newer adjunctive modalities for keloid management, including intralesional cryotherapy, in which a needle-based cryoprobe delivers freezing directly to the core of the keloid while sparing the overlying epidermis, and laser-assisted therapy using pulsed-dye or fractional devices, are increasingly incorporated into combination treatment protocols for particularly resistant or extensive keloids, though intralesional corticosteroid injection, alone or in combination with these newer modalities, remains the foundation of first-line management for the great majority of keloids given its long track record, low cost, and broad accessibility relative to these more specialized adjunctive options.

CAUTION: Surgical excision of a keloid without a planned adjuvant treatment strategy carries a high risk of recurrence, frequently producing a keloid larger than the one removed; any decision to pursue surgical management should be made jointly with the patient after a clear discussion of this risk and the specific adjuvant protocol planned to reduce it.

Hair and Scalp Disorders in Patients of African Descent

Central centrifugal cicatricial alopecia, the most common cause of scarring alopecia in women of African descent, presents with hair loss beginning at the vertex or crown of the scalp and gradually expanding centrifugally, often with an accompanying sensation of tenderness, itching, or a feeling of tightness preceding visible hair loss by months to years; because the condition causes permanent, scarring hair loss once established, early recognition and treatment, typically with anti-inflammatory agents including topical and intralesional corticosteroids and, in more active or extensive disease, oral anti-inflammatory or antifibrotic therapy, is essential to halt disease progression before extensive permanent scarring occurs, making patient and clinician awareness of the condition's early, sometimes subtle symptoms a critical component of preserving remaining hair. Traction alopecia, resulting from chronic tension on the hair shaft from tightly pulled hairstyles, braiding, or the sustained weight of hair extensions, characteristically affects the frontal and temporal hairline, and the "fringe sign," the retention of a thin row of vellus hairs along the anterior hairline despite more substantial hair loss just posterior to it, is a useful bedside clue supporting this diagnosis; early-stage traction alopecia, before scarring becomes established, is potentially reversible with reduction in traction-inducing hairstyling practices, but progression to a scarring phase produces permanent hair loss, again underscoring the clinical value of early recognition and intervention.

KEY POINT: Both central centrifugal cicatricial alopecia and traction alopecia are potentially reversible in their early, non-scarring phase but produce permanent hair loss once significant scarring has occurred; any patient presenting with vertex-predominant or hairline-predominant hair loss and a history or examination consistent with either condition should be counseled that timely treatment meaningfully affects the ultimate outcome.

Acne keloidalis nuchae, presenting as firm, follicular papules and, in more advanced disease, coalescing keloidal plaques at the posterior scalp and nape of the neck, occurs predominantly in men of African descent and is thought to relate to chronic follicular irritation, often exacerbated by close haircutting practices and tight shirt collars; management includes topical and intralesional corticosteroids for early inflammatory disease, oral antibiotics for papulopustular flares with an infectious component, and, for established fibrotic plaques that fail medical management, surgical excision, generally reserved for more advanced, medically refractory cases given the same keloid-prone healing tendency discussed above. Pseudofolliculitis barbae, resulting from curved hair follicles characteristic of tightly coiled hair curling back into the skin after shaving and provoking a foreign-body inflammatory reaction, is best managed by reducing shaving frequency or switching to a depilatory or, for patients desiring a longer-term solution, laser hair removal, which is particularly effective for this specific condition, though it requires the Fitzpatrick-appropriate technique modifications discussed in the following section to minimize pigmentary complications in the darker skin tones in which pseudofolliculitis barbae most commonly occurs.

Melasma

Melasma, presenting as symmetric, blotchy, tan to brown patches most commonly on the cheeks, forehead, and upper lip, occurs disproportionately in women with darker skin tones and is driven by a combination of ultraviolet exposure, hormonal influences including pregnancy and oral contraceptive use, and, in many patients, a genetic predisposition reflected in a frequently reported family history; the condition follows a notoriously treatment-resistant, chronic relapsing course, and setting realistic expectations regarding gradual improvement rather than complete clearance is an essential component of counseling, since patients who expect rapid, complete resolution are more likely to become frustrated and discontinue an otherwise appropriately structured treatment regimen. Strict, consistent broad-spectrum photoprotection, specifically including protection against visible light in addition to ultraviolet radiation given evidence that visible light itself can trigger and worsen melasma in darker skin tones, forms the essential foundation of any melasma treatment plan, and tinted mineral sunscreens containing iron oxide provide superior visible-light protection compared with untinted formulations for this specific reason. First-line topical therapy includes combination formulations containing hydroquinone, a topical retinoid, and a mild topical corticosteroid, most classically the triple combination cream, with tranexamic acid, both topical and, for more resistant cases, oral, emerging as a valuable additional treatment option; procedural treatments including chemical peels and certain laser modalities can provide additional benefit but carry a meaningful risk of rebound worsening or post-inflammatory hyperpigmentation if performed with inappropriate technique, making careful patient selection and conservative treatment parameters essential.

PATIENT EDUCATION: Melasma is a chronic condition that typically improves gradually with consistent treatment rather than resolving completely and permanently, and consistent daily broad-spectrum sun protection, including protection against visible light, is the single most important factor determining whether achieved improvement is maintained over time.

Dermoscopic and Structural Considerations in Darker Skin Tones

Dermoscopic examination in patients with darker skin tones requires an adjusted interpretive framework, since background pigmentation patterns that would be considered atypical or concerning in lightly pigmented skin, including more prominent and diffuse pigment network patterns, are frequently normal background findings in constitutively darker skin and should not, in isolation, prompt biopsy; dermoscopists experienced in evaluating patients with skin of color instead place correspondingly greater diagnostic weight on asymmetry of pigment distribution, architectural disorder, and the specific parallel ridge pattern on acral skin discussed above, rather than pigment network prominence alone. Basal cell carcinoma, while overall less common in patients with darker skin tones given the lower burden of cumulative ultraviolet-driven mutation, presents with a distinctly higher proportion of pigmented subtypes in this population compared with the classic pearly, telangiectatic, non-pigmented presentation emphasized in most textbook descriptions, and a pigmented basal cell carcinoma is frequently mistaken for a benign nevus or seborrheic keratosis, contributing to its own pattern of diagnostic delay analogous to that described for acral lentiginous melanoma above; dermoscopic features including arborizing telangiectasias and blue-gray ovoid nests remain useful distinguishing features of pigmented basal cell carcinoma regardless of the patient's underlying skin tone, and any pigmented lesion with these specific dermoscopic features occurring on a background of otherwise typical background pigmentation warrants biopsy.

CAUTION: A pigmented lesion in a patient with darker skin tones showing arborizing telangiectasias or blue-gray ovoid nests on dermoscopy should raise suspicion for pigmented basal cell carcinoma rather than being assumed to represent a benign nevus or seborrheic keratosis on the basis of its pigmented appearance alone.

Fitzpatrick-Appropriate Modifications for Laser and Energy-Based Procedures

Laser and energy-based device treatments carry a meaningfully elevated risk of pigmentary complications, both hyperpigmentation and hypopigmentation, and in some cases scarring, in patients with darker Fitzpatrick skin types, because melanin within the epidermis competes with the intended target chromophore for absorption of the laser energy, generating excess unwanted epidermal heating; this risk is not a reason to withhold beneficial procedures from patients with skin of color, but rather requires specific technique modifications to perform these procedures safely. General principles include selecting longer wavelengths that penetrate more deeply while being less strongly absorbed by epidermal melanin, using longer pulse durations to allow more time for epidermal cooling between energy delivery, employing lower fluence settings with a greater number of treatment passes rather than fewer higher-intensity passes, ensuring robust epidermal cooling through contact cooling devices or cryogen spray, and always performing a conservative test spot in an inconspicuous area before proceeding with full treatment in any patient with a darker skin tone or uncertain treatment response.

A structured pre-treatment risk assessment, incorporating Fitzpatrick skin type, recent sun exposure and tanning (which transiently increases epidermal melanin and correspondingly elevates procedural risk even in a patient with a lighter baseline skin type), and any personal or family history of post-inflammatory pigmentary change or keloid formation, should be documented before any laser or energy-based procedure, and patients should be counseled explicitly that the risk of pigmentary complication, while minimized through appropriate technique selection, cannot be reduced to zero, and that a conservative, more gradual treatment approach with lower per-session energy delivery is generally the safer strategy in this population even though it may require a greater total number of treatment sessions to achieve the desired result.

Hair removal lasers targeting the melanin within the hair follicle exemplify this challenge particularly clearly, since the same chromophore, melanin, is both the intended target within the hair follicle and the unwanted competing target within the epidermis; longer-wavelength devices, most notably the long-pulsed Nd:YAG laser, are generally preferred for hair removal in darker skin tones given their deeper penetration and relatively lower epidermal melanin absorption compared with shorter-wavelength alexandrite or diode devices, which, while highly effective in lighter skin tones, carry a substantially higher risk of epidermal pigmentary injury when used in patients with more deeply pigmented skin. Ablative and fractional resurfacing procedures similarly require conservative parameter selection and, frequently, pre- and post-procedure pigment-modulating skin care, given the well-recognized risk of post-procedural hyperpigmentation in darker skin tones undergoing these more aggressive resurfacing modalities. Non-ablative fractional resurfacing, which spares more of the epidermis while still stimulating dermal collagen remodeling, generally carries a lower pigmentary risk profile than fully ablative resurfacing and is frequently the preferred modality for patients with darker skin tones seeking improvement in scarring, texture, or photoaging, though even non-ablative devices still require the conservative parameter selection and appropriate cooling protocols described above rather than an assumption that the non-ablative modality alone eliminates pigmentary risk. Pre-treatment priming with a topical retinoid or hydroquinone-containing regimen for several weeks before a planned resurfacing procedure is a strategy used by some experienced clinicians to reduce the incidence of post-procedural hyperpigmentation in higher-risk patients, though the evidence supporting this specific practice remains more limited than the evidence supporting the core technique modifications, wavelength selection, and conservative fluence principles described throughout this section.

CAUTION: Laser and energy-based device treatment performed with parameters or wavelengths appropriate for lighter skin types, but applied without modification to a patient with a darker Fitzpatrick skin type, carries a substantially elevated risk of pigmentary complications and scarring; a conservative test spot and appropriately selected wavelength, pulse duration, and fluence are essential safety steps for every such procedure in this patient population.

Vitiligo and Its Distinct Psychosocial Impact in Skin of Color

Vitiligo, resulting from autoimmune destruction of melanocytes and producing sharply demarcated, depigmented macules and patches, occurs across all skin tones with similar incidence, but the depigmented patches are dramatically more visually apparent, and correspondingly more psychosocially distressing, in patients with darker skin tones given the greater contrast between the depigmented and surrounding normally pigmented skin; this heightened visibility translates into a well-documented, disproportionately greater impact on quality of life, self-esteem, and, in some cultural contexts, social and marriage prospects for patients with darker skin tones affected by vitiligo, making psychosocial assessment and support an especially important component of comprehensive care for this population, beyond the medical repigmentation therapies discussed in the dedicated pigmentation disorders chapter earlier in this text. Camouflage cosmetics specifically formulated to match a broader range of deeper skin tones, and connection to vitiligo-specific patient support organizations and communities, are valuable adjuncts that should be proactively offered rather than left for the patient to seek out independently, particularly given documented gaps in the availability of well-matched camouflage products for the deepest skin tones historically underserved by the cosmetic industry.

KEY POINT: The medical management of vitiligo does not differ fundamentally by skin tone, but the psychosocial impact and the practical challenge of finding well-matched camouflage cosmetics are both disproportionately greater for patients with darker skin tones, making proactive psychosocial support and camouflage resource referral a particularly important component of care for this population.

Photoprotection Counseling and Skin Cancer Risk Perception in Skin of Color

A persistent and clinically consequential misconception, held by both patients and, at times, clinicians, holds that patients with darker skin tones do not require sun protection given their higher baseline melanin content and correspondingly lower risk of ultraviolet-driven skin cancer; while it is true that the overall incidence of keratinocyte carcinoma and ultraviolet-driven melanoma subtypes is substantially lower in patients with darker skin tones, this population remains susceptible to photoaging, to ultraviolet-triggered worsening of melasma and post-inflammatory hyperpigmentation, discussed above, and, though less commonly, to skin cancer itself, making a blanket recommendation to forgo sun protection both clinically inaccurate and a missed opportunity to address the pigmentary concerns that are frequently the primary presenting complaint in this population. Sunscreen formulation preferences also warrant specific attention in this population: many patients with darker skin tones report dissatisfaction with the visible white or gray cast left by traditional mineral sunscreen formulations on deeper skin tones, a cosmetic concern that can meaningfully reduce consistent sunscreen use if not proactively addressed, and newer tinted mineral formulations and improved micronized or chemical-mineral hybrid formulations that minimize this visible cast should be specifically recommended to improve adherence in patients who have previously discontinued sunscreen use for this reason.

PATIENT EDUCATION: Sun protection remains clinically important for patients with all skin tones, including the darkest skin tones, primarily to prevent photoaging and worsening of pigmentary conditions such as melasma and post-inflammatory hyperpigmentation; patients who have previously found mineral sunscreens cosmetically unacceptable due to a visible white or gray cast should be offered tinted or reformulated alternatives rather than simply discontinuing sun protection altogether.

Systemic lupus erythematosus and other photosensitive connective tissue diseases, discussed in greater detail in the earlier chapter on connective tissue disease and the skin, also present distinct diagnostic considerations in patients with darker skin tones, where the malar erythema classically emphasized in descriptions of acute cutaneous lupus can be considerably more difficult to appreciate, and discoid lupus lesions more frequently produce clinically significant dyspigmentation, both hyperpigmentation at the active, inflamed border and hypopigmentation within longstanding, burnt-out lesions, that can itself become the patient's primary cosmetic concern independent of ongoing disease activity; early, aggressive treatment of active discoid lesions to prevent this pigmentary progression is therefore an especially important management priority in patients with darker skin tones.

Cosmetic Considerations and Common Patient Requests

Patients with skin of color present with a distinct set of common cosmetic concerns and procedural considerations beyond the pigmentary and laser-related issues discussed above. Chemical peels, a commonly requested procedure for overall skin texture and tone improvement, require careful depth and agent selection in darker skin tones, since deeper peels carry a meaningfully elevated risk of post-procedural dyschromia; superficial peels using glycolic acid, salicylic acid, or lactic acid are generally better tolerated and lower-risk first-line options in this population, with deeper peeling agents reserved for carefully selected patients and performed by clinicians experienced specifically in treating darker skin tones. Injectable neuromodulator and soft-tissue filler procedures do not carry the same pigmentary risk profile as laser and peel procedures, since they do not rely on selective chromophore targeting, but injection-site bruising, itself a form of transient discoloration, can be more visually prominent and slower to resolve in some patients with darker skin tones, warranting appropriate pre-procedure counseling regarding expected bruising duration and, when desired, use of adjunctive measures such as pre-treatment avoidance of blood-thinning supplements and post-treatment ice application to minimize this effect.

Hair care practices and product formulations also warrant specific clinical attention, since many common hair care practices among patients of African descent, including chemical relaxers, frequent heat styling, and certain protective hairstyles, carry their own recognized contribution to conditions including traction alopecia and, in the case of some chemical relaxer formulations, scalp irritation and, per some epidemiologic studies, other health associations that remain an active area of ongoing research; a nonjudgmental, collaborative discussion of a patient's hair care routine and its potential contribution to a presenting scalp or hair concern, rather than a reflexive recommendation to abandon culturally significant hairstyling practices altogether, generally yields a more productive and sustainable treatment partnership.

Melanoma and Diagnostic Delay in Patients With Skin of Color

As discussed in the dedicated melanoma chapter earlier in this text, patients with darker skin tones are diagnosed with melanoma at a later stage and experience worse melanoma-specific survival than patients with lighter skin tones, a disparity driven by several converging factors specific to this population: acral lentiginous melanoma, which occurs with a similar absolute incidence across skin tones but represents a proportionally much larger share of melanoma diagnoses in patients with darker skin given the comparatively lower incidence of ultraviolet-driven melanoma subtypes in this population, is less familiar to both patients and some clinicians and is more frequently mistaken for trauma, a subungual hematoma, or a benign process, contributing to diagnostic delay; lower perceived personal risk among both patients and clinicians, reflecting an outdated but persistent assumption that melanoma is predominantly a disease of lightly pigmented skin, reduces both patient self-surveillance behavior and clinician index of suspicion; and reduced access to dermatologic care in some patient populations further compounds these diagnostic delays. Deliberate attention to the acral surfaces, nail units, and mucosal surfaces during full-body skin examinations, and explicit patient education that melanoma, while less common overall in patients with darker skin tones, still occurs and preferentially affects these specific anatomic sites in this population, are practical steps that directly address this well-documented disparity.

Clinical Case: A Persistent Dark Patch Mistaken for a Bruise

A 58-year-old woman with Fitzpatrick skin type VI presented for evaluation of a dark, irregularly bordered patch on her right heel that she had first noticed approximately eight months earlier and had assumed represented a bruise from an unremembered minor injury, given her recollection of occasionally bumping her foot against furniture; the lesion had not resolved over this extended timeframe as an ordinary bruise would be expected to, prompting her eventual presentation. Examination revealed an irregularly bordered, variably pigmented brown-black patch measuring approximately 1.8 centimeters on the plantar heel, with dermoscopic examination showing a parallel ridge pattern, a finding recognized as concerning for acral lentiginous melanoma when identified on volar skin.

Biopsy confirmed acral lentiginous melanoma, and given the lesion's considerable size and the diagnostic delay that had already occurred, staging workup was pursued promptly, ultimately demonstrating disease still confined to the primary site without nodal or distant involvement. She underwent wide local excision with clear margins and sentinel lymph node biopsy, which was negative, and was counseled extensively, with sensitivity to her understandable frustration at the diagnostic delay, that acral lentiginous melanoma is frequently initially mistaken for a bruise or other minor traumatic finding precisely because it occurs on a body site not typically associated with melanoma risk in general patient and clinician awareness, and that her ongoing surveillance would specifically include careful examination of her palms, soles, and nail units at every future visit given both her personal history and the disproportionate representation of this melanoma subtype in patients with her skin tone.

Clinical Case: Progressive Hair Loss Dismissed as Ordinary Shedding

A 42-year-old woman presented with several years of gradually progressive hair loss beginning at the crown of her scalp, which she had attributed to stress and ordinary age-related thinning and had managed by adjusting her hairstyle to conceal the affected area; she reported intermittent scalp tenderness and an occasional burning sensation over the involved area that had been present for even longer than the visible hair loss itself, though she had not previously mentioned these symptoms to a clinician, assuming they were unrelated. Examination revealed centrally located hair loss at the vertex with smooth, shiny skin and loss of visible follicular ostia in the affected area, surrounded by a peripheral zone of more subtle thinning, findings consistent with central centrifugal cicatricial alopecia.

A scalp biopsy confirmed the diagnosis, showing perifollicular fibrosis and a reduced follicular density consistent with established scarring alopecia, and she was counseled that the smooth, follicle-free central area represented permanent, irreversible hair loss, but that prompt treatment could halt further centrifugal progression and preserve her remaining hair in the surrounding, still-active zone of disease. She was started on a combination of intralesional corticosteroid injections to the active peripheral zone, an oral anti-inflammatory agent, and a topical anti-inflammatory regimen for daily use, along with specific counseling regarding hairstyling practices that reduce ongoing traction and thermal or chemical trauma to the scalp. At follow-up over the subsequent year, her disease progression had halted, and this case prompted a broader discussion in her care about the importance of asking specifically about scalp symptoms, tenderness, itching, and burning, in patients of African descent even when hair loss is not the presenting complaint, given how commonly these prodromal symptoms precede visible hair loss in this condition and how easily they can be dismissed by both patient and clinician as nonspecific or unrelated.

THE MORPHOLOGY-TO-MANAGEMENT SYSTEM — Recalibrating the Pattern for the Full Range of Skin Tones

---

Pattern Introduced This Chapter: The violaceous rather than pink-red inflammatory plaque, the persistent pigmentary change that outlasts and outweighs the original inflammatory concern, and the acral dark patch mistaken for an ordinary bruise.

Cross-Cutting Anchor: Every classic dermatologic description in this text emphasizing erythema, redness, or pink coloration must be mentally recalibrated toward violaceous, gray-brown, or simply darker-than-surrounding-skin discoloration when examining a patient with a darker skin tone, and pigmentary sequelae and site-specific disease patterns unique to skin of color must be actively anticipated rather than incidentally noticed.

Summary and Key Concepts

Erythema and inflammation present as violaceous, gray-brown, or darker discoloration rather than classic pink-red color in more deeply pigmented skin, making palpation and scale assessment proportionately more important diagnostic tools.

Post-inflammatory hyperpigmentation is frequently the most distressing concern for patients with skin of color and requires early inflammatory control, strict photoprotection, and dedicated pigment-directed therapy.

Keloids extend beyond original wound margins and occur disproportionately in darker skin tones, and surgical excision without planned adjuvant therapy carries a high recurrence risk.

Central centrifugal cicatricial alopecia and traction alopecia are potentially reversible in early, non-scarring stages but cause permanent hair loss once scarring is established, making early recognition essential.

Melasma requires strict broad-spectrum and visible-light photoprotection alongside pigment-directed topical therapy, with realistic expectations set for gradual rather than complete improvement.

Laser and energy-based procedures require longer wavelengths, longer pulse durations, lower fluences, and conservative test spots in darker skin tones to minimize pigmentary complications, and melanoma diagnostic delay in patients with skin of color reflects underrecognition of acral lentiginous subtypes.

CHAPTER 23: GENITAL, MUCOSAL, AND ANOGENITAL DERMATOSES

Learning Objectives

1. Recognize lichen sclerosus and distinguish it from its common mimics, including vitiligo and lichen planus.
2. Construct an evidence-based approach to the evaluation of genital ulcers, distinguishing infectious from non-infectious causes.
3. Diagnose and manage the common causes of balanitis and vulvar dermatitis.
4. Recognize oral lichen planus and the other major inflammatory conditions affecting the oral mucosa.
5. Identify vulvar and penile intraepithelial neoplasia and understand the appropriate biopsy and surveillance approach.
6. Apply an evidence-based framework to the evaluation and management of vulvodynia and other chronic genital pain syndromes.

Dermatologic conditions affecting the genital, anogenital, and oral mucosal surfaces present distinct diagnostic challenges that set them apart from disease occurring on keratinized skin elsewhere on the body: the thinner, more delicate, non-keratinized or minimally keratinized epithelium at these sites alters the classic morphologic appearance of many otherwise familiar dermatoses, chronic moisture and occlusion favor a distinct set of infectious and irritant contributors, and the substantial psychosocial and sexual health dimensions of disease at these sites require a particularly sensitive, unhurried clinical approach. This chapter addresses the inflammatory, neoplastic, and idiopathic conditions of the genital and oral mucosal surfaces not already covered in detail elsewhere in this text, with particular attention to the diagnostic pitfalls that most commonly lead to delayed or incorrect diagnosis at these anatomically and psychologically sensitive sites.

Lichen Sclerosus

Lichen sclerosus is a chronic, inflammatory condition most commonly affecting the anogenital skin, presenting as porcelain-white, atrophic, often crinkled or "cigarette paper"-textured plaques classically distributed in a figure-of-eight pattern encompassing the vulva and perianal skin in women, or affecting the glans and foreskin in men, where it is often referred to by the clinical synonym balanitis xerotica obliterans; the condition occurs across a wide age range, including a well-recognized prepubertal presentation in girls that is sometimes mistakenly attributed to sexual abuse given the anogenital location and associated purpura, a mimic that requires careful clinical distinction and sensitive family communication. Chronic untreated lichen sclerosus produces progressive scarring with architectural changes including labial resorption, clitoral hood fusion burying the clitoris, and introital narrowing in women, and phimosis, meatal stenosis, and urethral stricture in men, complications that make early, adequately potent treatment essential rather than optional, since these architectural changes are generally irreversible once established even with subsequent successful disease control.

Ultra-high-potency topical corticosteroids, most commonly clobetasol propionate ointment, applied on a structured induction-then-maintenance schedule, remain the first-line treatment for lichen sclerosus and are highly effective at controlling symptoms and halting architectural progression when used consistently and at adequate potency; a common and clinically significant error is underdosing this condition out of an excessive, generalized concern about corticosteroid-related atrophy on genital skin, a concern that, while appropriately applied to many other genital dermatoses, does not apply in the same way to lichen sclerosus, where the disease process itself, not the ultra-high-potency corticosteroid treatment, is the primary driver of the atrophic, sclerotic skin changes, and adequately treated lichen sclerosus in fact typically shows histologic and clinical improvement in skin texture with successful treatment rather than progressive atrophy from the medication itself.

KEY POINT: Contrary to a common misconception, ultra-high-potency topical corticosteroids are the appropriate and necessary first-line treatment for lichen sclerosus, and underdosing out of excessive caution regarding steroid atrophy allows the disease's own irreversible scarring process to progress unchecked; the treating clinician should distinguish disease-related atrophy, which improves with adequate treatment, from a truly excessive treatment-related concern, which is uncommon at appropriate treatment durations and monitored follow-up intervals.

Lichen sclerosus carries a well-documented, though modest in absolute terms, increased risk of vulvar and penile squamous cell carcinoma arising within chronically affected skin, making long-term surveillance, generally at six- to twelve-month intervals, an essential component of ongoing management even once symptoms are well controlled, and any area of persistent thickening, ulceration, or a new nodule arising within a background of otherwise stable lichen sclerosus warrants prompt biopsy to exclude malignant transformation rather than being attributed reflexively to the underlying benign disease process.

Genital Lichen Planus

Genital lichen planus can present as the classic violaceous, flat-topped papules described in the chapter on papulosquamous disorders elsewhere in this text, but more distinctively and more challengingly presents in an erosive form, particularly affecting the vulvovaginal mucosa, producing painful, well-demarcated erosions with a surrounding whitish, lacy Wickham striae-like border; erosive vulvovaginal lichen planus frequently coexists with erosive disease of the oral mucosa and, less commonly, the gingiva, a combination sometimes referred to as the vulvovaginal-gingival syndrome, and recognition of this multi-site pattern should prompt a thorough examination of all three mucosal sites whenever erosive disease is identified at any one of them. Erosive genital lichen planus carries a substantial risk of progressive vaginal and vulvar scarring, including vaginal synechiae and introital stenosis, if inadequately treated, again underscoring the importance of adequately potent topical or, for more severe or treatment-resistant disease, systemic immunosuppressive therapy, together with the use of vaginal dilators in appropriately selected patients to help preserve vaginal caliber during the active treatment period.

CAUTION: Erosive vulvovaginal lichen planus is frequently misdiagnosed initially as recurrent candidiasis or an atrophic, hormonally mediated process given its erosive, sometimes ill-defined appearance, leading to a prolonged trial of ineffective antifungal or hormonal therapy; a well-demarcated erosion with a lacy white border, particularly when accompanied by oral mucosal disease, should prompt biopsy for confirmation rather than continued empiric treatment for these more common alternative diagnoses.

Balanitis and Vulvar Dermatitis

Balanitis, inflammation of the glans penis, encompasses a range of underlying causes that are usefully distinguished by their characteristic morphology and associated features. Candidal balanitis presents with erythema and superficial pustules or erosions, often with a fine white surface exudate, and is more common in uncircumcised men and those with diabetes mellitus, making a fasting glucose or hemoglobin A1c a reasonable component of the workup for recurrent or treatment-resistant candidal balanitis in a patient without a previously established diabetes diagnosis. Zoon balanitis (plasma cell balanitis), an idiopathic inflammatory condition most common in uncircumcised, middle-aged to older men, presents as a well-demarcated, glistening, orange-red plaque on the glans, classically described as having a "cayenne pepper" stippled appearance on closer inspection reflecting extravasated erythrocytes and plasma cell infiltration seen on biopsy, and is generally responsive to topical corticosteroids or topical calcineurin inhibitors, with circumcision serving as a definitive, curative option for treatment-resistant or recurrent disease given the condition's strong association with the chronic moisture and friction of the uncircumcised state.

Vulvar dermatitis, whether irritant, allergic contact, or seborrheic in etiology, frequently presents with a nonspecific pattern of erythema, lichenification from chronic scratching, and fissuring that can be challenging to definitively subclassify on clinical grounds alone; a careful history focused on potential irritant or allergen exposures, including feminine hygiene products, laundry detergents, topical medications previously applied to the area, and even chronic friction from tight clothing, is often more diagnostically productive than physical examination alone, and patch testing should be considered for presumed allergic contact dermatitis that persists despite removal of the most commonly implicated irritants. Given the considerable morphologic overlap among the various causes of vulvar dermatitis, and the potential for lichen sclerosus, lichen planus, and even early vulvar intraepithelial neoplasia to mimic a more benign inflammatory dermatitis, a low threshold for biopsy of any vulvar eruption that fails to respond to an appropriate empiric treatment trial within several weeks is a prudent general practice.

Fixed drug eruption affecting the genital skin deserves specific mention as an underrecognized cause of recurrent genital erosion, since patients and clinicians alike frequently fail to connect a recurring genital lesion to an oral medication taken for an unrelated indication; common culprit medications include nonsteroidal anti-inflammatory drugs, certain antibiotics, and some over-the-counter analgesics, and a history specifically probing for any medication taken in the day or two preceding each episode, cross-referenced against prior episodes, can reveal the causative agent even when the patient had not previously suspected a medication-related cause.

KEY POINT: Candidal balanitis and Zoon balanitis are distinguished primarily by morphology, superficial pustules and white exudate for candidal balanitis versus a well-demarcated, glistening orange-red "cayenne pepper" plaque for Zoon balanitis, and confirming the diagnosis with a potassium hydroxide preparation or biopsy avoids an unnecessary and ineffective prolonged course of antifungal treatment for a patient who in fact has Zoon balanitis.

Anatomic Variants Frequently Mistaken for Disease

Several entirely normal anatomic variants of the genital skin are commonly mistaken by patients, and occasionally by clinicians unfamiliar with their characteristic appearance, for warts or another sexually transmitted infection, and confident recognition of these variants prevents unnecessary anxiety, unnecessary treatment, and, at times, significant relationship distress stemming from an incorrect presumptive diagnosis. Pearly penile papules present as small, uniform, dome-shaped to filiform papules arranged in one or more rows circumferentially around the corona of the glans penis, are entirely asymptomatic, and represent a normal anatomic variant rather than a human papillomavirus-related growth; their regular, symmetric, circumferential arrangement, in contrast to the more irregular, variably sized, and randomly distributed appearance of genital warts, is the key distinguishing feature, and no treatment is medically necessary, though removal can be considered for patients with significant cosmetic concern. Vestibular papillomatosis, the analogous normal variant in women, presents as small, soft, symmetric papillae on the vulvar vestibule, similarly requiring only reassurance once distinguished from condyloma acuminata by its soft, non-coalescing, symmetric appearance.

Fordyce spots (ectopic sebaceous glands), presenting as small, grouped, yellowish-white papules on the labia, penile shaft, or oral mucosa, and angiokeratomas of Fordyce, presenting as small, dark red to violaceous, slightly keratotic papules most common on the scrotum and vulva in older adults, are two further entirely benign anatomic and vascular variants that are frequently mistaken by patients for a wart, molluscum, or other concerning growth; both are readily distinguished from these mimics on clinical examination alone in the substantial majority of cases, and patient reassurance, delivered with a clear explanation of the specific benign entity identified, is the appropriate management for both findings in the absence of associated symptoms or diagnostic uncertainty.

KEY POINT: Pearly penile papules, vestibular papillomatosis, Fordyce spots, and angiokeratomas of Fordyce are among the most common sources of patient anxiety and misdiagnosis in genital dermatology precisely because each can superficially resemble a wart or other sexually transmitted infection; confident recognition and clear patient education prevent unnecessary treatment and considerable unwarranted distress.

Anogenital Warts and Their Differentiation From Benign Variants

Condyloma acuminata, caused by low-risk human papillomavirus subtypes, present as soft, flesh-colored to hyperpigmented, exophytic papules with a characteristically irregular, cauliflower-like or filiform surface texture, in variable numbers and often coalescing into larger plaques with progressive growth, a morphology that, unlike the anatomic variants discussed above, is genuinely irregular and asymmetric in its distribution rather than following the uniform, symmetric, circumferential or grouped pattern of a benign anatomic variant. Application of dilute acetic acid, producing acetowhitening of infected epithelium, can assist in identifying subclinical lesions and in distinguishing condyloma from surrounding normal tissue, though this test lacks perfect specificity and should be interpreted within the overall clinical context rather than relied upon in isolation. Treatment options include patient-applied topical therapies such as imiquimod, podophyllotoxin, and sinecatechins, and clinician-administered treatments including cryotherapy, trichloroacetic acid, and surgical or laser removal for more extensive disease, with the choice guided by lesion number, location, and patient preference, and human papillomavirus vaccination should be discussed with all age-eligible patients presenting with anogenital warts, both to reduce the risk of future new lesions from additional vaccine-covered subtypes and to reduce the risk of the high-risk oncogenic human papillomavirus subtypes responsible for cervical, anal, and oropharyngeal dysplasia and carcinoma.

Condylomata lata, an important and distinct mimic of condyloma acuminata occurring in secondary syphilis, present as smooth, moist, flat-topped, often broad-based papules and plaques rather than the irregular, papillomatous surface texture of condyloma acuminata, and this distinction carries substantial clinical importance, since condylomata lata are highly infectious and their recognition should prompt immediate syphilis serologic testing and, if confirmed, treatment with the same protocols used for other stages of syphilis rather than any of the wart-directed treatments described above, which have no role in this infectious, syphilis-related condition.

CAUTION: A broad-based, smooth-surfaced, moist genital plaque should raise suspicion for condylomata lata of secondary syphilis rather than being reflexively treated as ordinary condyloma acuminata; confirmatory syphilis serology should be obtained whenever this morphology is encountered, given the substantially different treatment implications and the highly infectious nature of untreated secondary syphilis.

Genital Ulcers: An Evaluation Framework

A genital ulcer requires a systematic evaluation that considers both infectious and non-infectious causes, since the clinical appearance of ulcers from different etiologies frequently overlaps considerably more than classic textbook descriptions suggest. Herpes simplex virus infection, the most common infectious cause, typically presents with grouped vesicles progressing to shallow, painful erosions, often recurrent at the same anatomic site, while primary syphilis presents with a classically painless, indurated ulcer (chancre) with a clean base, and chancroid, caused by Haemophilus ducreyi and considerably less common in most developed-world settings, presents with a painful, ragged-edged ulcer often accompanied by tender suppurative inguinal lymphadenopathy; because clinical appearance alone is an unreliable means of distinguishing among these and other infectious causes, and because coinfection with more than one causative organism is not uncommon, a genital ulcer evaluation should include, at minimum, herpes simplex virus polymerase chain reaction or viral culture and syphilis serology, with additional infectious testing guided by the specific clinical context, exposure history, and local disease prevalence.

Non-infectious causes of genital ulceration, though considerably less common overall, are important to recognize given their distinct management implications. Aphthous-type genital ulcers, morphologically similar to oral aphthous ulcers, can occur as an isolated finding or in association with Behçet disease, discussed further below, and fixed drug eruption, presenting as a sharply demarcated, often dusky-violaceous erosive or ulcerated plaque recurring at the identical anatomic site with each re-exposure to the causative medication, is an important and sometimes overlooked non-infectious cause that should prompt a careful medication history, with particular attention to any new or recently resumed medication preceding the most recent episode. A genital ulcer that fails to heal within the expected timeframe for its presumed cause, or that fails to respond to appropriate treatment directed at that presumed cause, warrants biopsy to exclude a neoplastic process, including squamous cell carcinoma arising within a background of lichen sclerosus or lichen planus as discussed above.

A thorough sexual history, obtained privately and non-judgmentally, is an essential component of every genital ulcer evaluation, since the specific exposure history meaningfully informs both the pretest probability of the various infectious causes and the appropriate scope of additional sexually transmitted infection screening, including human immunodeficiency virus testing, which should be offered as a routine component of the evaluation given the well-established association between genital ulcerative disease and increased human immunodeficiency virus transmission risk; this discussion should be conducted with the same clinical neutrality and confidentiality afforded to any other component of the medical history, since a patient who senses judgment is considerably less likely to provide the accurate exposure history needed to guide appropriate testing and treatment.

CAUTION: The clinical appearance of a genital ulcer, whether painful or painless, indurated or soft-based, is an unreliable means of confidently distinguishing among infectious causes; herpes simplex virus testing and syphilis serology should be pursued for essentially every genital ulcer evaluation regardless of its apparent classic or atypical clinical appearance, given the substantial and well-documented overlap in presentation among these conditions.

Behçet Disease

Behçet disease is a systemic vasculitis characterized by the classic triad of recurrent oral aphthous ulcers, genital ulcers, and uveitis, though the full clinical spectrum extends considerably further to include cutaneous findings such as erythema nodosum-like lesions and pathergy (the development of a sterile pustule at the site of minor skin trauma such as a needle prick, a finding with reasonable diagnostic specificity when formally tested), together with a range of potential systemic vascular, neurologic, and gastrointestinal manifestations that determine much of the disease's overall morbidity; the disease shows a distinctive geographic distribution with substantially higher prevalence along the historic Silk Road region extending from East Asia through the Mediterranean, a pattern that has prompted extensive investigation into shared genetic and possibly environmental contributors across these populations. Oral and genital ulcers in Behçet disease closely resemble simple aphthous ulcers in isolation, making the diagnosis fundamentally a clinical one requiring recognition of the broader symptom complex and its characteristic recurrent, multi-system pattern over time rather than any single specific diagnostic test, and management requires close coordination with rheumatology and ophthalmology given the disease's potential for serious ocular and systemic vascular complications extending well beyond the mucocutaneous findings that often bring the patient to initial dermatologic attention.

Oral Mucosal Disease

Oral lichen planus, the mucosal counterpart of the more familiar cutaneous condition, presents in several recognized patterns: reticular disease, the most common and generally asymptomatic pattern, showing the characteristic lacy, white Wickham striae most often on the buccal mucosa; erosive disease, presenting with painful erosions and ulceration that can substantially impair eating and oral hygiene; and, less commonly, a plaque-like or atrophic pattern. Erosive oral lichen planus carries a small but recognized risk of malignant transformation to oral squamous cell carcinoma, making periodic surveillance and biopsy of any area of persistent ulceration, induration, or a new mass arising within a background of established oral lichen planus an essential long-term management practice, generally coordinated with oral medicine or otolaryngology specialists experienced in the surveillance of this specific condition. Recurrent aphthous stomatitis, considerably more common than oral lichen planus, presents with recurrent, painful, shallow ulcers with a grayish-white base and an erythematous halo, most often on non-keratinized oral mucosa, and while the majority of cases are idiopathic and self-limited, recurrent or unusually severe aphthous stomatitis should prompt consideration of associated systemic conditions, including inflammatory bowel disease, celiac disease, nutritional deficiencies (most notably iron, vitamin B12, and folate), and, as discussed above, Behçet disease when accompanied by genital ulceration or other suggestive systemic features.

Geographic tongue (benign migratory glossitis), presenting as well-demarcated, map-like areas of depapillation on the dorsal tongue surface that characteristically change in size, shape, and location over days to weeks, is an entirely benign, asymptomatic or mildly symptomatic finding requiring only patient reassurance regarding its benign nature once the classically migratory, changing pattern has been confirmed on serial observation or history, distinguishing it from more concerning fixed leukoplakic or erythroplakic mucosal lesions that do not show this same migratory behavior and that warrant a fundamentally different diagnostic approach given their own potential association with dysplasia or malignancy, discussed further below.

Angular cheilitis, presenting as erythema, fissuring, and maceration at the oral commissures, most commonly reflects chronic moisture accumulation and secondary candidal or bacterial colonization at this site, frequently related to age-associated changes in oral commissure architecture, ill-fitting dentures, or exaggerated perioral skin folds, and management combines a topical antifungal or, when bacterial superinfection is present, a combination antifungal-antibacterial preparation with correction of the underlying anatomic or mechanical contributor whenever feasible, since treatment directed at the superficial infection alone without addressing the underlying moisture-trapping anatomy frequently yields only temporary improvement before recurrence.

KEY POINT: A well-demarcated white or red oral mucosal lesion that does not migrate or change over serial observation, in contrast to the classic migratory pattern of geographic tongue, should be considered leukoplakia or erythroplakia until proven otherwise and warrants biopsy given the recognized association of both findings with mucosal dysplasia and squamous cell carcinoma.

Vulvar and Penile Intraepithelial Neoplasia

Vulvar and penile intraepithelial neoplasia represent precursor lesions to invasive squamous cell carcinoma at these sites and are broadly divided into human papillomavirus-associated disease, most common in younger patients and closely related to the same high-risk human papillomavirus subtypes responsible for cervical dysplasia, and differentiated-type intraepithelial neoplasia, which is not human papillomavirus-driven and instead arises within a background of chronic inflammatory dermatoses, most notably lichen sclerosus and lichen planus as discussed above, typically in older patients and carrying a distinct, generally more rapid progression to invasive carcinoma than the human papillomavirus-associated subtype. Clinical presentation is variable and can include white, red, or pigmented plaques or papules, sometimes with a verrucous or eroded surface, and given this considerable morphologic overlap with a range of benign inflammatory and infectious conditions discussed throughout this chapter, biopsy is required for definitive diagnosis whenever a persistent, atypical, or treatment-resistant vulvar or penile lesion is identified, particularly in a patient with an established background of lichen sclerosus or lichen planus given the meaningfully elevated risk in this specific clinical context.

CAUTION: Differentiated-type vulvar and penile intraepithelial neoplasia arising within a background of lichen sclerosus or lichen planus can progress to invasive squamous cell carcinoma more rapidly than human papillomavirus-associated intraepithelial neoplasia, and any new area of thickening, persistent erosion, or a distinct nodule within chronically affected skin in a patient with either underlying condition warrants prompt biopsy rather than continued observation.

Anogenital Involvement of Hidradenitis Suppurativa

Hidradenitis suppurativa, a chronic inflammatory condition of the follicular unit within apocrine gland-bearing skin, frequently involves the genital, perianal, and inguinal folds in addition to its more classically emphasized axillary and inframammary predilection, and anogenital involvement carries its own specific diagnostic and management considerations worth highlighting in this chapter dedicated to genital and anogenital disease. Painful, deep-seated nodules, abscesses, and, in more advanced disease, interconnected sinus tracts draining malodorous purulent material in the groin, perianal, and perivulvar or perineal skin can be mistaken for a simple furuncle, an anorectal fistula of Crohn disease, or a sexually transmitted infection, and the distinguishing features, a chronic, relapsing course over months to years, bilateral or multifocal involvement, and the characteristic double-headed or bridged comedones seen in more advanced disease, should prompt consideration of hidradenitis suppurativa rather than a presumption of an isolated acute infectious process. Anogenital hidradenitis suppurativa in particular carries a well-documented, though not fully explained, association with an increased risk of squamous cell carcinoma arising within chronically inflamed sinus tracts in long-standing, severe disease, making any area of new induration, non-healing ulceration, or unusually rapid change within longstanding perianal or genital hidradenitis suppurativa an indication for prompt biopsy.

Management of anogenital hidradenitis suppurativa follows the same general stage-based treatment framework used elsewhere on the body, incorporating topical and systemic antibiotics, hormonal therapy in appropriately selected patients, biologic therapy targeting tumor necrosis factor-alpha or other inflammatory pathways for moderate to severe disease, and surgical management, including wide local excision of chronically involved tissue, for the most severe, treatment-resistant disease; the genital and perianal location introduces additional practical considerations regarding wound healing, continence, and sexual function that should be discussed explicitly and sensitively when surgical management is being considered at these anatomically and psychologically significant sites, and a colorectal surgery consultation is frequently warranted when perianal disease raises concern for a coexisting or confounding anorectal fistula given the considerable clinical overlap between these two conditions in this location.

Special Populations: Pediatric and Postmenopausal Considerations

Beyond the prepubertal presentation of lichen sclerosus discussed in the clinical case below, several additional pediatric-specific considerations warrant attention in genital dermatology. Labial adhesions, a common finding in young girls resulting from fusion of the labia minora in the setting of low estrogen levels, low-grade chronic irritation, or both, typically resolve spontaneously with the onset of puberty and estrogenization, and treatment, when required for associated urinary symptoms, generally begins with a conservative trial of topical estrogen cream rather than surgical separation, which carries a high recurrence rate when performed on adhesions that have not first been given an adequate trial of medical management. In postmenopausal women, the genitourinary syndrome of menopause, resulting from declining estrogen levels, produces vulvovaginal atrophy, dryness, and thinning that can itself mimic or coexist with several of the inflammatory conditions discussed in this chapter, and distinguishing atrophy-related symptoms from a superimposed inflammatory dermatosis such as lichen sclerosus or lichen planus, both of which also occur with increased frequency in the postmenopausal population, often requires careful clinical correlation and, when diagnostic uncertainty persists, biopsy; topical vaginal estrogen therapy, when not contraindicated, can meaningfully improve genitourinary syndrome of menopause symptoms and should be considered as an adjunct to, though not a replacement for, disease-specific treatment when a coexisting inflammatory dermatosis is identified.

Vulvodynia and Chronic Genital Pain

Vulvodynia, defined as chronic vulvar pain of at least three months' duration without a clearly identifiable underlying cause on examination, represents a diagnosis of exclusion reached only after the specific dermatoses and infectious causes discussed throughout this chapter, along with musculoskeletal, neurologic, and psychological contributors, have been appropriately considered and excluded through a thorough history and examination; the condition is subclassified based on whether the pain is provoked (typically by touch or attempted penetration) or unprovoked, and localized (most often to the vulvar vestibule) or generalized, a classification framework that meaningfully guides the selection of subsequent management strategies. Management is necessarily multidisciplinary and individualized, incorporating pelvic floor physical therapy given the frequent contribution of pelvic floor muscle hypertonicity to the pain experience, topical or oral neuropathic pain agents, and, for many patients, psychological support addressing the substantial impact chronic genital pain has on sexual function, relationships, and overall quality of life; validating the patient's pain experience explicitly and early, rather than implying that a normal-appearing examination means the pain is not real or not significant, is an essential component of building the therapeutic relationship required for this often protracted, multidisciplinary treatment process.

PATIENT EDUCATION: A normal-appearing genital examination in the setting of chronic genital pain does not mean the pain is not real or is psychological in origin; vulvodynia is a recognized medical condition with an evolving understanding of its underlying neurologic and muscular contributors, and effective, evidence-based multidisciplinary treatment options exist even when no specific visible abnormality is identified on examination.

Clinical Case: Anogenital Purpura Concerning for Abuse

A 6-year-old girl was brought in by her mother for evaluation of vulvar itching and, more concerningly to the family, several areas of purpura noted around the vulva and perianal skin, raising immediate parental concern for possible sexual abuse and considerable family distress. Examination revealed porcelain-white, atrophic plaques in a classic figure-of-eight distribution encompassing the vulva and perianal skin, with several areas of purpura and mild fissuring superimposed on the atrophic plaques but no other examination findings suggestive of trauma, and a careful, sensitively conducted history revealed no behavioral or historical features raising independent concern for abuse.

The clinical presentation was recognized as consistent with prepubertal vulvar lichen sclerosus, a well-described entity in which the characteristic skin fragility of the disease itself predisposes to spontaneous or minor-trauma-related purpura and fissuring that can be visually alarming and, without specific familiarity with this presentation, mistakenly attributed to abuse; the family was counseled thoroughly and sensitively on this distinction, and the diagnosis was confirmed on histopathology from a small, carefully performed biopsy. Treatment with an appropriately potent topical corticosteroid under close pediatric dermatology follow-up produced substantial symptomatic improvement over the following weeks, and the family was counseled regarding the chronic nature of the condition, the importance of long-term surveillance into adulthood, and the specific reassurance that the purpura she had presented with was a recognized direct consequence of the skin fragility inherent to lichen sclerosus itself rather than a sign of abuse, a distinction that meaningfully eased the family's considerable initial distress.

Clinical Case: Painful Oral and Genital Ulcers With a Delayed Unifying Diagnosis

A 26-year-old man presented with a two-year history of recurrent, painful oral ulcers, treated intermittently by his primary care physician and dentist as ordinary aphthous stomatitis, and, over the preceding eight months, several episodes of similarly painful ulcers on the scrotum that he had not previously connected to his oral symptoms or mentioned to any of his treating clinicians given embarrassment about the genital location. He additionally reported an episode of eye redness and pain approximately four months earlier that had been evaluated and treated by an outside ophthalmologist as anterior uveitis, again without any clinician having yet connected these three separate symptom episodes into a single unifying diagnosis.

A more complete, specifically directed history obtained during this visit revealed the full triad of recurrent oral ulcers, genital ulcers, and uveitis, together with a positive pathergy test performed in clinic, in which a sterile needle prick to the forearm produced a small pustule at twenty-four hours, supporting a clinical diagnosis of Behçet disease. He was referred urgently to rheumatology and ophthalmology for coordinated multidisciplinary management, and colchicine was initiated for his mucocutaneous symptoms while further systemic evaluation proceeded to assess for other potential vascular or systemic manifestations of the disease. This case was used as a teaching point for the broader lesson that recurrent oral and genital ulceration evaluated separately, by different clinicians, and without an explicitly obtained combined history, can each be individually misattributed to a common, isolated benign process for a considerable period of time before the underlying systemic, unifying diagnosis becomes apparent, underscoring the importance of directly and specifically asking about oral, genital, and ocular symptoms together whenever any one of the three is the presenting concern.

THE MORPHOLOGY-TO-MANAGEMENT SYSTEM — Reading the Mucosal Surface on Its Own Terms

---

Pattern Introduced This Chapter: The porcelain-white figure-of-eight plaque mistaken for abuse, the erosive genital lichen planus mistaken for recurrent candidiasis, and the migratory geographic tongue mistaken for a fixed, concerning mucosal lesion.

Cross-Cutting Anchor: Genital and oral mucosal disease must be read against its own distinct set of expected patterns, distribution, and disease behavior rather than through the morphologic expectations built from keratinized skin elsewhere on the body, and a low threshold for biopsy is warranted whenever a genital or oral mucosal finding fails to fit its presumed diagnosis cleanly or fails to respond to appropriate empiric treatment.

Summary and Key Concepts

Lichen sclerosus requires adequately potent, ultra-high-potency topical corticosteroid treatment to prevent irreversible architectural scarring, and underdosing out of excessive atrophy concern allows disease-driven scarring to progress unchecked.

Erosive vulvovaginal and oral lichen planus is frequently mistaken for candidiasis or an atrophic process and carries a risk of progressive scarring if not adequately treated with appropriately potent anti-inflammatory therapy.

Candidal balanitis and Zoon balanitis are distinguished by morphology and confirmed with a potassium hydroxide preparation or biopsy, avoiding an ineffective prolonged antifungal trial.

Every genital ulcer evaluation should include herpes simplex virus testing and syphilis serology regardless of clinical appearance, given substantial overlap in presentation among infectious causes.

Differentiated-type vulvar and penile intraepithelial neoplasia arises within lichen sclerosus or lichen planus and can progress to invasive carcinoma more rapidly than human papillomavirus-associated disease, warranting a low threshold for biopsy of atypical lesions.

Vulvodynia is a diagnosis of exclusion managed with a multidisciplinary approach including pelvic floor physical therapy and neuropathic pain agents, and patient validation is essential even when examination findings are normal.

CHAPTER 24: DERMATOLOGIC EMERGENCIES

Learning Objectives

1. Recognize Stevens-Johnson syndrome and toxic epidermal necrolysis, distinguish them from their mimics, and initiate appropriate emergency management.
2. Diagnose drug reaction with eosinophilia and systemic symptoms and understand its characteristic delayed onset and multisystem involvement.
3. Construct a systematic differential diagnosis for erythroderma and identify the historical and examination features that narrow this differential.
4. Distinguish necrotizing fasciitis from cellulitis and recognize the clinical features that mandate emergent surgical evaluation.
5. Recognize staphylococcal scalded skin syndrome and purpura fulminans and understand their distinct pathophysiology and management priorities.
6. Apply an evidence-based approach to the recognition and emergent management of angioedema and anaphylaxis with prominent cutaneous involvement.

A small but critically important subset of dermatologic presentations represents a true medical emergency in which delayed recognition directly translates into increased morbidity and mortality, and this chapter is organized around the central clinical skill of rapid pattern recognition under time pressure: identifying the specific combination of skin findings, systemic symptoms, and historical context that should trigger an immediate escalation in the pace and intensity of evaluation and treatment, in clear contrast to the more measured diagnostic approach appropriate for the majority of conditions discussed elsewhere in this text. Every condition addressed in this chapter shares a common thread: each can, at least in its early stages, resemble a far more mundane process, and the clinical skill of distinguishing early dermatologic emergency from benign mimic under genuine time pressure is the unifying pedagogical purpose of this final core clinical chapter.

Stevens-Johnson Syndrome and Toxic Epidermal Necrolysis

Stevens-Johnson syndrome and toxic epidermal necrolysis represent a single disease spectrum, distinguished from one another primarily by the extent of body surface area affected by epidermal detachment, with Stevens-Johnson syndrome involving less than ten percent of body surface area, toxic epidermal necrolysis involving greater than thirty percent, and an overlap category occupying the intermediate range; the disease is most commonly triggered by a medication reaction, with certain drug classes carrying particularly well-established risk, including anticonvulsants (most notably aromatic anticonvulsants and lamotrigine), allopurinol, sulfonamide antibiotics, and certain nonsteroidal anti-inflammatory drugs, with onset typically occurring within one to eight weeks of starting the causative agent. The clinical presentation begins with a prodrome of fever, malaise, and mucosal discomfort, followed by the development of dusky, erythematous to violaceous macules and targetoid lesions that progress to flaccid bullae and, characteristically, sheet-like epidermal detachment; a positive Nikolsky sign, in which gentle lateral pressure on seemingly uninvolved skin produces immediate epidermal sliding and detachment, is a valuable bedside confirmatory finding, and mucosal involvement, affecting the oral, ocular, and genital mucosa in the substantial majority of cases, is an essential and highly characteristic diagnostic feature that helps distinguish this disease from its mimics.

CAUTION: Any patient presenting with fever, mucosal erosions, and a spreading dusky or targetoid eruption, particularly with a recent new medication started within the preceding several weeks, requires immediate discontinuation of all non-essential medications, urgent dermatology consultation, and assessment of body surface area involvement; delay in recognition directly increases the extent of epidermal detachment and associated mortality risk.

Several conditions can mimic the early presentation of Stevens-Johnson syndrome and toxic epidermal necrolysis and warrant consideration during initial evaluation: staphylococcal scalded skin syndrome, discussed in detail below, is distinguished primarily by its characteristic sparing of the mucosal surfaces; erythema multiforme major, though historically grouped with Stevens-Johnson syndrome in some classification schemes, is now recognized as a distinct entity most often triggered by herpes simplex virus infection rather than medication exposure, typically follows a more favorable course, and presents with more classically targetoid, symmetric acral lesions rather than the more widespread, confluent, dusky macules typical of Stevens-Johnson syndrome; and generalized bullous fixed drug eruption, while it can appear clinically similar, generally shows a less pronounced prodromal illness and a more favorable overall prognosis. Distinguishing among these conditions relies on a combination of clinical morphology, the presence or absence of a preceding herpes simplex virus infection, and, when the diagnosis remains uncertain, skin biopsy with frozen section, which can be obtained emergently to help guide the appropriate level of care while the more detailed permanent histologic sections are still being processed.

Immediate management centers on prompt identification and discontinuation of the causative medication, since continued exposure is strongly associated with worse outcomes, together with supportive care functionally analogous to that provided for a major burn, including fluid and electrolyte management, meticulous wound care, infection surveillance, and nutritional support, ideally provided within a burn unit or intensive care setting experienced in managing this specific disease given the combination of skin barrier failure and the risk of secondary infection and fluid loss; ophthalmology consultation should be obtained urgently given the substantial risk of long-term ocular complications, including corneal scarring and vision loss, from ocular mucosal involvement, and aggressive ocular surface care from the earliest recognition of the disease meaningfully reduces this long-term risk. Systemic immunomodulatory therapy, including intravenous immunoglobulin, cyclosporine, or systemic corticosteroids, is used at many specialized centers, though the evidence supporting any single specific agent remains less definitive than the evidence supporting prompt causative drug discontinuation and excellent supportive care, which together remain the most consistently emphasized priorities across published management guidelines.

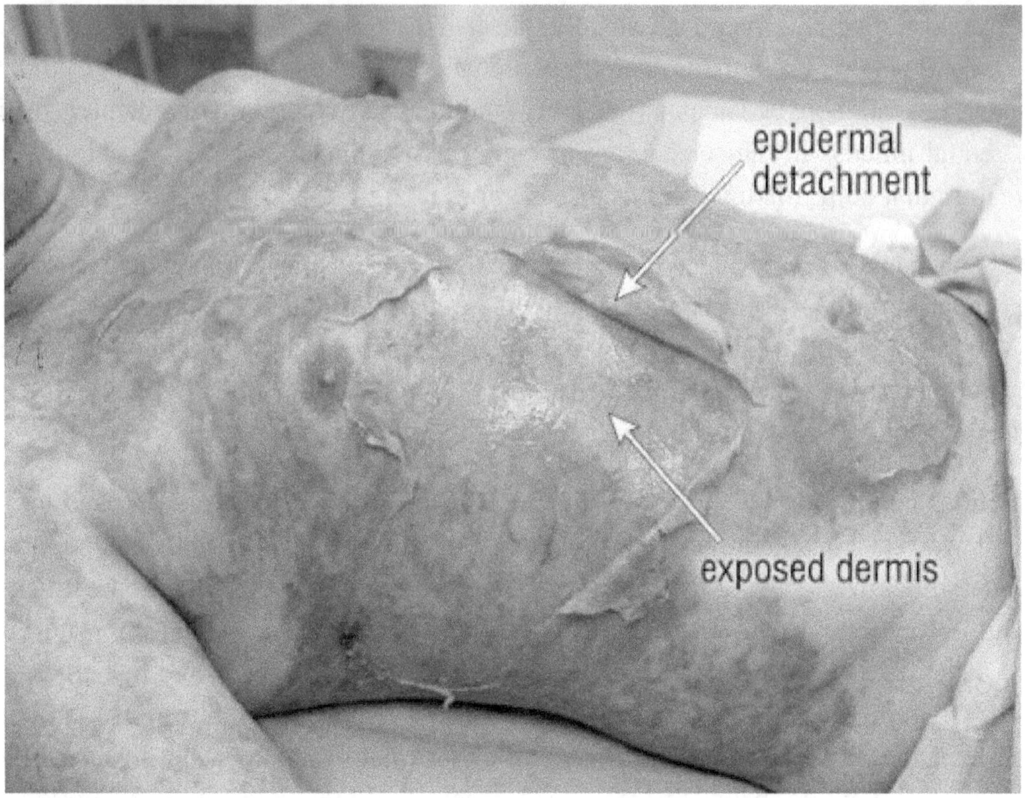

Long-term sequelae of Stevens-Johnson syndrome and toxic epidermal necrolysis extend well beyond the acute hospitalization and warrant proactive, coordinated long term follow-up: chronic ocular surface disease, including dry eye, symblepharon formation, and, in the most severe cases, progressive vision loss, can develop or continue to progress for months to years after the acute illness has resolved, making sustained ophthalmology follow-up essential rather than a single post-hospitalization visit; genital and, in women, vaginal scarring can similarly develop over time, and proactive gynecologic or urologic follow-up with early intervention, including the use of vaginal dilators when appropriate, can help prevent or reduce long-term architectural complications analogous to those discussed for erosive genital lichen planus in the preceding chapter.

KEY POINT: The SCORTEN severity-of-illness score, incorporating age, presence of malignancy, heart rate, initial body surface area of epidermal detachment, serum urea, serum bicarbonate, and serum glucose, provides a validated, structured tool for estimating mortality risk in toxic epidermal necrolysis and can help guide triage decisions regarding the appropriate level of care, though it is calculated as a supportive tool alongside, not a replacement for, ongoing clinical judgment and reassessment.

Drug Reaction With Eosinophilia and Systemic Symptoms

Drug reaction with eosinophilia and systemic symptoms, commonly abbreviated DRESS syndrome, is distinguished from most other severe cutaneous adverse drug reactions by its characteristically delayed onset, typically two to eight weeks after starting the causative medication, considerably longer than the more rapid onset typical of Stevens-Johnson syndrome and toxic epidermal necrolysis, a timing difference that can itself mislead both patient and clinician away from suspecting a medication as the cause given the substantial interval since the medication was started. Commonly implicated medications include aromatic anticonvulsants, allopurinol, and sulfonamide antibiotics, an overlapping list with the medications implicated in Stevens-Johnson syndrome and toxic epidermal necrolysis, and the clinical presentation includes a widespread morbilliform eruption, often with striking facial edema that can be an early and distinctive clue, fever, lymphadenopathy, and, critically, systemic organ involvement, most commonly hepatitis, but also potentially involving the kidneys, lungs, heart, and other organs, together with a peripheral eosinophilia that gives the syndrome its name, though eosinophilia can be absent or only modest, particularly early in the disease course.

Because the systemic organ involvement, rather than the cutaneous eruption itself, drives the majority of DRESS syndrome morbidity and the rare but real mortality risk, comprehensive laboratory evaluation including liver function tests, renal function, complete blood count with differential, and additional organ-specific testing guided by the clinical presentation is essential once the diagnosis is suspected, and this evaluation should be repeated serially over the following weeks, since organ involvement can evolve or new organ systems can become involved even after the causative medication has been discontinued and the cutaneous findings have begun to improve; systemic corticosteroids remain the mainstay of treatment for significant organ involvement, with the treatment course often required for a protracted period given the disease's well-recognized tendency to flare during corticosteroid tapering.

CAUTION: DRESS syndrome can flare, including with new or worsening organ involvement, during corticosteroid tapering or even weeks after apparent clinical resolution, and patients require extended follow-up with serial laboratory monitoring well beyond the point at which the cutaneous eruption has visibly improved, since cutaneous improvement does not reliably indicate that systemic disease activity has fully resolved.

Erythroderma: A Differential Diagnosis Framework

Erythroderma, defined as erythema and scaling involving greater than ninety percent of the body surface area, represents a final common cutaneous pathway for a diverse group of underlying conditions rather than a single disease entity, and the systemic physiologic consequences of erythroderma itself, including impaired thermoregulation, substantial insensible fluid loss, high-output cardiac strain, and an increased risk of secondary infection given the compromised skin barrier, can be life-threatening regardless of the specific underlying cause, making prompt recognition and supportive stabilization a priority even before the underlying etiology has been definitively established. A systematic approach to identifying the underlying cause incorporates a detailed history focused on preexisting skin disease (psoriasis and atopic dermatitis are among the most common underlying causes when a pre-existing dermatosis undergoes erythrodermic flare), new medications within a timeframe consistent with a drug reaction, and any personal or family history suggestive of cutaneous T-cell lymphoma, discussed in the earlier chapter on cutaneous lymphoma, given Sezary syndrome's characteristic erythrodermic presentation.

Ichthyosiform erythroderma and other genodermatoses discussed in the earlier chapter on pediatric dermatology can present with erythroderma from birth or early infancy, an important consideration distinguishing the congenital, lifelong erythrodermic presentations of severe congenital ichthyosis from the acquired, typically adult-onset erythroderma discussed throughout the remainder of this section, and a careful history establishing whether the erythroderma has been present since birth versus representing a new, acquired finding is itself one of the most useful initial branch points in narrowing this broad differential diagnosis.

Physical examination should specifically assess for lymphadenopathy, palmoplantar keratoderma, ectropion, and nail changes, each of which can help point toward a specific underlying cause, and skin biopsy, while sometimes nonspecific in the setting of erythroderma given the tendency of severe, prolonged inflammation to obscure the original disease-specific histologic features, remains a valuable component of the workup, particularly when performed at more than one time point or from more than one anatomic site if the initial biopsy is non-diagnostic; peripheral blood flow cytometry for a Sezary cell count and T-cell receptor gene rearrangement studies should be pursued when cutaneous T-cell lymphoma is a diagnostic consideration, as discussed in the earlier chapter on cutaneous lymphoma. Regardless of the ultimately identified underlying cause, initial supportive management is similar across etiologies and includes careful attention to fluid and electrolyte balance, temperature regulation given the significant thermoregulatory impairment erythroderma produces, bland emollients, and monitoring for secondary infection, with disease-specific therapy layered on once the underlying cause has been identified.

KEY POINT: Erythroderma is a physiologic emergency in its own right, independent of the underlying cause, given the risks of thermoregulatory failure, high-output cardiac strain, and substantial insensible fluid loss through the compromised skin barrier; supportive stabilization should proceed in parallel with, not be delayed by, the diagnostic workup to identify the specific underlying etiology.

Necrotizing Fasciitis and Severe Soft Tissue Infection

Necrotizing fasciitis is a rapidly progressive, life-threatening soft tissue infection extending along fascial planes that requires emergent surgical debridement as its primary, life-saving treatment, and distinguishing it from ordinary cellulitis at initial presentation, when the two conditions can appear deceptively similar, is one of the most consequential diagnostic tasks in this entire chapter given the disease's capacity to progress from subtle initial findings to fulminant, life-threatening illness within hours. Clinical features that should raise concern for necrotizing fasciitis rather than simple cellulitis include pain markedly out of proportion to the visible examination findings, a finding considered one of the single most reliable early clues to this diagnosis; rapid progression of erythema and swelling over a period of hours rather than the more gradual progression typical of ordinary cellulitis; the development of hemorrhagic bullae, dusky discoloration, or cutaneous anesthesia (reflecting destruction of cutaneous nerves within the advancing infection) within the affected area; and systemic toxicity, including fever, tachycardia, and hypotension, that appears disproportionate to the visible extent of the cutaneous findings.

CAUTION: Pain markedly out of proportion to examination findings, in a patient with an apparently ordinary cellulitis, is one of the most important and most frequently under-recognized early clues to necrotizing fasciitis; this specific historical detail should prompt urgent surgical consultation and consideration of imaging, rather than reassurance and discharge with standard oral antibiotics for presumed simple cellulitis.

Necrotizing fasciitis is further subclassified microbiologically into type I, a polymicrobial infection typically involving a mixture of aerobic and anaerobic organisms and most common in patients with diabetes, peripheral vascular disease, or a recent surgical or traumatic wound, and type II, a monomicrobial infection most classically caused by Streptococcus pyogenes and capable of occurring even in previously healthy individuals without an obvious portal of entry, a distinction with practical implications for empiric antibiotic selection, which should provide broad coverage for both possibilities pending culture results given the substantial overlap in initial clinical presentation between the two subtypes.

Laboratory findings, including an elevated white blood cell count, elevated C-reactive protein, and evidence of renal dysfunction, can support the diagnosis, and the LRINEC (Laboratory Risk Indicator for Necrotizing Fasciitis) score, incorporating C-reactive protein, white blood cell count, hemoglobin, sodium, creatinine, and glucose, provides a validated though imperfect risk-stratification tool that should never be used to definitively rule out the diagnosis in a patient with a strongly suggestive clinical picture; imaging, including computed tomography or magnetic resonance imaging, can demonstrate fascial thickening and gas within soft tissue when present, but imaging should never delay emergent surgical consultation in a patient with a high clinical suspicion, since surgical exploration itself remains both the definitive diagnostic test, through direct visualization of grayish, non-bleeding, easily dissectible fascia, and the primary life-saving treatment, and delayed debridement is one of the most consistently identified predictors of increased mortality across published outcome studies of this disease.

Staphylococcal Scalded Skin Syndrome

Staphylococcal scalded skin syndrome results from circulating exfoliative toxins produced by toxin-producing strains of Staphylococcus aureus, typically originating from a localized, sometimes clinically inapparent infection elsewhere in the body, that cleave desmoglein 1 within the superficial epidermis, producing widespread superficial epidermal detachment; the condition occurs predominantly in infants and young children, who have both a less mature renal clearance mechanism for the circulating toxin and lower levels of protective antitoxin antibodies compared with older children and adults, presenting with fever, marked skin tenderness, and a diffuse erythema that rapidly progresses to superficial flaccid bullae and sheet-like desquamation, characteristically sparing the mucosal surfaces, a critical distinguishing feature from Stevens-Johnson syndrome and toxic epidermal necrolysis discussed above, in which mucosal involvement is a defining, near-universal feature. Because the epidermal split in staphylococcal scalded skin syndrome occurs at a very superficial level, within the granular layer, rather than at the dermal-epidermal junction as in toxic epidermal necrolysis, the disease, despite its dramatic and alarming clinical appearance, generally carries a considerably better prognosis than toxic epidermal necrolysis when promptly recognized and treated, and a bedside distinction between the two, beyond the presence or absence of mucosal involvement, can be aided by a skin biopsy with frozen section when the diagnosis remains uncertain, given the very different level of tissue cleavage between the two conditions.

KEY POINT: Mucosal sparing is the single most useful bedside feature distinguishing staphylococcal scalded skin syndrome from Stevens-Johnson syndrome and toxic epidermal necrolysis; a young child with fever, skin tenderness, and superficial desquamation but entirely normal oral, ocular, and genital mucosa should be strongly suspected of having staphylococcal scalded skin syndrome rather than a severe cutaneous drug reaction.

Staphylococcal scalded skin syndrome is considerably less common in healthy adults than in infants and young children given the more mature renal clearance and greater accumulated antitoxin antibody levels typical of adulthood, but it can occur in adults with impaired renal function or immunosuppression, in whom the disease tends to carry a meaningfully higher mortality risk than the generally favorable prognosis seen in affected infants and children, an important distinction to bear in mind when an adult patient presents with a clinical picture suggestive of this diagnosis, since the same reassuring prognosis typically quoted for pediatric disease does not directly apply to this smaller but higher-risk adult population.

Management centers on prompt identification and treatment of the underlying staphylococcal source, most often with an anti-staphylococcal or, given increasing methicillin-resistant Staphylococcus aureus prevalence in some regions, appropriately broader-spectrum systemic antibiotic therapy pending culture results, together with supportive skin care and careful fluid and electrolyte monitoring given the insensible fluid losses that accompany the superficial desquamation, generally in a monitored inpatient setting for affected infants and young children given both the fluid management needs and the importance of prompt identification and treatment of the underlying infectious source.

Purpura Fulminans

Purpura fulminans is a rare, rapidly progressive syndrome of cutaneous hemorrhage and necrosis resulting from disseminated intravascular coagulation and dermal vascular thrombosis, most classically encountered in the setting of severe meningococcemia but also occurring with other severe bacterial infections and, less commonly, in association with inherited or acquired protein C or protein S deficiency; the clinical presentation begins with well-demarcated, painful, rapidly expanding purpuric patches that progress within hours to hemorrhagic bullae and frank cutaneous necrosis, most often affecting the extremities, and the speed of this progression, often visibly worsening over a period of just a few hours, is itself one of the most important clues distinguishing this disease from other, more slowly evolving purpuric or vasculitic presentations discussed in the earlier chapter on cutaneous vasculitis. Purpura fulminans in the setting of infection represents a true multisystem emergency requiring immediate broad-spectrum antibiotic therapy, aggressive hemodynamic support, and correction of the underlying coagulopathy, generally in an intensive care setting, and the cutaneous findings, while visually dramatic and clinically important as a diagnostic clue, are best understood as the visible surface manifestation of an underlying systemic process, sepsis and disseminated intravascular coagulation, that itself directly drives the disease's substantial mortality risk and that must be treated with the same urgency as any other source of septic shock.

CAUTION: Rapidly expanding purpuric patches evolving toward hemorrhagic bullae and necrosis over a period of hours, particularly in an acutely ill-appearing patient with fever, should prompt immediate consideration of purpura fulminans and meningococcemia, immediate empiric broad-spectrum antibiotic administration, and critical care evaluation, since any delay directly increases mortality risk in this rapidly progressive condition.

Toxic Shock Syndrome

Toxic shock syndrome, resulting from superantigen toxin production by toxigenic strains of Staphylococcus aureus or, in a distinct but clinically overlapping presentation, Streptococcus pyogenes, produces a syndrome of fever, hypotension, and a diffuse, sunburn-like macular erythema classically followed one to two weeks later by desquamation, most prominent on the palms and soles, together with multiorgan involvement that can affect the gastrointestinal, renal, hepatic, muscular, and central nervous systems; the historically emphasized association with tampon use represents only one of several recognized clinical contexts, and toxic shock syndrome should be considered in any patient with an appropriate constellation of fever, hypotension, diffuse erythema, and multiorgan involvement following a surgical procedure, a wound infection, or a postpartum infection, regardless of tampon use or menstrual status. Streptococcal toxic shock syndrome in particular is frequently associated with an identifiable, sometimes rapidly progressive soft tissue infection, including necrotizing fasciitis as discussed above, and any patient presenting with features suggestive of toxic shock syndrome should undergo a careful search for a focal source of infection requiring source control, including surgical debridement or removal of retained foreign material such as a tampon or nasal packing, since source control together with appropriate antibiotic therapy, typically combining a beta-lactam with clindamycin given the latter's protein synthesis-inhibiting effect on toxin production, is essential to a favorable outcome and cannot be achieved with antibiotics alone in the presence of an undrained or undebrided focal source.

CAUTION: Toxic shock syndrome should be considered in any patient with fever, hypotension, and diffuse erythema following a surgical procedure, wound infection, or postpartum period, not only in the context of tampon use; a thorough search for a focal, drainable or debridable source of infection is an essential component of management, since antibiotic therapy alone, without source control, is frequently insufficient to halt ongoing toxin production.

Acute Generalized Exanthematous Pustulosis

Acute generalized exanthematous pustulosis is a severe cutaneous adverse drug reaction characterized by the rapid onset, typically within one to two days of exposure to the causative medication, of numerous small, non-follicular, sterile pustules arising on a background of diffuse edematous erythema, most prominent in the intertriginous folds before spreading more generally, accompanied by fever and, frequently, a mild peripheral neutrophilia; commonly implicated medications include aminopenicillins, macrolide antibiotics, and calcium channel blockers, and the considerably more rapid onset of this condition, often within a day or two of drug exposure, contrasts sharply with the more delayed onset typical of DRESS syndrome and provides a useful distinguishing historical feature between these two drug-induced conditions when the clinical distinction is otherwise uncertain. Despite its dramatic and sometimes alarming clinical appearance, acute generalized exanthematous pustulosis generally follows a self-limited course once the causative medication is discontinued, with resolution over one to two weeks accompanied by characteristic post-pustular desquamation, and the primary diagnostic challenge is distinguishing this drug-induced, generally favorable-prognosis condition from generalized pustular psoriasis, a considerably more severe and potentially life-threatening condition with a similar pustular morphology but a fundamentally different underlying pathophysiology and treatment approach; a personal or family history of psoriasis, a more gradual onset, and, when biopsy is performed, specific histologic differences can help distinguish between these two important pustular mimics.

KEY POINT: The considerably more rapid onset of acute generalized exanthematous pustulosis, typically within one to two days of the causative medication, compared with the two-to-eight-week onset typical of DRESS syndrome, is a key historical feature distinguishing these two drug-induced conditions, both of which can otherwise present with overlapping fever and cutaneous findings.

Calciphylaxis

Calciphylaxis is a rare but life-threatening condition of vascular calcification and thrombosis within the small and medium-sized dermal and subcutaneous vessels, occurring predominantly in patients with end-stage renal disease on dialysis, though it can also occur, less commonly, in patients without renal failure who have other risk factors including obesity, warfarin use, and hypercoagulable states; the clinical presentation begins with painful, mottled, violaceous, net-like (livedo-like) plaques that progress to well-demarcated areas of cutaneous necrosis and non-healing ulceration, most commonly affecting areas with a higher proportion of subcutaneous adipose tissue, including the abdomen, thighs, and buttocks, and the pain associated with calciphylaxis is characteristically severe and frequently out of proportion to the visible extent of cutaneous involvement, particularly in the disease's earlier stages before frank necrosis has developed. Calciphylaxis carries a strikingly high mortality rate, driven substantially by secondary infection of the necrotic, poorly perfused tissue and by the severe, difficult-to-control pain that can itself contribute to a downward clinical spiral, and management requires a coordinated multidisciplinary approach incorporating aggressive wound care, meticulous pain management, optimization of the underlying mineral and bone metabolism abnormalities in coordination with nephrology, sodium thiosulfate therapy, which has become a mainstay of medical treatment despite an incompletely understood mechanism of action, and avoidance of further precipitating factors including warfarin, which should generally be discontinued and replaced with an alternative anticoagulation strategy when calciphylaxis is diagnosed in a patient taking this medication.

CAUTION: Calciphylaxis should be suspected in a dialysis-dependent patient presenting with new, exquisitely painful, net-like violaceous plaques, particularly on the abdomen, thighs, or buttocks, and warrants urgent multidisciplinary evaluation given the condition's substantial mortality risk, which is driven significantly by secondary infection of poorly perfused, necrotic tissue.

Angioedema and Anaphylaxis With Cutaneous Involvement

Angioedema, presenting as non-pitting, often asymmetric swelling of the deep dermis and subcutaneous tissue, most commonly affecting the lips, periorbital area, tongue, and, in its most dangerous presentation, the airway, requires urgent clinical distinction between mast cell-mediated (histaminergic) angioedema, typically associated with urticaria and responsive to antihistamines, epinephrine, and corticosteroids, and bradykinin-mediated angioedema, including hereditary angioedema resulting from C1 esterase inhibitor deficiency and angiotensin-converting enzyme inhibitor-induced angioedema, neither of which reliably responds to antihistamines, epinephrine, or corticosteroids given their fundamentally different underlying mediator pathway; recognizing this distinction is clinically essential because a patient with bradykinin-mediated angioedema who is treated only with the standard histaminergic angioedema protocol may not improve, and specific bradykinin pathway-targeted therapies, including C1 esterase inhibitor concentrate, icatibant, or ecallantide, should be considered for patients with a known diagnosis of hereditary angioedema or a strong clinical suspicion for a bradykinin-mediated mechanism, particularly when there is no accompanying urticaria and no response to an initial trial of standard histaminergic treatment.

Any airway involvement in the setting of angioedema, evidenced by voice change, stridor, drooling, or subjective difficulty breathing or swallowing, constitutes an immediate airway emergency requiring prompt airway assessment and, when indicated, early, proactive airway management, given the well-recognized potential for rapid progression to complete airway obstruction; anaphylaxis, when accompanied by cutaneous findings including urticaria, flushing, or angioedema alongside respiratory or cardiovascular compromise, requires immediate intramuscular epinephrine as the first-line, unequivocally indicated treatment, and any hesitation to administer epinephrine out of concern for its cardiovascular side effects is a well-documented and clinically significant source of preventable anaphylaxis mortality, since the risk of withholding epinephrine in true anaphylaxis substantially exceeds the risk of appropriately administering it.

KEY POINT: Angiotensin-converting enzyme inhibitor-induced angioedema, a bradykinin-mediated process, does not respond reliably to antihistamines, epinephrine, or corticosteroids, and management centers on prompt discontinuation of the causative medication and airway protection when indicated; a patient with recurrent angioedema who has previously received one of these medications without improvement should prompt reconsideration of the underlying mechanism rather than repeated administration of the same ineffective treatment.

Clinical Case: A Rapidly Spreading Leg Infection With Disproportionate Pain

A 54-year-old man with poorly controlled diabetes presented to the emergency department with a two-day history of a spreading area of erythema and swelling on his lower leg, initially treated by an urgent care clinic the previous day as cellulitis with oral antibiotics, but he returned given severe, worsening pain that he described as far more severe than the visible redness seemed to warrant, along with new fever and confusion noted by his family. Examination revealed dusky, violaceous discoloration at the periphery of the erythematous area, a small hemorrhagic bulla, and an area of reduced sensation to light touch within the affected skin, together with tachycardia and hypotension.

Given the disproportionate pain, hemorrhagic bullae, cutaneous anesthesia, and systemic toxicity, necrotizing fasciitis was strongly suspected, and emergent surgical consultation was obtained without delay for confirmatory imaging, given the high pretest clinical probability and the well-established mortality risk associated with any delay in surgical source control. He was taken emergently to the operating room, where surgical exploration confirmed grayish, edematous, easily dissectible fascia with minimal bleeding, consistent with necrotizing fasciitis, and extensive debridement was performed along with initiation of broad-spectrum antibiotics and intensive care unit admission for hemodynamic support. He required two additional debridement procedures over the following week but survived his hospitalization, and this case was used within the treating institution as a teaching example of the critical importance of recognizing pain out of proportion to examination findings as a red flag prompting urgent reassessment, even in a patient who had already been evaluated and started on treatment for a presumed more benign diagnosis less than twenty-four hours earlier.

Clinical Case: Facial Swelling Unresponsive to Standard Allergy Treatment

A 46-year-old woman with hypertension presented to the emergency department with acute swelling of her lips and tongue that had developed over the preceding two hours, without any associated urticaria, itching, or known new food or environmental exposure; she had been started on lisinopril for blood pressure control approximately fourteen months earlier and had tolerated it without apparent issue until this presentation. She was initially treated in a community emergency department with intramuscular epinephrine, intravenous diphenhydramine, and intravenous corticosteroids under a presumed diagnosis of allergic angioedema, but her swelling continued to progress over the following hour without improvement, prompting transfer to a tertiary care facility.

On reassessment, the absence of urticaria, the temporal association with a long-standing angiotensin-converting enzyme inhibitor, and the lack of any response to standard histaminergic angioedema treatment together raised suspicion for angiotensin-converting enzyme inhibitor-induced, bradykinin-mediated angioedema, a diagnosis that can develop even after many months to years of previously well-tolerated use of the causative medication, a delayed-onset pattern that is not widely appreciated and that had contributed to the medication not being initially suspected as the cause. Lisinopril was discontinued immediately, otolaryngology was consulted given ongoing concern for progressive tongue and airway swelling, and she was admitted for close airway monitoring; her swelling gradually improved over the following forty-eight hours without requiring airway intervention, and she was discharged with explicit counseling that she should never again receive any medication in the angiotensin-converting enzyme inhibitor class, along with clear documentation of this reaction in her medical record and a recommendation for a medical alert bracelet, given the risk of a more severe or airway-threatening recurrence with any future exposure to this drug class.

THE MORPHOLOGY-TO-MANAGEMENT SYSTEM — Recognizing the Skin Finding That Cannot Wait

Pattern Introduced This Chapter: The targetoid, mucosa-involving eruption racing toward sheet-like detachment, the cellulitis whose pain outpaces its appearance, and the purpuric patch expanding visibly within hours.

Cross-Cutting Anchor: Every condition in this chapter is distinguished from its far more common, benign mimic by a specific combination of disproportionate severity, a defining associated feature (mucosal involvement, cutaneous anesthesia, mucosal sparing, or a systemic mediator pathway), and a pace of progression measured in hours rather than days; recognizing this combination, rather than the isolated skin finding alone, is what separates a true dermatologic emergency from routine care delivered too slowly.

Summary and Key Concepts

Stevens-Johnson syndrome and toxic epidermal necrolysis are distinguished by percentage body surface area of epidermal detachment, require immediate causative drug discontinuation and burn-unit-level supportive care, and demand urgent ophthalmology involvement given the risk of long-term ocular complications.

DRESS syndrome has a characteristically delayed onset of two to eight weeks after the causative medication and can flare with new organ involvement during corticosteroid tapering, requiring extended serial monitoring.

Erythroderma is a physiologic emergency independent of its underlying cause, requiring supportive stabilization for thermoregulatory failure and fluid loss in parallel with the diagnostic workup for the specific etiology.

Necrotizing fasciitis is distinguished from cellulitis by pain out of proportion to examination findings, rapid progression, hemorrhagic bullae, and cutaneous anesthesia, and requires emergent surgical debridement without diagnostic delay.

Staphylococcal scalded skin syndrome spares mucosal surfaces, distinguishing it from toxic epidermal necrolysis, and carries a better prognosis given its more superficial plane of epidermal cleavage.

Bradykinin-mediated angioedema does not respond to antihistamines, epinephrine, or corticosteroids, and anaphylaxis with cutaneous findings requires immediate intramuscular epinephrine without hesitation.

CHAPTER 25: OFFICE-BASED DERMATOLOGIC PROCEDURES

Learning Objectives

1. Select the appropriate biopsy technique, shave, punch, or excisional, for a given clinical scenario and lesion characteristic.
2. Apply the principles of local anesthesia, including appropriate agent and dose selection, for common office-based dermatologic procedures.
3. Construct an evidence-based perioperative approach to anticoagulation and antiplatelet medication management before a planned procedure.
4. Perform the technical steps of cryotherapy and electrodesiccation and curettage and identify the lesions appropriate for each modality.
5. Recognize and manage the common complications of office-based dermatologic procedures, including bleeding, infection, and dehiscence.
6. Apply appropriate technique for common nail unit procedures, including partial and complete nail avulsion and chemical matrixectomy.

Office-based procedural dermatology encompasses the practical technical skills that translate the diagnostic and management principles discussed throughout this text into direct patient care, and proficiency in these core procedures, biopsy technique, excision, cryotherapy, electrodesiccation and curettage, intralesional injection, and basic nail surgery, is foundational to the practice of clinical dermatology regardless of subspecialty focus. This chapter addresses the technical principles, appropriate lesion and patient selection, and complication management relevant to the procedures most commonly performed in a general dermatology office setting, building directly on the diagnostic frameworks established throughout the preceding chapters of this text.

Biopsy Technique Selection

Shave biopsy, in which a superficial layer of tissue is removed using a flexible razor blade or similar instrument, is well suited to lesions believed to be confined to the epidermis or superficial dermis, including most suspected basal cell carcinomas, superficial squamous cell carcinomas, and many benign epidermal and melanocytic lesions, but is generally inappropriate for a lesion in which invasive depth assessment is clinically important, since a shave biopsy that transects the base of an unexpectedly deeper lesion, most critically a melanoma, can compromise accurate Breslow depth measurement, a parameter with direct staging and prognostic implications as discussed in the earlier chapter on melanoma; any pigmented lesion with even a moderate degree of clinical suspicion for melanoma should instead be biopsied with a technique capturing the full depth of the lesion, discussed below, unless the lesion is small enough for the shave to reliably capture the full depth with an adequately deep pass.

Punch biopsy, using a circular cutting instrument to obtain a cylindrical, full-thickness core of skin extending into the subcutaneous fat, is the preferred technique for most inflammatory dermatoses, since adequate depth including subcutaneous fat is often necessary for confident histologic diagnosis of panniculitis and other deeper inflammatory processes, and is also frequently used for smaller pigmented lesions where excisional biopsy is not immediately feasible, though a punch biopsy of an irregularly shaped pigmented lesion risks incomplete sampling of the most atypical area if the punch is not carefully positioned over the most concerning region identified on clinical or dermoscopic examination. Excisional biopsy, removing the entire lesion with a margin of surrounding normal tissue down to and including the subcutaneous fat, remains the preferred technique for any lesion with substantial clinical suspicion for melanoma, since it provides the most reliable, complete assessment of Breslow depth and other histologic parameters without any of the sampling limitations inherent to a partial biopsy technique.

Curettage alone, without a preceding formal biopsy, is sometimes used as an initial diagnostic and therapeutic maneuver for a lesion with a very high pretest clinical probability of representing a straightforward seborrheic keratosis or similar unambiguously benign process, but this approach should be reserved for lesions with minimal diagnostic uncertainty, since curettage alone does not provide the intact architectural tissue sample needed for confident histologic subclassification of a more atypical or ambiguous lesion, and any lesion with even modest diagnostic uncertainty warrants a formal biopsy technique, discussed throughout this section, that preserves adequate tissue architecture for the pathologist.

CAUTION: A shave biopsy that transects the base of an unexpectedly invasive melanoma compromises accurate Breslow depth measurement, with direct downstream consequences for staging, prognosis, and treatment planning; any pigmented lesion with a meaningful degree of clinical or dermoscopic suspicion for melanoma should be biopsied with a full-thickness technique, excisional biopsy when feasible or a deep punch biopsy positioned over the most atypical area when excision is not immediately practical.

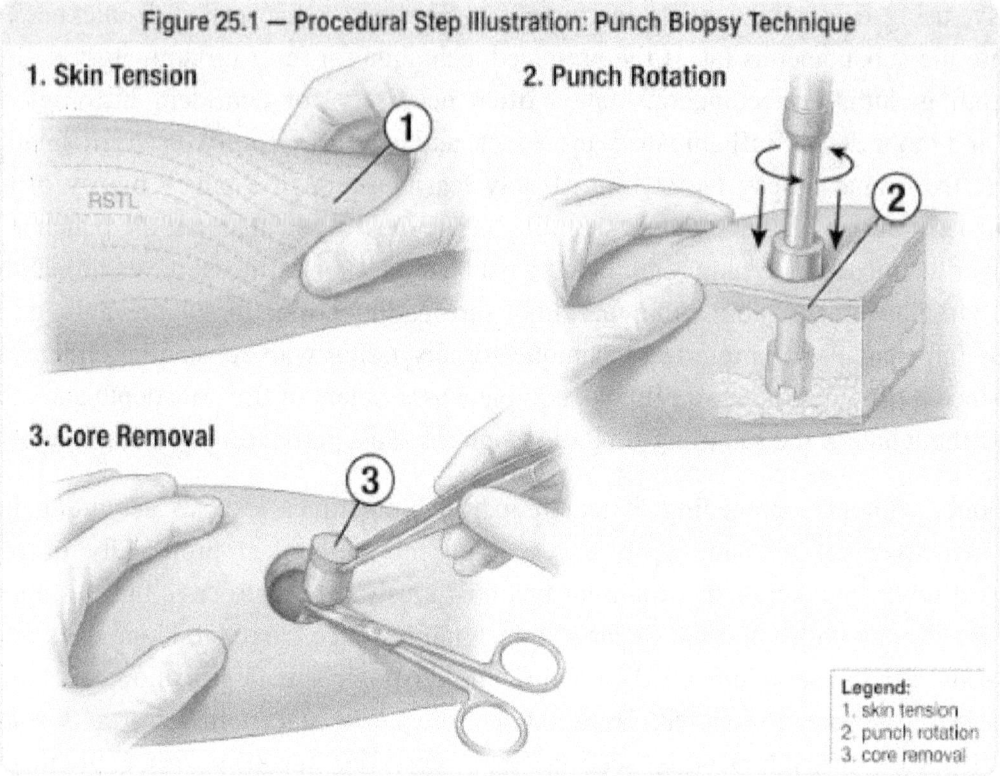

Local Anesthesia

Lidocaine with epinephrine remains the most commonly used local anesthetic for office-based dermatologic procedures, with the epinephrine component providing meaningful vasoconstriction that reduces intraoperative bleeding and prolongs the duration of anesthesia; the historical concern regarding epinephrine use on the digits, nose, ears, and penis, based on older case reports of digital ischemia, has been substantially reassessed by more recent, larger studies, and epinephrine-containing local anesthetic is now considered safe for use at these acral sites in patients without significant peripheral vascular disease when used at standard concentrations and appropriately conservative volumes, though many experienced clinicians continue to exercise particular caution and use conservative volumes at these sites given the theoretical, if now substantially reassessed, concern. Maximum safe dosing of lidocaine is calculated on a milligram-per-kilogram basis, with a commonly cited maximum of 4.5 milligrams per kilogram for lidocaine alone and up to 7 milligrams per kilogram when combined with epinephrine, and this calculation becomes particularly important for larger procedures involving substantial anesthetic volume, including extensive excisions or multiple simultaneous procedures performed in a single visit, where cumulative dosing should be tracked carefully to avoid systemic lidocaine toxicity, which can present with perioral numbness, tinnitus, and, at higher levels, seizures and cardiac arrhythmia.

KEY POINT: Epinephrine-containing local anesthetic is safe for use on the digits, nose, ears, and penis in patients without significant peripheral vascular disease at standard concentrations, a reassessment of an older, now largely outdated clinical teaching; cumulative lidocaine dosing should nonetheless be tracked using weight-based maximum dose calculations for any procedure requiring substantial anesthetic volume.

Topical anesthetic agents, including compounded lidocaine-prilocaine cream and topical tetracaine, can meaningfully reduce the discomfort of subsequent injectable anesthetic administration when applied under occlusion for a sufficient dwell time before the procedure, typically twenty to sixty minutes depending on the specific formulation, and this approach is particularly valuable for pediatric patients and for adults with significant needle-related anxiety; excessive application of topical anesthetic over a large body surface area, however, carries its own risk of systemic toxicity, most notably methemoglobinemia with prilocaine-containing formulations, and appropriate dose limits based on treated surface area and patient weight should be observed even for this seemingly lower-risk, non-injected route of anesthetic administration.

Buffering local anesthetic with sodium bicarbonate, typically in a ratio of approximately one part bicarbonate to nine or ten parts lidocaine, meaningfully reduces the burning sensation associated with injection by raising the solution's pH closer to physiologic range, and this simple, low-cost modification is increasingly used by procedurally focused dermatologists as a routine measure to improve patient comfort, particularly for larger volume injections or for patients undergoing multiple sequential procedures in a single visit.

Perioperative Anticoagulation Management

Current evidence-based guidance for most office-based dermatologic procedures, including biopsy, excision, and electrodesiccation and curettage, favors continuing anticoagulant and antiplatelet medications, including warfarin, direct oral anticoagulants, and aspirin, rather than discontinuing them perioperatively, since the risk of a thromboembolic event, stroke, or cardiac event resulting from medication discontinuation generally exceeds the risk of a bleeding complication that can typically be managed with local hemostatic measures alone; this represents a meaningful shift from older, more conservative practice patterns that favored routine perioperative discontinuation, and clinicians should be aware of this evidence-based shift when counseling patients and coordinating with prescribing physicians regarding perioperative medication management. Discontinuation of these medications should generally be reserved for the specific, less common circumstances in which a genuinely more extensive procedure with substantially elevated bleeding risk is planned, and any decision to discontinue an anticoagulant or antiplatelet medication for a planned dermatologic procedure should be made in direct coordination with the prescribing physician, weighing the specific procedure's bleeding risk against the individual patient's thromboembolic risk, rather than as a reflexive, one-size-fits-all default practice.

CAUTION: Reflexive discontinuation of warfarin, a direct oral anticoagulant, or aspirin before a routine office-based dermatologic procedure is generally not supported by current evidence and can expose the patient to an avoidable thromboembolic risk; continuation of these medications, combined with adequate local hemostatic technique, is the preferred default approach for the great majority of standard office-based procedures.

Cryotherapy

Cryotherapy, most commonly using liquid nitrogen delivered by spray or direct contact probe, produces tissue destruction through intracellular and extracellular ice crystal formation and subsequent cellular injury upon thawing, and is well suited to a range of benign and precancerous lesions, including actinic keratoses, seborrheic keratoses, common warts, and molluscum contagiosum, discussed in the earlier chapters on actinic damage and pediatric dermatology respectively; treatment depth and freeze duration should be calibrated to the specific lesion being treated, with thinner, more superficial lesions such as actinic keratoses generally requiring a shorter freeze time than thicker, more hyperkeratotic lesions such as common warts. Cryotherapy carries a well-recognized risk of both hypopigmentation and hyperpigmentation at the treatment site, an important consideration in patients with darker skin tones as discussed in the earlier chapter on diagnosis and management across skin tones, and patients should be counseled explicitly regarding this pigmentary risk, along with the expected post-treatment blister or crust formation and the typical healing timeline, before treatment is performed, particularly for cosmetically sensitive locations such as the face.

PATIENT EDUCATION: Cryotherapy commonly produces a blister at the treatment site within the first day or two, followed by crusting and healing over one to several weeks depending on treatment depth and body location; patients should be counseled to avoid intentionally rupturing an intact blister, keep the area clean, and expect the possibility of temporary or, less commonly, permanent pigmentary change at the treatment site, which is more likely to be cosmetically noticeable in patients with darker skin tones.

Electrodesiccation and Curettage

Electrodesiccation and curettage, a technique combining sharp curettage to mechanically debulk friable tumor tissue with electrodesiccation to achieve hemostasis and provide additional tumor destruction at the base and margins, is a well-established, efficient treatment option for appropriately selected superficial and nodular basal cell carcinomas and superficial squamous cell carcinomas in low-risk anatomic locations, as discussed in the earlier chapter on actinic damage and keratinocyte carcinoma; the technique relies on the characteristic friable, easily curetted texture of most basal cell and superficial squamous cell carcinomas relative to the firmer surrounding normal dermis, a textural difference the experienced clinician uses to help judge adequate treatment margins during the procedure itself. The technique is generally not appropriate for morpheaform or infiltrative basal cell carcinoma subtypes, for recurrent tumors, or for high-risk anatomic locations including the central face, given both the less reliable textural distinction between tumor and normal tissue in these more infiltrative subtypes and the less favorable cosmetic outcome of the resulting scar in cosmetically sensitive locations compared with a carefully planned surgical excision or Mohs micrographic surgery.

Excision and Suturing Principles

Surgical excision should be planned along or parallel to the relaxed skin tension lines whenever possible to optimize the eventual cosmetic outcome of the resulting scar, and the classic elliptical excision design, with a length-to-width ratio of approximately three to one, allows primary closure without excessive tissue bunching ("dog-ears") at the ends of the closure; appropriate margins for excision of a confirmed malignancy should be selected based on the specific tumor type and any available risk-stratification information, as detailed in the earlier chapters addressing keratinocyte carcinoma and melanoma specifically, and margins for a purely diagnostic or cosmetic excision of a benign lesion can generally be considerably narrower given the absence of any oncologic margin requirement. Layered wound closure, incorporating a deep, absorbable suture layer to reduce tension on the skin surface and reapproximate the deeper wound edges, followed by a superficial, typically non-absorbable or fast-absorbing suture layer for precise skin edge approximation, generally produces a more favorable cosmetic outcome than a single-layer closure for any wound under meaningful tension, and appropriate suture removal timing varies by anatomic location, with facial sutures typically removed earlier, around five to seven days, given the face's excellent blood supply and lower tension, and sutures on the trunk or extremities, particularly over joints, typically left in place longer, up to two weeks or more, given the higher tension and slower healing at these sites.

KEY POINT: Suture removal timing should be tailored to anatomic location rather than applied as a single uniform interval across all surgical sites: earlier removal on the face minimizes the risk of visible suture track marks given the face's excellent blood supply, while later removal on higher-tension sites such as the back or over a joint reduces the risk of wound dehiscence.

Intralesional Injection Technique

Intralesional corticosteroid injection, most commonly using triamcinolone acetonide at a concentration selected based on the specific lesion and anatomic site being treated, is used throughout this text for conditions including keloids, alopecia areata, discoid lupus, and numerous other inflammatory dermatoses requiring targeted, higher-concentration local therapy than topical treatment alone can achieve; injection technique should aim to distribute the medication evenly throughout the dermal or lesional target while avoiding excessive volume or concentration that risks iatrogenic skin or subcutaneous atrophy, a well-recognized complication that is generally more likely with higher concentrations, larger injected volumes, and more superficial injection technique. Appropriate dilution of the injected corticosteroid concentration for thinner-skinned anatomic sites, including the face, and correspondingly higher concentrations for thicker, more fibrotic lesions such as an established keloid, reflects the same basic principle applied throughout this text regarding topical corticosteroid potency selection: matching treatment intensity to the specific tissue characteristics and disease process being treated, rather than applying a single default concentration and volume across all clinical scenarios.

CAUTION: Excessive concentration or volume of intralesional corticosteroid, or overly superficial injection technique, risks iatrogenic skin and subcutaneous atrophy that can itself become a source of patient dissatisfaction independent of the original condition being treated; injection technique and concentration should be tailored to the specific anatomic site and lesion characteristics rather than applied uniformly.

Incision and Drainage of Cutaneous Abscesses

Incision and drainage remains the primary, essential treatment for a fluctuant cutaneous abscess, with systemic antibiotic therapy serving as an adjunct rather than a substitute for adequate mechanical drainage, since antibiotics alone typically fail to adequately penetrate and resolve a well-formed abscess cavity regardless of the causative organism's antibiotic susceptibility; adjunctive systemic antibiotics are generally reserved for abscesses with surrounding cellulitis, systemic signs of infection, immunosuppression, or other specific risk factors for treatment failure with drainage alone, reflecting current evidence-based practice that has moved away from reflexive antibiotic prescription for every drained abscess regardless of these accompanying features. Technique involves a linear incision at the point of maximum fluctuance, sized adequately to allow thorough drainage and, when indicated, blunt digital or instrument exploration to break up loculations within the abscess cavity that could otherwise allow the abscess to persist or recur despite an apparently adequate initial incision; packing the resulting cavity with gauze, when the abscess is large enough to warrant packing, helps maintain drainage and prevent premature superficial closure of the incision before the deeper cavity has had adequate opportunity to heal from the base outward, and packing is typically changed at intervals of one to two days until the cavity has substantially decreased in size.

KEY POINT: Incision and drainage, not systemic antibiotics, is the primary treatment for a fluctuant abscess; antibiotics are a useful adjunct for abscesses accompanied by surrounding cellulitis, systemic signs of infection, or specific host risk factors, but do not substitute for adequate mechanical drainage of the abscess cavity itself.

Wound Dressing Selection and Post-Procedure Care

Appropriate wound dressing selection is guided by the specific wound type, its location, and its expected healing course: a simple, sutured surgical wound generally requires only a basic non-adherent dressing and petrolatum-based ointment to maintain a moist healing environment, which has been consistently shown to promote faster epithelialization and reduce scarring compared with allowing a wound to dry and form a scab, a practice that runs counter to a persistent but outdated lay belief that wounds heal better when left uncovered and allowed to dry. Wounds healing by secondary intention, including those resulting from electrodesiccation and curettage, larger biopsy sites, or a dehisced or packed abscess cavity, require a more involved dressing regimen, typically incorporating daily cleansing, application of petrolatum or a specialized moisture-retentive dressing, and, for deeper wounds, appropriate packing material, continued until the wound has fully re-epithelialized from the base and margins inward, a process that can take considerably longer, often several weeks to months depending on wound size and location, than the healing time for a primarily closed surgical incision.

Patients should receive clear, specific written wound care instructions before leaving the office following any procedure, including expected normal healing appearance, warning signs that should prompt a return visit (increasing pain, spreading erythema, purulent drainage, fever, or wound dehiscence), activity restrictions appropriate to the specific procedure and anatomic location, and an explicit timeline for suture removal or follow-up when applicable; patients undergoing a procedure at a cosmetically or functionally significant site, including the face, hands, or a site overlying a joint, benefit from particularly detailed counseling given the greater consequence of a suboptimal healing outcome at these locations.

PATIENT EDUCATION: A moist wound healing environment, maintained with a non-adherent dressing and petrolatum-based ointment, promotes faster healing and reduces scarring compared with allowing a wound to dry and scab over; patients should be explicitly counseled against the common misconception that exposing a healing wound to air produces a better outcome.

Electrosurgery Safety Considerations: Cardiac Implantable Devices

Electrosurgical devices, used for electrodesiccation and curettage, hemostasis during excisional surgery, and several other common office-based procedures, generate electromagnetic interference that carries a theoretical risk of disrupting the function of implanted cardiac devices, including pacemakers and implantable cardioverter-defibrillators, most notably through inappropriate device inhibition or, for a defibrillator, inappropriate shock delivery triggered by misinterpreted electrical interference; the overall risk for brief, low-energy, superficial dermatologic electrosurgical procedures is considered low, particularly with bipolar rather than monopolar electrosurgical technique and with the grounding pad, when used, positioned to direct current flow away from the device, but a specific risk assessment, including consultation with the patient's cardiology team for higher-risk device configurations or more extensive planned electrosurgical use, is a reasonable precaution for any patient with a known cardiac implantable device undergoing a planned procedure involving substantial electrosurgical energy delivery. Bipolar electrosurgery, in which current passes only between the two tips of the instrument itself rather than through the patient's body to a distant grounding pad, is generally preferred over monopolar technique in patients with a cardiac implantable device given its more localized, lower-risk current pathway, and brief, superficial procedures using battery-powered, low-energy hyfrecation for minor lesion destruction are generally considered lower risk than more extensive monopolar electrosurgical procedures.

CAUTION: Patients with a cardiac implantable device undergoing a planned procedure involving substantial electrosurgical energy delivery should have this history specifically identified before the procedure, with consideration given to bipolar rather than monopolar technique and, for higher-risk scenarios, consultation with the patient's cardiology team, given the theoretical risk of device interference from electrosurgical electromagnetic energy.

Nail Unit Procedures

Partial or complete nail avulsion, in which the nail plate is separated from the underlying nail bed and removed, provides direct access for biopsy of the nail bed or matrix when a subungual lesion, onychomycosis unresponsive to standard treatment, or another nail unit abnormality requires histologic evaluation, and is also frequently performed as a therapeutic procedure for ingrown toenails and severe onychomycosis; the procedure requires an appropriately administered digital block, most commonly performed using a plain local anesthetic without epinephrine at the base of the digit, historically reflecting the same digital ischemia concern discussed above regarding epinephrine use at acral sites, though as noted, more recent evidence has reassessed this concern, and either approach, with appropriate technique and conservative volume, is now considered acceptable by many experienced proceduralists. Digital tourniquet use during nail unit procedures provides a bloodless surgical field that meaningfully improves visualization of the nail bed and matrix during biopsy or matrixectomy, but the tourniquet must be removed promptly at the conclusion of the procedure and documented clearly to avoid the rare but serious complication of prolonged digital ischemia from an inadvertently retained tourniquet, a well-recognized and entirely preventable procedural error that underscores the importance of a specific, deliberate tourniquet removal step built into the standard procedural checklist for any nail unit procedure. Chemical matrixectomy, most commonly performed using phenol applied directly to the lateral nail matrix following partial nail avulsion, provides definitive, longer-term treatment for recurrent ingrown toenails by permanently ablating the portion of the nail matrix responsible for generating the problematic lateral nail plate segment, and appropriate technique, including adequate hemostasis before phenol application to prevent the phenol from being diluted or washed away by ongoing bleeding, and thorough post-application irrigation to remove residual phenol and limit collateral tissue damage, is essential to both procedural success and minimizing postoperative complications including prolonged drainage and delayed healing.

Informed Consent and Scar Expectation Setting

Informed consent for any office-based dermatologic procedure should include a clear, specific discussion of the procedure's purpose, alternative approaches when reasonable alternatives exist, and expected risks, including bleeding, infection, and, for essentially any procedure that breaches the epidermis, some degree of permanent scarring, since even an optimally performed, uncomplicated procedure leaves some visible mark in the great majority of cases, a reality that should be explicitly communicated before the procedure rather than only addressed if the patient later expresses dissatisfaction with the resulting scar appearance. Patients with a personal or family history of keloid formation, discussed in the earlier chapter on diagnosis and management across skin tones, warrant a specifically tailored consent discussion addressing this elevated risk, and for elective, non-medically necessary procedures in a keloid-prone patient, this discussion should include the patient's own assessment of whether the anticipated benefit of the procedure justifies this meaningfully elevated risk, since the ultimate decision belongs to an adequately informed patient rather than being made unilaterally by the treating clinician.

Setting realistic expectations regarding the scar maturation timeline is an important component of postoperative counseling that is sometimes underemphasized relative to the immediate procedural and wound care instructions: a fresh surgical scar typically appears pink to red and can feel firm or slightly raised for the first several months after a procedure, and this appearance, while sometimes concerning to patients unfamiliar with the normal scar maturation process, generally represents an entirely expected stage of healing rather than a poor outcome, with most scars continuing to soften, flatten, and fade in color over a period extending up to twelve to eighteen months after the original procedure; patients who are counseled about this extended timeline in advance are considerably less likely to seek premature, sometimes unnecessary scar revision consultation during this still-evolving early maturation period.

Recognizing and Managing Procedural Complications

Postoperative bleeding, the most common complication of office-based dermatologic procedures, is generally managed with direct pressure applied for an adequate duration, typically at least ten to fifteen minutes of continuous, uninterrupted pressure, since intermittent checking that repeatedly interrupts pressure formation is a common and easily correctable technique error that prolongs the time to hemostasis; a hematoma developing beneath a surgical closure, evidenced by a firm, tender, expanding fluctuant swelling, generally requires prompt evacuation, either through gentle opening of a portion of the closure or needle aspiration depending on the hematoma's size and the timing relative to the original procedure, since an unevacuated hematoma increases the risk of wound dehiscence, infection, and a less favorable cosmetic outcome. Surgical site infection, presenting with increasing pain, erythema, warmth, and purulent drainage typically beginning several days after the procedure, should be distinguished from the expected mild inflammatory response present in the first day or two after any surgical procedure, and any surgical site with clinical features suggestive of true infection warrants appropriate wound culture and empiric antibiotic therapy directed at the most likely causative organisms, generally Staphylococcus aureus and Streptococcus species, pending culture results.

Contact dermatitis to a topical antibiotic ointment, most notably bacitracin or neomycin, applied to a healing surgical wound is a commonly encountered and frequently misattributed complication, since the resulting periwound erythema, itching, and vesiculation can be mistaken for surgical site infection, prompting an unnecessary course of oral antibiotics when the correct management is simply discontinuation of the offending topical agent and substitution with plain petrolatum, which provides equivalent wound care benefit without the corresponding contact allergy risk; distinguishing allergic contact dermatitis from true infection relies on the absence of purulent drainage and systemic signs of infection, the characteristically pruritic rather than painful quality of the periwound reaction, and, when the distinction remains uncertain, the eruption's response to simple discontinuation of the topical agent rather than to antibiotic therapy.

Wound dehiscence, the separation of a previously closed surgical wound, most commonly results from excessive tension on the closure, premature suture removal, infection, or a combination of these factors, and management depends on the timing and extent of the dehiscence: a small, early dehiscence without evidence of infection can sometimes be managed with prompt resuturing, while a more extensive dehiscence, or one complicated by infection, is generally better managed by allowing healing by secondary intention with appropriate wound care, given the higher risk of recurrent dehiscence if the wound is resutured under the same excessive tension or in the presence of ongoing infection that contributed to the original complication.

KEY POINT: Sustained, uninterrupted direct pressure for at least ten to fifteen minutes is the most important and most commonly underused technique for managing postoperative bleeding; repeatedly lifting the pressure dressing to check for ongoing bleeding disrupts clot formation and paradoxically prolongs the time to hemostasis.

Clinical Case: A Shave Biopsy That Complicated Melanoma Staging

A 61-year-old man was referred for evaluation of a pigmented lesion on his back that had been biopsied by his primary care physician using a shave technique approximately two weeks earlier, given its irregular border and variable color, with the biopsy report returning as melanoma but noting that the deep margin of the specimen was transected, meaning that a definitive Breslow depth measurement could not be reliably established from the available tissue. This ambiguity created a substantial downstream clinical challenge, since the appropriate re-excision margin and the decision regarding whether sentinel lymph node biopsy was indicated both depend directly on an accurate Breslow depth measurement, as discussed in the earlier chapter on melanoma.

Given the transected deep margin, a wide local re-excision was planned using a margin appropriate for the deepest possible Breslow depth consistent with the available partial pathology information, an approach that necessarily erred toward a wider margin than might have been required had the original biopsy provided a definitive, reliable depth measurement, and the patient was counseled regarding this diagnostic uncertainty and its direct impact on his surgical planning. This case was used within the referring practice as a specific teaching example reinforcing the principle, discussed earlier in this chapter, that any pigmented lesion carrying even moderate clinical suspicion for melanoma should be biopsied using a full-thickness technique, excisional biopsy when feasible, capturing the complete depth of the lesion, precisely to avoid the type of diagnostic ambiguity and resulting treatment complexity this patient subsequently experienced.

Clinical Case: An Anticoagulated Patient Referred for Unnecessary Bridging

A 72-year-old man on warfarin for a mechanical mitral valve was referred for excision of a biopsy-confirmed squamous cell carcinoma on his forearm; his cardiologist's office had recommended holding warfarin for five days before the procedure and bridging with a heparin injection regimen in the interim, a plan that both the patient and his cardiologist assumed was the standard, expected approach for any surgical procedure regardless of its scope, and the patient presented to his preoperative dermatology visit already anxious about the logistics and cost of the recommended bridging regimen.

A review of current evidence-based guidance for office-based dermatologic excision confirmed that continuation of warfarin, rather than discontinuation with bridging, was the appropriate approach for this specific, relatively limited procedure, given that the risk of a thromboembolic event from a mechanical mitral valve during even a brief anticoagulation interruption meaningfully exceeds the bleeding risk of a standard dermatologic excision performed with adequate local hemostatic technique. This recommendation, along with the relevant supporting evidence, was communicated directly to the patient's cardiologist, and the excision was performed successfully with the patient continuing his warfarin uninterrupted, achieving hemostasis through electrocautery and a layered closure without any bleeding complication. This case was used as a teaching example, both for trainees and for referring physicians in the local care network, illustrating that reflexive anticoagulation bridging protocols developed for major surgical procedures do not automatically apply to more limited office-based dermatologic procedures, and that direct, evidence-based communication between the dermatologist and the prescribing physician can prevent an unnecessary, costly, and logistically burdensome bridging regimen for the patient.

THE MORPHOLOGY-TO-MANAGEMENT SYSTEM — Matching the Procedure to the Pattern

Pattern Introduced This Chapter: The pigmented lesion whose Breslow depth was compromised by an overly superficial biopsy, the surgical site whose bleeding was prolonged by impatient, intermittent pressure, and the anticoagulated patient whose medication was needlessly discontinued against current evidence.

Cross-Cutting Anchor: Every procedure in this chapter succeeds or fails based on matching technique, depth, and perioperative management to the specific clinical situation rather than applying a single default approach across every lesion and every patient, and the most consequential procedural errors in this chapter, an inadequate biopsy depth, an interrupted pressure hold, an unnecessarily discontinued anticoagulant, all stem from exactly this kind of one-size-fits-all shortcut.

Summary and Key Concepts

Shave biopsy risks compromising Breslow depth assessment for a lesion with unexpected invasive depth, making full-thickness biopsy technique essential for any pigmented lesion with meaningful melanoma suspicion.

Epinephrine-containing local anesthetic is safe at standard concentrations on the digits, nose, ears, and penis in patients without significant peripheral vascular disease, reassessing older, more restrictive teaching.

Current evidence favors continuing anticoagulant and antiplatelet medications for most office-based dermatologic procedures rather than routine perioperative discontinuation, given that thromboembolic risk generally exceeds manageable bleeding risk.

Electrodesiccation and curettage is appropriate for select superficial and nodular basal cell and superficial squamous cell carcinomas in low-risk locations but not for morpheaform, infiltrative, or recurrent tumors.

Layered wound closure along relaxed skin tension lines, with suture removal timing tailored to anatomic location, optimizes cosmetic outcome and minimizes dehiscence risk.

Sustained, uninterrupted direct pressure for at least ten to fifteen minutes is the most effective and most commonly underused technique for managing postoperative bleeding, and hematomas, true infections, and dehiscence each require prompt, specific management.

THE MORPHOLOGY-TO-MANAGEMENT MASTER ATLAS

This Atlas consolidates every Pattern introduced through The Morphology-to-Management System across the preceding twenty-five chapters into a single, indexed, cross-referenced reference. Each entry restates the Pattern's Stem Signature, the definitive clinical Decision it triggers, and its Trap Logic, the look-alike presentations that must be actively ruled out, so that the reader can move directly from a bedside observation to a confident management pivot without paging back through the full chapter discussion. Entries are grouped by clinical category rather than by chapter sequence, since a clinician scanning this Atlas during clinic, on call, or before a rotation is more often searching by the pattern they are looking at than by chapter number. This Atlas is a pure pattern reference: it contains no questions, no drills, and no answer keys of any kind. The organizing insight behind every entry catalogued here is the same insight that runs throughout this entire textbook: the majority of diagnostic delay in clinical dermatology does not arise from a rare disease being genuinely impossible to recognize, but from a common, plausible, benign-appearing diagnosis being accepted for too long without adequate scrutiny of the specific detail, a treatment response pattern, a distribution nuance, a timeline inconsistency, that would have revealed the true underlying process. Reading this Atlas as a standalone reference, independent of any single chapter, is an intentional design choice: the patterns catalogued here are meant to travel with the reader into the clinic and onto the ward, functioning as a rapid mental checklist against which any new, unfamiliar, or treatment-resistant presentation can be measured.

Inflammatory and Papulosquamous Patterns

THE MORPHOLOGY-TO-MANAGEMENT SYSTEM — The Treatment-Resistant Plaque That Isn't What It Seems

The Pattern: A scaly, erythematous plaque presumed to be eczema or psoriasis that fails to respond fully, or responds only temporarily, to appropriate topical anti-inflammatory therapy.

Stem Signature: Partial, transient improvement with topical corticosteroids followed by prompt recurrence once treatment is tapered; an atypical surface texture, distribution, or associated symptom that does not quite fit the presumed diagnosis.

Trap Logic: This pattern spans an unusually wide range of underlying conditions, from ordinary treatment-resistant inflammatory disease to mycosis fungoides, cutaneous lupus, and other mimics discussed throughout this text; the trap is treating the presumed diagnosis indefinitely rather than reconsidering it.

The Decision: Biopsy any plaque that fails to clear completely and durably within an appropriate treatment trial, particularly when the response pattern is described as partial or temporary rather than complete.

Pattern Anchor: Partial response followed by reliable recurrence, more than any single morphologic feature, is the anchor finding that should trigger diagnostic reconsideration across nearly every inflammatory-appearing dermatosis in this text.

THE MORPHOLOGY-TO-MANAGEMENT SYSTEM — The Violaceous Recalibration for Darker Skin Tones

The Pattern: Inflammatory disease presenting as violaceous, gray-brown, or simply darker-than-surrounding discoloration rather than the classic pink-red erythema emphasized in most morphologic descriptions.

Stem Signature: Subtle or absent visual erythema in a patient with a darker skin tone, with induration, warmth, or scale providing more reliable diagnostic signal than color alone.

Trap Logic: Reliance on visual erythema as the primary diagnostic cue, a habit built from erythema-centric textbook descriptions, systematically underestimates disease severity and delays diagnosis in patients with darker skin tones.

The Decision: Recalibrate the examination toward palpation, scale assessment, and patient-reported symptom severity whenever erythema is difficult to visually appreciate.

Pattern Anchor: Violaceous or gray-brown discoloration is the darker-skin-tone equivalent of classic erythema and should be actively sought rather than incidentally noticed. Cross-reference: Chapter 22.

THE MORPHOLOGY-TO-MANAGEMENT SYSTEM — The Acneiform Eruption with a Hidden Trigger

The Pattern: An acneiform eruption in an adult that fails to respond to standard acne therapy, or that develops abruptly in a patient without a prior history of acne.

Stem Signature: Monomorphic, rather than the classically varied, lesion morphology; a temporal relationship to a new medication, occlusive cosmetic product, or endocrine change; or a distribution atypical for ordinary acne vulgaris.

Trap Logic: Drug-induced acneiform eruptions, occlusion-related acne, and acne arising from an underlying endocrinopathy are each frequently treated as ordinary acne vulgaris, delaying recognition of the specific underlying trigger and leading to an ineffective standard treatment course.

The Decision: Take a directed history for new medications, cosmetic product changes, and hyperandrogenic symptoms whenever an acneiform eruption presents atypically or fails standard therapy, and address the underlying trigger directly rather than escalating standard acne treatment indefinitely.

Pattern Anchor: Monomorphic lesion morphology is the single most useful clue that an acneiform eruption is not ordinary acne vulgaris.

THE MORPHOLOGY-TO-MANAGEMENT SYSTEM — The Urticarial Lesion That Overstays Its Welcome

---

The Pattern: Individual urticarial wheals that persist beyond twenty-four hours at the same anatomic location, in contrast to the fleeting, migratory wheals of ordinary urticaria.

Stem Signature: Lesions that leave residual bruising, pigmentation, or purpura upon resolution, sometimes accompanied by burning or pain rather than the itching typical of ordinary urticaria.

Trap Logic: Persistent, fixed urticarial lesions are frequently treated with escalating doses of antihistamines intended for ordinary urticaria, when the correct diagnosis, urticarial vasculitis, requires an entirely different, biopsy-directed diagnostic and treatment pathway.

The Decision: Biopsy an urticarial lesion that persists beyond twenty-four hours at a fixed location, resolves with residual pigmentation or purpura, or is described as burning rather than itching.

Pattern Anchor: Fixed location beyond twenty-four hours, not lesion size or number, is what separates urticarial vasculitis from ordinary urticaria.

Bullous and Immunobullous Patterns

THE MORPHOLOGY-TO-MANAGEMENT SYSTEM — The Flaccid Bulla with a Positive Nikolsky Sign

---

The Pattern: Flaccid, easily ruptured bullae and erosions, often first appearing on mucosal surfaces before spreading to the skin, in an older adult.

Stem Signature: A positive Nikolsky sign (lateral pressure on seemingly normal skin produces sliding epidermal detachment) and predominant mucosal involvement preceding cutaneous disease.

Trap Logic: Early oral erosions are frequently mistaken for aphthous stomatitis or a dental problem, delaying recognition of the underlying autoimmune blistering disease.

The Decision: Perform biopsy for both routine histology and direct immunofluorescence from perilesional skin whenever an autoimmune blistering disease is suspected; initiate systemic immunosuppression promptly given the disease's potential severity.

Pattern Anchor: A positive Nikolsky sign with predominant mucosal involvement points toward pemphigus vulgaris rather than a subepidermal blistering disease. Cross-reference: Chapter 11.

THE MORPHOLOGY-TO-MANAGEMENT SYSTEM — The Tense Bulla That Spares the Mucosa

The Pattern: Tense, intact bullae arising on urticarial or eczematous-appearing erythematous plaques in an older adult, with minimal to no mucosal involvement.

Stem Signature: Bullae remain intact rather than rupturing easily, and a negative or minimal Nikolsky sign distinguishes this pattern from the pemphigus pattern above.

Trap Logic: A pre-bullous, purely urticarial or eczematous phase can precede frank blister formation by weeks, leading to a mistaken diagnosis of ordinary eczema or urticaria before the diagnostic bullae appear.

The Decision: Biopsy for histology and direct immunofluorescence at the edge of an active bulla or urticarial plaque; systemic corticosteroids or steroid-sparing agents form the backbone of treatment.

Pattern Anchor: Tense bullae with mucosal sparing and a negative Nikolsky sign point toward bullous pemphigoid rather than pemphigus vulgaris. Cross-reference: Chapter 11.

Infectious Disease Patterns

THE MORPHOLOGY-TO-MANAGEMENT SYSTEM — The Expanding Ring That Isn't Ringworm

The Pattern: An annular, expanding, erythematous plaque with central clearing, presumed at first glance to represent tinea corporis.

Stem Signature: A distinguishing feature that does not fit tinea corporis cleanly, an unusually large size, a targetoid rather than uniform ring, systemic symptoms, or a relevant exposure history, such as a tick bite in the case of erythema migrans.

Trap Logic: Erythema migrans, granuloma annulare, and tinea corporis can each present with a superficially similar annular morphology, and a reflexive diagnosis of ringworm without a potassium hydroxide preparation or further history can lead to a missed diagnosis with significant downstream consequences, particularly for early Lyme disease.

The Decision: Confirm the diagnosis with a potassium hydroxide preparation before committing to an antifungal treatment course, and take a specific exposure and systemic symptom history for any annular eruption before assuming it is tinea.

Pattern Anchor: Not every annular, ring-shaped eruption is tinea; confirm before treating.

THE MORPHOLOGY-TO-MANAGEMENT SYSTEM — The Furuncle That Fails to Resolve with Standard Care

---

The Pattern: A presumed furuncle or simple abscess treated with incision and drainage or oral antibiotics that fails to improve, recurs promptly, or is accompanied by disproportionate pain or systemic toxicity.

Stem Signature: Pain out of proportion to examination findings, rapid progression over hours, or systemic toxicity disproportionate to the visible extent of the cutaneous findings.

Trap Logic: A deeper, more aggressive soft tissue infection can be mistaken for and initially treated as a simple furuncle, delaying recognition of a surgical emergency.

The Decision: Escalate promptly to surgical evaluation whenever pain, progression rate, or systemic toxicity disproportionately exceeds what the visible cutaneous findings would suggest.

Pattern Anchor: Disproportionate pain and systemic toxicity, not the size of the visible lesion, are what separate a true surgical emergency from a simple furuncle. Cross-reference: Chapter 24.

Vasculitic, Reactive, and Connective Tissue Patterns

THE MORPHOLOGY-TO-MANAGEMENT SYSTEM — Palpable Purpura Demanding a Systemic Search

---

The Pattern: Palpable purpura, most often on the lower extremities, reflecting inflammation of small dermal vessels.

Stem Signature: Purpura that is raised rather than flat to palpation, often in crops, sometimes accompanied by systemic symptoms including joint pain, abdominal pain, or renal involvement.

Trap Logic: Palpable purpura is frequently dismissed as a simple bruising tendency or a benign skin finding rather than recognized as the visible marker of a systemic vasculitic process that may involve the kidneys, gut, or lungs.

The Decision: Pursue a systemic evaluation including urinalysis, renal function, and, when indicated, additional serologic and imaging workup for any patient with palpable purpura, rather than treating the skin finding in isolation.

Pattern Anchor: Palpability, not color or size, is what separates vasculitic purpura from ordinary bruising and is the anchor finding that should trigger systemic evaluation. Cross-reference: Chapter 12.

THE MORPHOLOGY-TO-MANAGEMENT SYSTEM — The Malar Rash That Hides Its Photosensitivity

The Pattern: Facial erythema in a malar distribution, with or without scarring discoid plaques elsewhere, in a patient with joint pain, fatigue, or other systemic symptoms.

Stem Signature: Sparing of the nasolabial folds in the classic malar pattern, photosensitivity with flares following sun exposure, and, in darker skin tones, dyspigmentation that can outlast the active inflammatory phase.

Trap Logic: Malar erythema is frequently mistaken for rosacea or a simple sunburn, delaying recognition of an underlying connective tissue disease, particularly when erythema is subtle in darker skin tones.

The Decision: Pursue autoimmune serologic testing and coordinate with rheumatology whenever malar erythema is accompanied by systemic symptoms or photosensitivity; treat active discoid lesions early and aggressively to prevent permanent scarring and dyspigmentation.

Pattern Anchor: Nasolabial fold sparing and photosensitivity distinguish lupus-related malar erythema from rosacea. Cross-reference: Chapter 13.

Pigmentary, Hair, and Nail Patterns

THE MORPHOLOGY-TO-MANAGEMENT SYSTEM — The Pigmentary Change That Outlasts the Original Disease

The Pattern: Persistent hyperpigmentation or hypopigmentation remaining at the site of a resolved inflammatory or traumatic skin event.

Stem Signature: Pigmentary change that becomes the patient's primary presenting concern, disproportionate to the severity of the original inflammatory trigger, and more pronounced and more distressing in darker skin tones.

Trap Logic: A treatment plan that successfully controls the original inflammatory condition but does not specifically address the resulting pigmentary change often leaves the patient feeling inadequately treated.

The Decision: Treat the underlying inflammatory trigger early and aggressively to limit pigmentary sequelae, combine strict photoprotection with pigment-directed topical therapy, and set explicit expectations regarding the extended timeline for pigmentary resolution.

Pattern Anchor: The pigmentary sequela, not the original inflammatory condition, is often what the patient most wants resolved. Cross-reference: Chapter 14; Chapter 22.

THE MORPHOLOGY-TO-MANAGEMENT SYSTEM — The Scalp Symptom That Precedes Visible Hair Loss

---

The Pattern: Vertex-predominant hair loss with preceding or accompanying scalp tenderness, itching, or burning, most common in women of African descent.

Stem Signature: Smooth, shiny skin with loss of visible follicular ostia at the center of the affected area, surrounded by a peripheral zone of active, still-treatable disease.

Trap Logic: Prodromal scalp symptoms often precede visible hair loss by months to years and are easily dismissed by both patient and clinician as nonspecific or unrelated.

The Decision: Treat promptly with anti-inflammatory therapy directed at the active peripheral zone to halt centrifugal progression; counsel that central, follicle-free areas represent permanent, irreversible loss.

Pattern Anchor: Early treatment preserves remaining hair; established scarring is permanent regardless of subsequent treatment. Cross-reference: Chapter 15; Chapter 22.

THE MORPHOLOGY-TO-MANAGEMENT SYSTEM — The Nail Finding That Reflects Disease Elsewhere

---

The Pattern: A nail unit abnormality, pitting, onycholysis, oil-drop discoloration, or a longitudinal pigmented band, presenting as an isolated finding without an obvious local cause.

Stem Signature: The specific nail finding pattern (pitting and oil drop discoloration for psoriatic nail disease; a widening, irregular pigmented band with periungual pigment extension, Hutchinson sign, for subungual melanoma) together with the absence of a clear local traumatic or infectious explanation.

Trap Logic: Nail findings are frequently attributed reflexively to onychomycosis without confirmatory testing, delaying recognition of psoriatic nail disease, subungual melanoma, or another systemic or neoplastic process reflected at the nail unit.

The Decision: Confirm suspected onychomycosis with potassium hydroxide preparation, culture, or histopathology before committing to prolonged antifungal therapy, and biopsy any longitudinal pigmented band with atypical features or periungual pigment extension.

Pattern Anchor: A nail finding without a clear local cause should prompt consideration of a systemic or neoplastic process before defaulting to a presumed fungal diagnosis. Cross-reference: Chapter 16.

Neoplastic and Oncologic Patterns

THE MORPHOLOGY-TO-MANAGEMENT SYSTEM — The Deceptively Innocuous Rapidly Growing Nodule

The Pattern: A firm, painless, red to violaceous, rapidly growing dome-shaped nodule on chronically sun-exposed skin of an older or immunosuppressed adult, meeting most of the AEIOU criteria.

Stem Signature: Painlessness and an unremarkable clinical appearance markedly discordant with an aggressive underlying growth rate.

Trap Logic: This presentation is frequently mistaken for a cyst, insect bite reaction, or benign vascular lesion, delaying urgent biopsy.

The Decision: Biopsy promptly; pursue sentinel lymph node biopsy given the high rate of occult nodal metastasis, and coordinate multidisciplinary treatment incorporating surgery, radiation, and, for advanced disease, immunotherapy.

Pattern Anchor: Meeting most of the AEIOU criteria should prompt urgent biopsy regardless of how benign the lesion appears. Cross-reference: Chapter 20.

THE MORPHOLOGY-TO-MANAGEMENT SYSTEM — The Bruise That Never Resolves

The Pattern: A persistent, irregularly bordered, dark patch on an acral surface (palm, sole, or nail unit) assumed to represent trauma or a bruise.

Stem Signature: Failure to resolve over the timeframe expected for an ordinary bruise, with a parallel ridge pattern on dermoscopy when present on volar skin.

Trap Logic: This pattern is disproportionately responsible for melanoma diagnostic delay in patients with darker skin tones, in whom acral lentiginous melanoma represents a larger relative share of melanoma diagnoses.

The Decision: Biopsy any acral pigmented lesion that fails to resolve over the expected timeframe for trauma; incorporate the acral surfaces, nail units, and mucosa into every full-body skin examination regardless of the patient's overall melanoma risk profile.

Pattern Anchor: A dark patch that does not resolve like an ordinary bruise is not a bruise. Cross-reference: Chapter 19; Chapter 22.

THE MORPHOLOGY-TO-MANAGEMENT SYSTEM — The Pigmented Lesion Whose Depth Cannot Be Recovered

The Pattern: A pigmented lesion with meaningful clinical suspicion for melanoma biopsied with a technique that transects its deep margin.

Stem Signature: A pathology report noting a transected deep margin and an unreliable or unreportable Breslow depth.

Trap Logic: Shave biopsy is an efficient, commonly used technique for most pigmented lesions, but its use on an unexpectedly invasive melanoma compromises the single most important staging and prognostic parameter in the entire disease.

The Decision: Use a full-thickness biopsy technique, excisional biopsy when feasible, for any pigmented lesion carrying meaningful melanoma suspicion, before the biopsy is ever performed.

Pattern Anchor: Breslow depth, once compromised by an inadequate biopsy, cannot be recovered by any subsequent procedure. Cross-reference: Chapter 19; Chapter 25.

THE MORPHOLOGY-TO-MANAGEMENT SYSTEM — The Pearly Papule That Bleeds and Never Heals

The Pattern: A slowly enlarging, pearly, translucent papule with overlying telangiectasias and a tendency to bleed with minor trauma or intermittently crust and scab without fully healing.

Stem Signature: A history of the lesion being present for months to years, intermittently noticed to bleed, and a personal report that "it never quite heals" despite the patient's own attempts at wound care.

Trap Logic: This pattern is frequently mistaken for a persistent pimple, an insect bite, or a slow-healing scratch, particularly when small, delaying biopsy for a considerable period; a pigmented variant can additionally be mistaken for a benign nevus or seborrheic keratosis, especially in patients with darker skin tones.

The Decision: Biopsy any papule with this "never quite heals" history regardless of its small size, and select a treatment modality, electrodesiccation and curettage, standard excision, or Mohs micrographic surgery, matched to the tumor's specific subtype and anatomic location.

Pattern Anchor: A lesion that intermittently bleeds and never fully heals over months is basal cell carcinoma until proven otherwise. Cross-reference: Chapter 18.

THE MORPHOLOGY-TO-MANAGEMENT SYSTEM — The Hyperkeratotic Papule Arising Within Sun-Damaged Skin

The Pattern: A firm, hyperkeratotic, often tender papule or nodule arising within a background of chronically sun-damaged skin, sometimes evolving from a preceding actinic keratosis.

Stem Signature: Tenderness to palpation, a more rapid growth rate than the surrounding actinic keratoses, and increasing induration at the base of the lesion.

Trap Logic: Progression from actinic keratosis to invasive squamous cell carcinoma can be gradual and easy to miss when a field of chronically sun-damaged skin is being followed for multiple actinic keratoses simultaneously, allowing one lesion's transformation to be overlooked among many similar-appearing neighbors.

The Decision: Biopsy any lesion within a field of actinic keratoses that becomes tender, more indurated, or more rapidly growing than its neighbors, and stratify subsequent treatment by the tumor's specific high-risk versus low-risk features.

Pattern Anchor: Tenderness and induration, not size alone, distinguish an evolving squamous cell carcinoma from its surrounding field of actinic keratoses. Cross-reference: Chapter 18.

Pediatric and Developmental Patterns

THE MORPHOLOGY-TO-MANAGEMENT SYSTEM — The Timeline That Reveals the Diagnosis

The Pattern: A pediatric eruption or growth whose correct interpretation depends more on its timeline relative to age and developmental stage than on its morphology in isolation.

Stem Signature: Onset timing (birth versus weeks versus months of age), growth pattern (proliferative-then-involuting versus proportionate-with-the-child), and fever-to-rash sequence each carry substantial diagnostic weight in pediatric dermatology.

Trap Logic: The same lesion or eruption can carry an entirely different significance depending on when in a child's development it appears; applying adult-derived pattern recognition without this developmental lens leads to systematic misdiagnosis.

The Decision: Anchor every pediatric dermatologic evaluation in a specific developmental timeline: age of onset, growth trajectory, and any preceding systemic symptoms.

Pattern Anchor: In pediatric dermatology, timeline is pattern. Cross-reference: Chapter 21.

THE MORPHOLOGY-TO-MANAGEMENT SYSTEM — The Vascular Lesion Racing Against a Developmental Window

The Pattern: A rapidly proliferating vascular lesion in an infant, located near the eye, airway, or lumbosacral spine, or noted to be growing unusually quickly.

Stem Signature: Absence or subtlety at birth followed by rapid growth over the first weeks of life, a proliferative-then-involuting natural history distinct from a vascular malformation, which is present at birth and grows only proportionately with the child.

Trap Logic: The generally favorable natural history of most infantile hemangiomas can lead to a default posture of observation even when the specific anatomic location carries a time-sensitive risk, most critically to visual development, that observation alone will not adequately address.

The Decision: Refer urgently to a specialist experienced in vascular anomalies for any hemangioma in a periocular, airway, or lumbosacral location, or any hemangioma showing ulceration, and treat promptly with oral propranolol when indicated rather than deferring to routine observation.

Pattern Anchor: Location, not size, determines urgency for an infantile hemangioma; a periocular hemangioma races against a developmental window that observation cannot pause. Cross-reference: Chapter 21.

Mucosal, Genital, and Anogenital Patterns

THE MORPHOLOGY-TO-MANAGEMENT SYSTEM — The Genital Plaque Mistaken for Simple Eczema

The Pattern: A persistent, well-demarcated, eczematous-appearing plaque in the vulvar, scrotal, or perianal region that fails to respond to appropriate topical treatment.

Stem Signature: Treatment resistance over several weeks despite an appropriate empiric regimen, sometimes with an atrophic, porcelain-white, or erosive quality distinguishing it from ordinary irritant or allergic dermatitis.

Trap Logic: Lichen sclerosus, erosive lichen planus, extramammary Paget disease, and differentiated-type intraepithelial neoplasia all mimic simple genital eczema and are each easily and commonly delayed in diagnosis for this reason.

The Decision: Biopsy any persistent, treatment-resistant genital plaque rather than escalating through an indefinite sequence of empiric topical treatments.

Pattern Anchor: Treatment resistance is the anchor finding that should trigger biopsy across nearly every genital and anogenital dermatosis. Cross-reference: Chapter 23.

THE MORPHOLOGY-TO-MANAGEMENT SYSTEM — The Oral, Genital, and Ocular Triad Evaluated in Isolation

The Pattern: Recurrent oral ulcers, genital ulcers, and ocular inflammation, each evaluated separately by different clinicians and never connected into a single unifying history.

Stem Signature: A patient history that, when specifically and directly elicited across all three mucosal and ocular sites in a single combined history, reveals a recurrent, multi-site pattern that no single treating clinician had previously assembled.

Trap Logic: Oral and genital ulceration evaluated in isolation, without a directly elicited combined history spanning all three affected sites, are each individually and plausibly misattributed to a common, isolated benign process, delaying recognition of the underlying systemic diagnosis for years.

The Decision: Ask directly and specifically about oral, genital, and ocular symptoms together whenever any one of the three is the presenting concern, and perform a pathergy test when the combined history is suggestive.

Pattern Anchor: The unifying diagnosis is often hiding in a history that has simply never been asked for as a single combined question. Cross-reference: Chapter 23.

Emergency Patterns

THE MORPHOLOGY-TO-MANAGEMENT SYSTEM — The Cellulitis Whose Pain Outpaces Its Appearance

The Pattern: An apparently ordinary cellulitis with pain that is markedly out of proportion to the visible examination findings.

Stem Signature: Rapid progression over hours, hemorrhagic bullae, dusky discoloration, or cutaneous anesthesia developing within the affected area.

Trap Logic: Early necrotizing fasciitis can appear deceptively similar to ordinary cellulitis, and reliance on visible examination findings alone, without weighing the patient's reported pain severity, is a well-documented contributor to fatal diagnostic delay.

The Decision: Obtain urgent surgical consultation for emergent evaluation and, when confirmed, immediate debridement; do not allow imaging to delay surgical consultation in a patient with a strongly suggestive clinical picture.

Pattern Anchor: Pain out of proportion to examination findings is the single most important early clue distinguishing necrotizing fasciitis from ordinary cellulitis. Cross-reference: Chapter 24.

THE MORPHOLOGY-TO-MANAGEMENT SYSTEM — The Targetoid Eruption Racing Toward Detachment

The Pattern: Fever, mucosal erosions, and a spreading dusky or targetoid eruption, typically within one to eight weeks of a new medication.

Stem Signature: A positive Nikolsky sign and mucosal involvement across at least two of the oral, ocular, and genital surfaces.

Trap Logic: Early lesions can resemble a viral exanthem or a hypersensitivity reaction, and staphylococcal scalded skin syndrome, which spares the mucosa, is an important mimic in the pediatric population.

The Decision: Discontinue all non-essential medications immediately, obtain urgent dermatology consultation, and manage in a burn-unit-capable setting with proactive ophthalmology involvement.

Pattern Anchor: Mucosal involvement, together with a positive Nikolsky sign, distinguishes this life-threatening drug reaction from its self-limited mimics. Cross-reference: Chapter 24.

Quick-Reference Index by Chapter

Pattern	Category	Chapter Cross-Reference
The Treatment-Resistant Plaque That Isn't What It Seems	Inflammatory / Papulosquamous	Multiple chapters; see Chapter 20 for the malignancy-specific variant
The Violaceous Recalibration for Darker Skin Tones	Skin of Color	Chapter 22
The Acneiform Eruption with a Hidden Trigger	Inflammatory	Foundational acne and adnexal disease chapters
The Urticarial Lesion That Overstays Its Welcome	Inflammatory / Vasculitis	Foundational urticaria chapters; Chapter 12
The Expanding Ring That Isn't Ringworm	Infectious	Foundational infectious dermatoses chapters
The Furuncle That Fails to Resolve with Standard Care	Infectious / Emergency	Chapter 24
The Flaccid Bulla with a Positive Nikolsky Sign	Immunobullous	Chapter 11
The Tense Bulla That Spares the Mucosa	Immunobullous	Chapter 11
Palpable Purpura Demanding a Systemic Search	Vasculitis	Chapter 12
The Malar Rash That Hides Its Photosensitivity	Connective Tissue Disease	Chapter 13

The Pigmentary Change That Outlasts the Original Disease	Pigmentation	Chapter 14; Chapter 22
The Scalp Symptom That Precedes Visible Hair Loss	Hair and Scalp	Chapter 15; Chapter 22
The Nail Finding That Reflects Disease Elsewhere	Nail	Chapter 16
The Pearly Papule That Bleeds and Never Heals	Oncology	Chapter 18
The Hyperkeratotic Papule Arising Within Sun-Damaged Skin	Oncology	Chapter 18
The Deceptively Innocuous Rapidly Growing Nodule	Oncology	Chapter 20
The Bruise That Never Resolves	Oncology	Chapter 19; Chapter 22
The Pigmented Lesion Whose Depth Cannot Be Recovered	Oncology / Procedural	Chapter 19; Chapter 25
The Timeline That Reveals the Diagnosis	Pediatric	Chapter 21
The Vascular Lesion Racing Against a Developmental Window	Pediatric	Chapter 21
The Genital Plaque Mistaken for Simple Eczema	Genital / Mucosal	Chapter 23
The Oral, Genital, and Ocular Triad Evaluated in Isolation	Genital / Mucosal	Chapter 23
The Cellulitis Whose Pain Outpaces Its Appearance	Emergency	Chapter 24
The Targetoid Eruption Racing Toward Detachment	Emergency	Chapter 24

Using This Atlas in Practice

This Atlas is intended as a living reference within the reader's own practice: as clinical experience accumulates with each pattern catalogued here, the reader is encouraged to annotate this section with additional discriminating features, local practice patterns, and personally encountered variations on each Trap Logic discussed above. The five-part structure used consistently throughout this text, Pattern, Stem Signature, Trap Logic, Decision, and Pattern Anchor, is designed to function as a portable cognitive scaffold that extends well beyond the specific conditions catalogued in this book, applicable to any new or unfamiliar dermatologic presentation the reader encounters over the course of clinical practice: name the pattern, identify its stem signature, actively rule out its trap logic mimics, commit to the decision that pattern demands, and anchor the lesson in a single memorable, high-yield clinical anchor.

Three practical scenarios illustrate how this Atlas is designed to be used in real time rather than read cover to cover. During a busy clinic session, a clinician evaluating a treatment-resistant plaque can scan the Inflammatory and Papulosquamous Patterns category to quickly check whether the specific response pattern being observed, a partial, temporary improvement followed by recurrence, matches a catalogued Trap Logic warranting biopsy before another treatment cycle is attempted. On call overnight, a clinician facing an unfamiliar, rapidly evolving eruption in an acutely ill patient can turn directly to the Emergency Patterns category to rapidly cross-check the specific combination of findings, disproportionate pain, mucosal involvement, or rapid purpuric progression, against the small set of genuinely time-critical patterns catalogued in this text, without needing to first identify which of the twenty-five chapters might be relevant. Before a rotation or clinical placement in a specific subspecialty area, a trainee can review the full category most relevant to that rotation, pediatric dermatology, skin of color, or procedural dermatology, as a rapid, structured refresher of the highest-yield diagnostic pitfalls awaiting them in that specific clinical context, in each case using the Atlas as a rapid decision-support tool that complements, rather than replaces, the deeper chapter-length discussion of pathophysiology, evidence, and management found earlier in this text.

Readers are encouraged to revisit this Atlas periodically rather than treating it as a single, one-time reference consulted only during initial study of this textbook. Clinical pattern recognition is a skill that sharpens with deliberate, repeated review, and the compact, indexed format of this Atlas is specifically designed to support that kind of recurring, spaced review far more efficiently than returning to the full narrative chapters each time a specific pattern needs to be refreshed in memory. Clinicians who find a particular Trap Logic personally challenging, whether because of an unusual case encountered in their own practice or because a specific mimic has proven difficult to distinguish reliably at the bedside, are encouraged to revisit that specific entry, and its corresponding full chapter discussion, more frequently than the others until the discriminating features described here become fully automatic in clinical practice.

CONCLUSION

This text set out to do more than catalogue the diseases of the skin, hair, nails, and mucosa; it set out to teach a way of looking. Twenty-five chapters and the preceding Atlas have moved across nearly the full breadth of clinical dermatology, from the molecular architecture of the epidermal barrier to the emergent management of toxic epidermal necrolysis, and the discipline itself resists easy summary precisely because it rewards close, patient observation more than any other field in medicine. What follows is not a restatement of that material but a reflection on the themes that ran beneath it, and on what remains true of dermatologic practice regardless of which chapter a reader turns to next.

The Discipline of Looking Closely

Every chapter in this book, whatever its organ system or disease category, has returned again and again to a single clinical habit: looking closely enough, and long enough, to notice the detail that separates a correct diagnosis from a plausible one. The treatment-resistant plaque that improves only partially with a topical corticosteroid before reliably recurring. The pain that outpaces the visible extent of an apparently ordinary cellulitis. The nodule that intermittently bleeds and never quite finishes healing. None of these findings requires exotic technology or rare expertise to recognize; each requires only the discipline of pausing before accepting the first, most comfortable explanation, and asking what a slightly closer look, or a slightly more skeptical one, might reveal. This is the quiet argument this entire textbook has been making: that diagnostic excellence in dermatology is built less from an ever-expanding list of memorized entities and more from a small number of transferable habits of attention, applied consistently across every organ system, every age, and every skin tone a clinician encounters.

That last qualifier, every skin tone, deserves to be restated plainly here rather than left as a single dedicated chapter's concern. A diagnostic habit that reliably catches disease in lightly pigmented skin but systematically misses the same disease in darker skin tones is not, in any meaningful sense, a complete diagnostic habit; it is a habit still under construction. The recalibration this text has asked of its reader, toward violaceous and gray-brown discoloration, toward palpation and scale when erythema is subtle, toward the acral surfaces where melanoma and pigmented basal cell carcinoma are disproportionately missed, is not a supplementary consideration bolted onto an otherwise complete clinical education. It is part of what a complete clinical education in dermatology now requires, and the persistence of diagnostic delay and worse outcomes for patients with skin of color across multiple conditions discussed in this book is a standing reminder that this recalibration remains unfinished work across the specialty as a whole, not only within the pages of a single textbook.

Pattern Recognition as a Living Skill

The Morphology-to-Management System that has run through every chapter of this book, and that stands consolidated in the preceding Atlas, was built on a specific wager: that a consistent five-part structure, naming the pattern, reading its stem signature, actively ruling out its trap logic, committing to the decision it demands, and fixing the lesson to a single memorable anchor, would prove more durable in a reader's memory, and more useful at the bedside under real time pressure, than either an unstructured list of facts or a rigid diagnostic algorithm applied mechanically regardless of context. Whether that wager has succeeded is, in the end, not something a book can determine from its own pages; it is something only demonstrated in the examination room, on the hospital ward, and during the unhurried moments of continuing education long after this book has been read once and set on a shelf. Pattern recognition of the kind this text has tried to teach is not a skill acquired once and then possessed permanently. It is a living skill, sharpened by every subsequent patient who presents with a familiar-looking rash that turns out to be something else entirely, and dulled, gradually and often imperceptibly, by years of pattern-matching against only the common and the straightforward. The most experienced clinicians are not those who have simply seen the most patients, but those who have remained curious enough, chapter after chapter and patient after patient, to keep asking whether the comfortable diagnosis in front of them is truly the correct one.

This is also why the preceding Atlas was built as an index rather than as a second set of chapters to be read once and filed away. A reference that lives at the back of a book, organized for rapid lookup by pattern rather than by chapter number, is only useful if it is actually returned to, repeatedly, over years of practice, each time a treatment-resistant plaque or an unfamiliar nodule prompts a moment of genuine diagnostic uncertainty. The clinical value of this text, and of any clinical reference of comparable ambition, is therefore not fully realized on a single first reading. It accumulates gradually, consultation by consultation, as the patterns catalogued here are tested, refined, and occasionally corrected against the individual variation every real patient inevitably presents.

The Physician-Patient Relationship Beneath the Morphology

It would be a disservice to close this book without returning to the patients themselves, who have appeared throughout these chapters not as abstract case presentations but as people navigating fear, uncertainty, and, not infrequently, a diagnosis that had eluded correct recognition for months or years before finally reaching the right clinician. The family whose child's vulvar purpura was mistaken, for a frightening interval, as a sign of abuse rather than lichen sclerosus. The man whose acral pigmented lesion had been dismissed as an ordinary bruise for the better part of a year. The patient with Behçet disease whose oral ulcers, genital ulcers, and uveitis were each evaluated in isolation by different clinicians before anyone thought to ask about all three together. Every one of these narratives is, at its core, a story about the cost of diagnostic delay, measured not only in disease progression but in the accumulated anxiety, frustration, and erosion of trust a patient experiences while waiting for someone to look closely enough to see what was, in retrospect, recognizable all along. The clinical skills this book has tried to teach exist in service of shortening that interval, and the satisfaction of dermatologic practice, at its best, comes precisely from the moment a correct diagnosis is finally named and a clear, evidence-based path forward is offered to a patient who has often been waiting a long time to hear it.

Patient communication, woven throughout this text in the Patient Education boxes accompanying nearly every chapter, deserves the same ongoing attention as diagnostic acuity itself. A correct diagnosis, delivered without adequate explanation of its natural history, its treatment timeline, and its realistic expectations, leaves a patient only partially served. Melasma that will not clear completely despite consistent treatment. Post-inflammatory pigmentary change that will take longer to resolve than the inflammatory condition that caused it. A scar that will look red and slightly raised for the better part of a year before settling into its final, flatter, paler appearance. Setting these expectations plainly and early, before frustration has a chance to take root, is not a peripheral communication skill layered on top of clinical dermatology. It is part of the clinical work itself, as essential to a successful outcome as the correct diagnosis and the correct prescription.

A Field That Continues to Evolve

Clinical dermatology has changed substantially even within the working lifetime of many practicing clinicians, and there is no reason to expect that pace of change to slow. Biologic and small-molecule systemic therapies have transformed the management of psoriasis, atopic dermatitis, and hidradenitis suppurativa in ways that would have seemed implausible a generation ago. Oral propranolol replaced systemic corticosteroids as first-line therapy for problematic infantile hemangiomas within a remarkably short interval once its efficacy was recognized. Immune checkpoint inhibitors have meaningfully extended survival for patients with advanced melanoma and Merkel cell carcinoma who, not long ago, faced a uniformly poor prognosis. The specific therapeutic details in this book, dosing conventions, treatment algorithms, and emerging agents, reflect the evidence and guidelines current at the time of writing, and the reader should expect, and actively seek out, continued evolution in each of these areas over the years following this book's publication. What is far less likely to change is the underlying clinical reasoning this book has tried to teach: the discipline of looking closely, the specific patterns that distinguish a benign process from its more consequential mimic, and the humility to reconsider a working diagnosis when the clinical picture does not evolve as expected. Therapeutics will continue to advance; the reasoning that determines which patient needs which therapy, and how urgently, changes far more slowly, and it is this reasoning, more than any specific drug or dose, that this book has tried above all to transmit.

KEY POINT: The specific therapeutic recommendations in this text reflect the evidence base current at the time of writing and will continue to evolve; the underlying diagnostic reasoning and pattern recognition skills this book has emphasized throughout are considerably more durable and should be treated as the lasting foundation on which future therapeutic knowledge is built.

Closing Thought

The skin is, among all the organs, uniquely positioned at the intersection of the visible and the systemic: a rash can be nothing more than a rash, or it can be the first visible sign of a connective tissue disease, an occult malignancy, or a life-threatening drug reaction, and the clinician's task, chapter after chapter, patient after patient, is to tell the difference reliably and in time. This book has tried to equip its reader, whether a medical student encountering these patterns for the first time, a resident refining clinical judgment under the pressure of a busy service, or an experienced practitioner returning to sharpen a specific area of practice, with both the depth of clinical knowledge and the disciplined habits of observation that task requires. The chapters close here, but the clinical reasoning they were written to cultivate is, by its nature, never finished; it continues to develop with every patient encountered, every pattern confirmed or revised, and every moment of looking a little more closely than the first glance alone would have required.

www.ingramcontent.com/pod-product-compliance
Lightning Source LLC
LaVergne TN
LVHW062034101126
852251LV00025B/330
* 9 7 8 0 5 5 7 9 7 6 2 7 0 *